UCLA Symposia on Molecular and Cellular Biology, New Series

Series Editor, C. Fred Fox

Please contact the publisher for information about previous titles in this series.

UCLA Symposia Board

Human Tumor Antigens and Specific Tumor Therapy

Human Tumor Antigens and Specific Tumor Therapy

Proceedings of a Cetus-Triton
Biosciences–UCLA Symposium
Held at Keystone, Colorado
April 23–30, 1988

Editors

Richard S. Metzgar
Department of Microbiology and Immunology
Duke University Medical Center
Durham, North Carolina

Malcolm S. Mitchell
Department of Medical Oncology
Comprehensive Cancer Center
University of Southern California
Los Angeles, California

Alan R. Liss, Inc. • **New York**

**Address all Inquiries to the Publisher
Alan R. Liss, Inc., 41 East 11th Street, New York, NY 10003**

While the authors, editors, and publisher believe that drug selection and dosage and the specifications and usage of equipment and devices, as set forth in this book, are in accord with current recommendations and practice at the time of publication, they accept no legal responsibility for any errors or omissions, and make no warranty, express or implied, with respect to material contained herein. In view of ongoing research, equipment modifications, changes in governmental regulations and the constant flow of information relating to drug therapy, drug reactions and the use of equipment and devices, the reader is urged to review and evaluate the information provided in the package insert or instructions for each drug, piece of equipment or device for, among other things, any changes in the instructions or indications of dosage or usage and for added warnings and precautions.

Library of Congress Cataloging-in-Publication Data

Cetrus-Triton Biosciences-UCLA Symposium on Human Tumor Antigens and Specific Tumor Therapy (1988: Keystone, Colo.)
Human tumor antigens and specific tumor therapy.

(UCLA symposia on molecular and cellular biology; new ser., vol. 99)
"Cetus-Triton Biosciences-UCLA Symposium on Human Tumor Antigens and Specific Tumor Therapy"—Pref.
Includes bibliographies and index.
1. Cancer—Immunotherapy—Congresses. 2. Tumor antigens—Congresses. I. Metzgar, Richard S. II. Mitchell, Malcolm S. III. Cetus Corporation. IV. Triton Biosciences, Inc. V. University of California, Los Angeles. VI. Title. VII. Series: UCLA symposia on molecular and cellular biology; new ser., v. 99. [DNLM: 1. Antibodies, Monoclonal—congresses. 2. Antigens, Neoplasm—congresses. 3. Immunotherapy—methods—congresses. 4. Neoplasms—therapy—congresses. W3 U17N new ser. v.99 / QZ 266 C423 1988h]
RC271.I45C47 1988   616.99'4061   83-32602
ISBN 0-8451-2698-9

Contents

Contributors

M. Abe, Department of Medicine, Dana-Farber Cancer Institute, Boston, MA 02115 [25]

Paul Abrams, NeoRx Corporation, Seattle, WA 98119 [191]

Julian Ambrus, Laboratory of Immunoregulation, National Institute of Allergy and Infectious Disease, National Institutes of Health, Bethesda, MD 20892 [231]

D.L. Barnd, Department of Microbiology and Immunology, Duke University, Durham, NC 27710 [157]

Paul Beaumier, NeoRx Corporation, Seattle, WA 98119 [191]

David Berd, Division of Medical Oncology, Thomas Jefferson University, Philadelphia, PA 19107 [297]

B. Bock, Institute for Immunology, University of Munich, D8000 Munich 2, Federal Republic of Germany [199]

Paula Boerner, University of California at San Diego, Cancer Center, La Jolla, CA 92093 [147]

R.L.H. Bolhuis, Dr. Daniel Den Hoed Cancer Center, 3075 EA Rotterdam, The Netherlands [221]

Ebo Bos, Organon International B.V., 5340 BH, Oss, The Netherlands [127]

C. Bruyns, Laboratoire de Physiologie Animale, U.L.B., 1640 Rhode-st-Genèse, Belgium [93]

Joy Burchell, Imperial Cancer Research Fund, London WC2A 3PX, England [11]

J-C. Bystryn, Kaplan Cancer Center, New York University School of Medicine, New York, NY 10016 [307]

Silvana Canevari, Division of Experimental Oncology E, Istituto Nazionale Tumori, 20133 Milano, Italy [181]

Danilo Canlapan, Immunotherapy Section, Department of Radiation Oncology, UCLA School of Medicine, Los Angeles, CA 90024 [317]

Walter P. Carney, Medical Products Department, E. I. Dupont, North Billerica, MA 01862 [53]

Patrizia Casalini, Division of Experimental Oncology E, Istituto Nazionale Tumori, 20133 Milano, Italy [181]

Peter J. Chandler, Division of Surgical Oncology, John Wayne Cancer Clinic, Jonsson Comprehensive Cancer Center, UCLA School of Medicine, Los Angeles, CA 90024 [115]

The numbers in brackets are the opening page numbers of the contributors' articles.

Jian-Jun Chen, IDEC Pharmaceuticals Corporation, La Jolla, CA 92037 [265]

Edward P. Cohen, Department of Microbiology and Immunology, University of Illinois College of Medicine, Chicago, IL 60680 [243]

Maria I. Colnaghi, Division of Experimental Oncology E, Istituto Nazionale Tumori, 20133 Milano, Italy [181]

Gabriella Della Torre, Division of Experimental Oncology E and A, Istituto Nazionale Tumori, 20133 Milano, Italy [181]

M. Dugan, Kaplan Cancer Center, New York University School of Medicine, New York, NY 10016 [307]

Trevor Duhig, Imperial Cancer Research Fund, London WC2A 3PX, England [11]

Mark C. Fagan, Center for Research in Periodontal Diseases and Oral Molecular Biology, University of Illinois at Chicago, Chicago, IL 60612 [35]

George C. Fareed, International Genetic Engineering, Inc. (INGENE), Santa Monica, CA 90404 [317]

Mehmet Fer, NeoRx Corporation, Seattle, WA 98119 [191]

Soldano Ferrone, Department of Microbiology and Immunology, New York Medical College, Valhalla, NY 10595 [35]

O.J. Finn, Department of Microbiology and Immunology, Duke University, Durham, NC 27710 [157]

G.J. Fleuren, Department of Pathology, Universiteit Leiden, 2300 RC Leiden, Zuid-Holland, The Netherlands [221]

Alan Fritzberg, NeoRx Corporation, Seattle, WA 98119 [191]

Takao Fujimori, Meiji Institute of Health Science, Odawara, Kanagawa 250, Japan [83]

I. Funke, Institute for Immunology, University of Munich, D8000 Munich 2, Federal Republic of Germany [199]

Sandra Gendler, Imperial Cancer Research Fund, London WC2A 3PX, England [11]

S.P. Goedegebuure, Dr. Daniel Den Hoed Cancer Center, 3075 EA Rotterdam, Zuid-Holland, The Netherlands [221]

Pradip Gosh-Dastidar, International Genetic Engineering, Inc. (INGENE), Santa Monica, CA 90404 [317]

Lloyd H. Graf, Jr., Center for Research in Periodontal Diseases and Oral Molecular Biology, and the Department of Physiology and Biophysics, University of Illinois at Chicago, Chicago, IL 60612 [35]

Peter J. Hamer, Medical Products Department, E. I. Dupont, North Billerica, MA 01862 [53]

Michael G. Hanna, Jr., Bionetics Research Institute/Organon Teknika, Rockville, MD 20850 [127,335]

M.N. Harris, Kaplan Cancer Center, New York University School of Medicine, New York, NY 10016 [307]

Martin V. Haspel, Bionetics Research Institute/Organon Teknika, Rockville, MD 20850 [127,335]

D. Hayes, Department of Medicine, Dana-Farber Cancer Institute, Boston, MA 02115 [25]

Bernhard Holzmann, Institute for Immunology, University of Munich, D8000 Munich 2, Federal Republic of Germany [73]

Herbert C. Hoover, Massachusetts General Hospital, Boston, MA 02114 [335]

Reiko F. Irie, Division of Surgical Oncology, John Wayne Cancer Clinic, Jonsson Comprehensive Cancer Center, UCLA School of Medicine, Los Angeles, CA 90024 [115]

James D. Irvin, Department of Chemistry, Southwest Texas State University, San Marcos, TX 78666 [231]

Carl Harald Janson, Department of Immunology, Karolinksa Institute, S-10401 Stockholm, Sweden [277]

Judith P. Johnson, Institute for Immunology, University of Munich, D8000 Munich 2, Federal Republic of Germany [45,73]

Guy J.F. Juillard, Immunotherapy Section, Department of Radiation Oncology, UCLA School of Medicine, Los Angeles, CA 90024 [317]

June Kan-Mitchell, Department of Microbiology, University of Southern California, Los Angeles, CA 90033 [105]

Sudhakar Kasina, NeoRx Corporation, Seattle, WA 98119 [191]

Ikuo Kawashima, Department of Oncology, Tokyo Metropolitan Institute of Medical Science, Bunkyo-ku, Tokyo 113, Japan [83]

L.A. Kerr, Department of Microbiology and Immunology, Duke University, Durham, NC 27710; present address: Department of Urology, Mayo Clinic, Rochester, MN 55902 [157]

Young S. Kim, Department of Microbiology and Immunology, University of Illinois College of Medicine, Chicago, IL 60680 [243]

Hiroshi Kobayashi, Laboratory of Pathology, Cancer Institute, Hokkaido University School of Medicine, Sapporo, Hokkaido 060, Japan [255]

Heinz Kohler, IDEC Pharmaceuticals Corporation, La Jolla, CA 92037 [265]

Karen A. Kozlowski, Center for Research in Periodontal Diseases and Oral Molecular Biology, University of Illinois at Chicago, Chicago, IL 60612 [35]

D. Kufe, Department of Medicine, Dana-Farber Cancer Institute, Boston, MA 02115 [25]

Michael S. Lan, Department of Microbiology and Immunology, Duke University Medical Center, Durham, NC 27710 [1]

Joyce LaVecchio, Medical Products Department, E. I. Dupont, North Billerica, MA 01862 [53]

Jar-How Lee, International Genetic Engineering, Inc. (INGENE), Santa Monica, CA 90404 [317]

Jürgen M. Lehmann, Institute of Immunology, University of Munich, D8000 Munich 2, Federal Republic of Germany [45]

Alvin Liu, International Genetic Engineering, Inc. (INGENE), Santa Monica, CA 90404 [317]

Philip O. Livingston, Memorial Sloan-Kettering Cancer Center, New York, NY 10021 [287]

Michael T. Lotze, Surgery Branch, National Cancer Institute, National Institutes of Health, Bethesda, MD 20892 [167]

Valeria Mancino, Center for Research in Periodontal Diseases and Oral Molecular Biology, University of Illinois at Chicago, Chicago, IL 60612 [35]

M. Marechal, AZ-VUB, Jette Hospital, Brussels, Belgium **[93]**

William H. McBride, Immunotherapy Section, Department of Radiation Oncology, UCLA School of Medicine, Los Angeles, CA 90024 **[317]**

Richard P. McCabe, Bionetics Research Institute/Organon Teknika, Rockville, MD 20850 **[127,335]**

Håkan Mellstedt, Radiumhemmet and Immunological Research Laboratory, Karolinksa Hospital, S-10401 Stockholm, Sweden **[277]**

Richard S. Metzgar, Department of Microbiology and Immunology, Duke University Medical Center, Durham, NC 27710 **[xvii, 1,157]**

Delia Mezzanzanica, Division of Experimental Oncology E, Istituto Nazionale Tumori, 20133 Milano, Italy **[181]**

M.C. Miceli, Department of Microbiology and Immunology, Duke University, Durham, NC 27710 **[157]**

Malcolm S. Mitchell, Department of Medical Oncology, Comprehensive Cancer Center, University of Southern California, Los Angeles, CA 90033 **[xvii, 345]**

A. Charles Morgan, NeoRx Corporation, Seattle, WA 98119 **[191]**

Donald L. Morton, Division of Surgical Oncology, John Wayne Cancer Clinic, Jonsson Comprehensive Cancer Center, UCLA School of Medicine, Los Angeles, CA 90024 **[115]**

James H. Murray, Bionetics Research Institute/Organon Teknika, Rockville, MD 20850 **[127]**

Dorothea Myers, Tumor Immunology Laboratory, Department of Therapeutic Radiology, University of Minnesota, Minneapolis, MN 55455 **[231]**

Simon Ng, Medical Products Department, E. I. Dupont, North Billerica, MA 01862 **[53]**

Lloyd J. Old, Samuel Freeman Laboratory, Memorial Sloan-Kettering Cancer Center, New York, NY 10021 **[63,137]**

R. Oratz, Kaplan Cancer Center, New York University School of Medicine, New York, NY 10016 **[307]**

Daniel Padua, Immunotherapy Section, Department of Radiation Oncology, UCLA School of Medicine, Los Angeles, CA 90024 **[317]**

Debra Petit, Medical Products Department, E. I. Dupont, North Billerica, MA 01862 **[53]**

Nicholas Pomato, Bionetics Research Institute/Organon Teknika, Rockville, MD 20850 **[127,335]**

Thaddeus G. Pullano, Medical Products Department, E. I. Dupont, North Billerica, MA 01862 **[53]**

Syamal Raychaudhuri, IDEC Pharmaceuticals Corporation, La Jolla, CA 92037 **[265]**

John Reno, NeoRx Corporation, Seattle, WA 98119 **[191]**

Gert Riethmüller, Institute of Immunology, University of Munich, D8000 Munich 2, Federal Republic of Germany **[45,73,199]**

Charles D. Rosenberg, Cornell University Graduate School of Medical Sciences, New York, NY 10021 **[35]**

Steven A. Rosenberg, Surgery Branch, National Cancer Institute, National Institutes of Health, Bethesda, MD 20892 **[167]**

D.F. Roses, Kaplan Cancer Center, New York University School of Medicine, New York, NY 10016 **[307]**

Ivor Royston, University of California at San Diego, Cancer Center, La Jolla, CA 92093 [147]

Yukihiko Saeki, IDEC Pharmaceuticals Corporation, La Jolla, CA 92037 [265]

Darrell Salk, NeoRx Corporation, Seattle, WA 98119 [191]

Dirk Schadendorf, Memorial Sloan-Kettering Cancer Center, New York, NY 10021 [137]

G. Schlimok, Institute for Immunology, University of Munich, D8000 Munich 2, Federal Republic of Germany [199]

James P. Schrementi, Center for Research in Periodontal Diseases and Oral Molecular Biology, University of Illinois at Chicago, Chicago, IL 60612 [35]

Robert Schroff, NeoRx Corporation, Seattle, WA 98119 [191]

T. Schuurs, Organon International, Oss, The Netherlands [93]

B. Schweiberer, Institute for Immunology, University of Munich, D8000 Munich 2, Federal Republic of Germany [199]

Christine Sers, Institute of Immunology, University of Munich, D8000 Munich 2, Federal Republic of Germany [45]

J. Siddiqui, Department of Medicine, Dana-Farber Cancer Institute, Boston, MA 02115 [25]

Gowsala Sivam, NeoRx Corporation, Seattle, WA 98119 [191]

M. Slaoui, Laboratoire de Physiologie Animale, U.L.B., 1640 Rhode-st-Genèse, Belgium [93]

Ryszard Slomski, Department of Microbiology and Immunology, University of Illinois College of Medicine, Chicago, IL 60680; present address: Institute of Human Genetics, Polish Academy of Sciences, Poznan, Poland [243]

J. Speyer, Kaplan Cancer Center, New York University School of Medicine, New York, NY 10016 [307]

A. Srinivasan, NeoRx Corporation, Seattle, WA 98119 [191]

Pramod K. Srivastava, Samuel Freeman Laboratory, Memorial Sloan-Kettering Cancer Center, New York, NY 10021 [63,137]

Barbara G. Stade, Institute for Immunology, University of Munich, D8000 Munich 2, Federal Republic of Germany [73]

Uwe D. Staerz, Bascl Institute for Immunology, Basel, Switzerland [209]

Nobuhiko Tada, Department of Pathology, Tokai University School of Medicine, Isehara, Kanagawa 250-11, Japan [83]

Tadashi Tai, Department of Oncology, Tokyo Metropolitan Institute of Medical Science, Bunkyo-ku, Tokyo 113, Japan [83]

Joyce Taylor-Papadimitriou, Imperial Cancer Research Fund, London WC2A 3PX, England [11]

Mahmood J. Tehrani, Department of Immunology, Karolinksa Institute, S-10401 Stockholm, Sweden [277]

K. Thielemans, AZ-VUB, Jette Hospital, Brussels, Belgium [93]

Shohken Tomita, Surgery Branch, National Cancer Institute, National Institutes of Health, Bethesda, MD 20892 [167]

Kevin L. Trimpe, Medical Products Department, E. I. Dupont, North Billerica, MA 01862 [53]

Fatih M. Uckun, Tumor Immunology Laboratory, Department of Therapeutic Radiology, University of Minnesota, Minneapolis, MN 55455 [231]

J. Urbain, Laboratoire de Physiologie Animale, U.L.B., 1640 Rhode-st-Genèse, Belgium [93]

R. J. van de Griend, Department of Pathology, Universiteit Leiden, 2300 RC Leiden, Zuid-Holland, The Netherlands [221]

J-L Vanderheyden, NeoRx Corporation, Seattle, WA 98119 [191]

J. van Dijk, Department of Pathology, Universiteit Leiden, 2300 RC Leiden, Zuid-Holland, The Netherlands [221]

Thomas H. Weisenburger, Immunotherapy Section, Department of Radiation Oncology, UCLA School of Medicine, Los Angeles, CA 90024 [317]

Hans Wigzell, Department of Immunology, Karolinska Institute, S-10401 Stockholm, Sweden [277]

D. Scott Wilbur, NeoRx Corporation, Seattle, WA 98119 [191]

Hiroshi Yamaguchi, Memorial Sloan-Kettering Cancer Center, New York, NY 10021 [137]

Preface

The Cetus–Triton Biosciences–UCLA Symposium on **Human Tumor Antigens and Specific Tumor Therapy** was held at Keystone, Colorado, April 23–30, 1988, concurrently with a symposium on **Mechanisms of Action of Therapeutic Applications of Biologicals in Cancer and Immune Deficiency Disorders**, which was intended to discuss complementary topics. A joint session covering the use of combination therapies was held on the final evening. These conferences, which were attended by several hundred scientists, were an attempt to present in a coherent way a broad range of scientific investigations into biomodulation as a treatment for human cancer. Although some animal models of human disease were discussed, the emphasis in both meetings was on studies of human cancer.

The symposium on **Human Tumor Antigens and Specific Tumor Therapy** first focused on the strides that have been made into the identification, molecular characterization, and cloning of human tumor-associated antigens. It is clear that monoclonal antibodies have facilitated isolation of some tumor-associated antigens, leading to a determination of their nature and their relationship to antigens present in homologous and different normal tissues. Among these antigens were glycoproteins and glycolipids in melanoma, and high molecular weight mucins in adenocarcinomas. The latter have received substantial attention in several laboratories, and studies have begun to clarify the roles of these difficult-to-purify substances as target antigens through molecular biology as well as classical biochemistry and immunology. In fact, genes for several antigens have already been cloned, which may make predefined tumor vaccines possible in the not-too-distant future.

Human monoclonal antibodies, although still in their infancy, have nevertheless begun to contribute to our knowledge of tumor-associated antigens and have the special potential of indicating which of those antigens are immunogenic in man. In particular, studies with human monoclonal antibodies have shown that antigens on both the outer surface of the plasma membrane of tumor cells and on the interior of the cell are immunogenic. This is unlike findings with antigens to mouse antibodies. Murine monoclonal antibodies, as well as murine-human chimeric or human antibodies, offer potential for highly specific targeted treatment with chemotherapy, toxins, or radionuclides, of which we heard several promising reports.

It has been possible, even with incomplete knowledge of which antigens are the ones most important to include as immunogens in "tumor vaccines," to begin tests of active specific immunotherapy against human cancers. Immunological studies on treated patients have provided evidence for dominant immunogens, and research continues on strategies for increasing the degree of response to what are intrinsically weak immunogens. These do not differ from antigens on normal host tissues as widely as an immunologist-clinician might hope. In addition to antibodies, cytolytic lymphocytes directed against tumor-associated antigens also have been identified in human beings. The specificity of cloned cytolytic lymphocytes derived from several types of cancer patients is being elucidated. This should provide further evidence that is needed to construct more appropriate and useful vaccines. Antiidiotypic antibodies provide an alternative strategy, and they have led to a better understanding of the fundamental controls of the immune response regardless of their ultimate role in active immunization.

Integration of immunological therapies into the standard practice of oncologists is already being accomplished. Combination treatment involving chemotherapy and biological therapy are under investigation at many universities. Since biomodulation of cancer depends upon an intact immune response, combining this modality with chemotherapy is problematical because most chemotherapeutic compounds are immunosuppressive. It is clear that combined modalytic treatments will be common very soon, at first with cytokines, but ultimately with active immunization as well.

Immunologists have been particularly intrigued with the possibility of using specific immunization as a means of treating cancer, and of preventing recurrence after initial surgery. It is even more appealing to consider active specific immunization as a means for preventing the occurrence of cancer. Stimulating the tumor-bearing host to reject a tumor is a far more physiological process than trying to eradicate a tumor with purely cytotoxic approaches. Moreover, there is far less attendant toxicity. Only our insufficient, though increasing, knowledge of which immunogens to select, and how best to administer them stand in the way of far-reaching gains from active immunotherapy. This symposium has highlighted major advances in that endeavor, and we trust will be only the first of many UCLA Symposia to address active specific immunotherapy as an important anti-tumor treatment.

We thank Cetus Corporation and Triton Biosciences, Inc., for their generous co-sponsorship of this symposium. We also acknowledge additional support from: Organon Teknika/Bionetics Research, Inc.; Cytogen Corporation; NeoRx Corporation; E.I. DuPont, Oncogen Research Group; and

Xoma Corporation. As always, the staff of the UCLA Symposia made the task of the chairmen largely ceremonial through their attention to every detail at the conference site. Finally, the impressive ability of the speakers and audience to handle the ski slopes by afternoon and the intricacies of science in the morning and evening lent renewed emphasis to Juvenal's concept of *"mens sana in corpore sano."*

Malcolm S. Mitchell
Richard S. Metzgar

Human Tumor Antigens and Specific Tumor Therapy, pages 1–9
© 1989 Alan R. Liss, Inc.

MOLECULAR STUDIES OF A PANCREATIC TUMOR MUCIN, DU-PAN-2[1]

Michael S. Lan and Richard S. Metzgar

Department of Microbiology and Immunology
Duke University Medical Center, Durham, NC 27710

ABSTRACT   The DU-PAN-2 mucin demonstrates molecular
heterogeneity by polyacrylamide and agarose gel electrophoresis as well as by gel-filtration chromatography. The
DU-PAN-2 murine monoclonal antibody reacts with the glycosylated molecule but fails to react with the DU-PAN-2
apomucin prepared by trifluoromethane sulfonic acid (TFMS)
treatment. The epitope recognized by the DU-PAN-2 monoclonal
antibody is difficult to define since chemical and enzymatic
treatments that fragment the molecule result in loss of
antigenicity. Both neuraminidase and some protease digestions
of the molecule can destroy antigenicity. A rabbit antiserum to TFMS deglycosylated DU-PAN-2 antigen reacts with
the apomucin but not the fully glycosylated molecule. This
antiserum is able to detect precursors to the DU-PAN-2 mucin
in lysates of some adenocarcinoma cell lines.

INTRODUCTION

DU-PAN-2 is a mucin antigen of pancreatic tumor cells
identified by an IgM murine monoclonal antibody (1,2). The
antigen is secreted by pancreatic tumor cells and tumor cell
lines and can be readily detected in the body fluids of many
patients with pancreatic cancer (3). The DU-PAN-2 mucin is
also a marker of differentiation in pancreatic tumor cells
(4) and is expressed on some normal ductal cells of the
pancreas and liver (4,5). Although the DU-PAN-2 antigen is

[1]This work was supported by grant IM-472 from the
American Cancer Society and grants CA 40044 and CA 32672
from the National Cancer Institute. Michael S. Lan is a
recipient of a postdoctoral fellowship from the National
Cancer Center.

present in low concentration in normal pancreatic secretions
(6), elevated levels of the antigen can be detected in the
serum of some patients with non-malignant hepatobiliary
diseases (5). In order to better understand the functional
role of the DU-PAN-2 antigen in differentiation and perhaps
transformation, the molecular properties of the mucin must
be defined. The purpose of this report is to summarize our
progress on the characterization of the DU-PAN-2 mucin and
its peptide.

Purified DU-PAN-2 mucin antigen as defined by the murine
IgM monoclonal antibody (DU-PAN-2) has been purified from
human ascites fluid and from spent medium of a pancreatic
tumor tissue culture cell line, HPAF, according to the scheme
in Figure 1. The HPAF cell line was established from the
same patient that provided the ascites fluid used for these
studies. The apomucin of the DU-PAN-2 antigen was prepared
by treatment with TFMS according to the procedure of Edge
et al. (7).

FIGURE 1
SCHEMATIC OF DU-PAN-2 ANTIGEN PURIFICATION

HPAF tissue culture   Ascites from pancreatic
supernatant and/or   adenocarcinoma patient
cell lysate

50-75% ammonium sulfate
fractionation

Sepharose CL-6B gel filtration
chromatography

Monoclonal antibody affinity
chromatography

CsCl density gradient ultracentrifugation (in the presence
of 4M guanidine-HCl)

TFMS reaction

CHARACTERIZATION OF THE DU-PAN-2 Epitope

Although the mucin properties of the DU-PAN-2
molecule have been well described (2), the nature of the epitope defined by the original murine monoclonal antibody is
still not characterized. Unlike some other tumor associated
mucin antigens, we have been unable to detect the DU-PAN-2
epitope on glycolipids. Evidence from enzymatic and chemical
modifications of the DU-PAN-2 antigen have suggested that
both protein and carbohydrate parts of the molecule play a
role in antibody binding (Table 1).

TABLE 1
ENZYMATIC AND CHEMICAL MODIFICATION OF DU-PAN-2
ANTIGEN (Ag)

Component	Treatment or Agent	Effect
Affinity purified [1]Desialylation 3H-GlcNAc labeled DU-PAN-2 Ag		14.4% sialic acid re- covered, no detectable Ag activity
Affinity purified [2]Trypsin 3H-GlcNAc labeled Chymotrypsin DU-PAN-2 Ag		No detectable size change or loss of Ag activity
Affinity purified Pronase 3H-GlcNAc labeled Pepsin DU-PAN-2 Ag Papain		Ag fragmented and most of activity lost
Affinity purified [4]Periodate DU-PAN-2 Ag reaction		No detectable Ag activity
Affinity purified Heating at DU-PAN-2 Ag 100°C, 15 min		No loss of Ag activity

[1] Reaction was carried out in 1mU of neuraminidase on 50 mM
   sodium acetate, 5mM calcium chloride, pH 5.5.
[2] Protease treatment was performed in 1 mg enzyme/ml at 37°C
   for 24 hours in appropriate buffer system.
[3] DU-PAN-2 Ag was determined by passing through the Sephadex
   G-200 column before and after enzyme treatment.
[4] The reaction was carried out at room temperature for one
   hour by adding 50 mM sodium periodate.

Neuraminidase treatment of ^{3}H-glucosamine labeled DU-PAN-2 antigen resulted in a loss of antigenic activity within 20 minutes and release of 2/3 of the sialic acid residues in this time period (Figure 2). This data suggests that sialic acid plays an essential role in maintaining antigenic activity. However, the studies do not distinguish between sialic acid playing a role in conformation of the molecule versus this sugar being an integral component of the epitope.

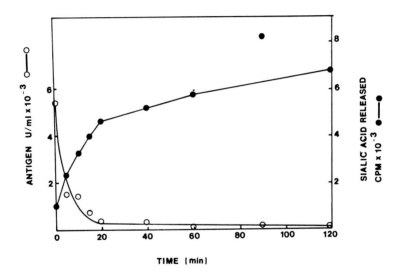

Figure 2. Enzymatic release of sialic acid. Radio-labeled DU-PAN-2 antigen was incubated with neuraminidase (0.1 mU/ml) in 50 mM sodium acetate buffer containing 5 mM calcium chloride, pH 5.5 at 37°C for various time intervals. Enzyme activity was destroyed by boiling the mixture at 100°C for 10 minutes. Released sialic acid was measured by counting the dialyzable radioactive material. Residual DU-PAN-2 activity was determined by competition RIA.

Affinity purified DU-PAN-2 antigen also was subjected to mild alkaline reductive β-elimination (Table 2). Following β-elimination, 75% of the galactosamine was converted to

galactosaminitol which indicated O-glycosidical linkage of
the mucin molecule. The DU-PAN-2 antigen activity dramatically
decreased after alkaline reductive β-elimination. Less than
1.5% of the total antigen activity was recovered although 90%
of the total labeled sugars were accounted for and could be
fractionated by ion exchange chromatography (data not shown).

TABLE 2
ALKALINE REDUCTIVE β-ELIMINATION REACTION

Component	Antigen (units) reactivity[a]	Radioactivity	Hexosamine ratio[b]
DU-PAN-2 antigen	108,800 units	3.6×10^6 cpm	$GlcNH_2:GalNH_2$ (6.5:1)
β-elimination product	1,602 units	3.2×10^6 cpm	$GlcNH_2:GalNH_2:$ GalOH (8.5:0.35:1)
			$GlcNH_2:(GalNH_2+$ GalOH) (6.3:1)

[a] DU-PAN-2 antigen units was determined by RIA (3).

[b] Hexosamine ratios were measured by radioactivities recovered from an amino acid analyzer according to the method
of Spiro (8).

The potential role of carbohydrates in the DU-PAN-2
epitope was supported by the heat resistance properties of
the antigen and its sensitivity to periodate treatment
(Table 1).
A possible role of the peptide backbone of the mucin in
the DU-PAN-2 epitope was suggested by the ability of certain
proteases (pepsin, papain and pronase) to alter antibody
binding. Gel filtration chromatography experiments further
demonstrated that digestion with some proteases altered the
molecular size and shifted the antigen migration pattern
from the excluded to the included volume of the Sephadex
G-200 column. The molecular size changes caused by proteolytic digestion were not surprising since a dispersed naked
peptide region has been proposed for mucin structures (9).
Although the effect of the proteases could cause conform-

ational changes in the molecule as has been suggested for neuraminidase, a significant decrease in antigen activity would not be anticipated for a mucin epitope consisting of only sugar structures. The possibility also exists that both protein and carbohydrate components are involved in the epitope. The participation of antibody binding in both protein and carbohydrate structures has been clearly demonstrated in the M-N blood group antigen system (10).

DU-PAN-2 APOMUCIN STUDIES

In an effort to characterize and identify the DU-PAN-2 peptide, we subjected the affinity purified antigen to deglycosylation by the TFMS procedure (Figure 1 and reference 7). The procedure resulted in recovery of 65-75% of metabolically labeled DU-PAN-2 protein core and loss of more than 95% of ^{3}H-GlcNAC labeled saccharides (11). Rabbit antisera to the purified glycosylated DU-PAN-2 antigen and the TFMS treated antigen apomucin were produced and characterized. The 1% agarose gel western immunoblot reactivity of the polyclonal rabbit antisera and the original DU-PAN-2 monoclonal antibody with the glycosylated affinity purified DU-PAN-2 antigen, the TFMS deglycosylated antigen and an NP40 extracted lysate of HPAF cells is shown in Figure 3. The DU-PAN-2 monoclonal antibody failed to react with the deglycosylated antigen (B,2) but reacted as previously described with the purified DU-PAN-2 antigen (B,1) and with the HPAF lysate (B,3). In contrast, the rabbit antiserum 67 reacted with the apomucin (C,2) but failed to react with the fully glycosylated DU-PAN-2 antigen (C,1). The reactivity of the HPAF lysate with rabbit antiserum 67 to the deglycosylated DU-PAN-2 antigen (C,3) indicated that there are intracellular forms of apomucin which are not yet glycosylated to a degree which interferes with antibody binding.

We further evaluated the reactivities and specificities of the DU-PAN-2 monoclonal antibody and the rabbit antisera to the DU-PAN-2 mucin and apomucin with lysates of various tumor cell lines by immunodot blot analysis (Table 3). The apomucin was detected in most of the pancreatic adenocarcinoma cell lines and a breast carcinoma cell line BT-20. Rabbit antisera to the DU-PAN-2 apomucin was consistently detected when the glycosylated molecule could be detected by the rabbit antiserum 68 raised against the DU-PAN-2 mucin. However, the DU-PAN-2 monoclonal antibody could only detect mucins by HPAF, T3M4 and Panc-1 cell lines. The rabbit poly-

clonal antibodies might recognize cross reactive determinants
or not recognized by the mouse monoclonal antibody or the
immunodot blot analysis was not sensitive enough to detect
antigen with the monoclonal antibody compared to the rabbit
antiserum.

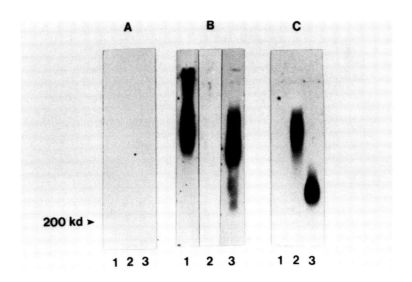

FIGURE 3. Agarose gel immunoblot. Affinity purified
DU-PAN-2 antigen (lane 1), deglycosylated DU-PAN-2 antigen
(lane 2) and HPAF cell lysate (lane 3) were electrophoresed
in 1% agarose gel and immunoblotted with normal rabbit serum
or control monoclonal antibody (A), DU-PAN-2 murine monoclonal antibody (B), and rabbit antiserum against deglycosylated DU-PAN-2 antigen (C).

Recently, monoclonal antibodies to the DU-PAN-2 peptide
core have been generated and are being characterized. In
addition, the rabbit antiserum to the apomucin is being used
to screen an HPAF λgt11 cDNA expression library. These
studies should elucidate further understanding of the bio-
synthesis and molecular structure of these mucin type glycoproteins of pancreatic tumors.

TABLE 3
REACTIVITY OF DU-PAN-2 ANTIBODIES WITH TUMOR CELL LINES

Cell Lines	Immunoblot Reactivity		
Pancreatic Adenocarcinoma	R#68 DU-PAN-2[1]	R#68 αDU-PAN-2 mucin[2]	R#67 α-apomucin[3]
HPAF	+++[4]	++++	++
T3M4	+	+	+++
SW979	−	++++	++++
Panc-1	±	−	±
BxPC3	−	++++	+
Colon Carcinoma	−	−	−
Melanoma			
DM-6	−	−	−
SKMEL	−	−	−
Breast Carcinoma			
SKBR3	−	−	−
BT-20	−	++	+++

[1] DU-PAN-2 murine monoclonal IgM antibody
[2] Rabbit antisera 68 was generated by immunization with affinity purified DU-PAN-2 glycosylated antigen.
[3] Rabbit antiserum 67 was generated by immunization with deglycosylated DU-PAN-2 apomucin.
[4] Intensity was scored according to the degree of reactivity of rabbit antisera with various tumor cell lysates by immunodot blots.

REFERENCES

1.   Lan MS, Finn OJ, Fernsten PD, Metzgar RS (1985). Isolation and properties of a human pancreatic adeno-carcinoma-associated antigen, DU-PAN-2. Cancer Res 45:305.
2.   Lan MS, Khorrami A, Kaufman B, Metzgar RS (1987). Molecular characterization of a mucin-type antigen associated with human pancreatic cancer. J Biol Chem 262:12863.

3. Metzgar RS, Rodriguez N, Finn OJ, Lan MS, Daasch VN, Fernsten PD, Meyers WC, Sindelar WF, Sandler RS, Seigler HF (1984). Detection of a pancreatic cancer-associated antigen (DU-PAN-2 antigen) in serum and ascites of patients with adenocarcinoma. Proc Natl Acad Sci. 81:5242.

4. Metzgar RS, Mahvi DV, Borowitz MJ, Lan MS, Meyers WC, Seigler HF, Finn OJ (1985). DU-PAN-2: A pancreatic adenocarcinoma associated antigen. In Monoclonal Antibodies and Cancer Therapy, Alan R. Liss, Inc. p.63.

5. Haviland AE, Borowitz MJ, Killenberg PG, Lan MS, Metzgar RS (1988). Detection of an oncofetal antigen (DU-PAN-2) in the sera of patients with non-malignant hepatobiliary diseases and hepatomas. Int. J. Cancer (In Press).

6. Mahvi DM, Seigler HF, Meyers WC, Kalthoff H, Schmiegel WH, Metzgar RS (1988). DU-PAN-2 levels in serum and pancreatic ductal fluids of patients with benign and malignant pancreatic disease. Pancreas (In Press).

7. Edge ASB, Faltynek CR, Hof L, Reichert JR., LE, Weber P (1981). Deglycosylation of glycoproteins by trifluoromethane sulfonic acid. Analytical Biochem 118:131.

8. Spiro RG (1972). The carbohydrates of glycoproteins. Methods in Enzymology 28:11.

9. Carlstedt I, Sheehan JK (1984). Macromolecular properties and polymeric structure of mucus glycoproteins. In Mucus and Mucosa, Pitman, London (Ciba Foundation Symposium 109) p. 157.

10. Lisowska E, Kordowicz M (1976). 5th International Convocation on Immunology, S. Karger, Basel p. 188.

11. Metzgar RS, Lan MS, Kim YW, Koriwchak MJ, Mullins TD, Hollingsworth MA (1988). DU-PAN-2 mucin type differentiation antigen of normal and malignant pancreatic ductal cells. In Immunity to Cancer II, Alan R. Liss Inc. (In Press).

Human Tumor Antigens and Specific Tumor Therapy, pages 11–23
© 1989 Alan R. Liss, Inc.

A POLYMORPHIC EPITHELIAL MUCIN EXPRESSED
BY BREAST AND OTHER CARCINOMAS:
IMMUNOLOGICAL AND MOLECULAR STUDIES[1]

Sandra Gendler, Joyce Taylor-Papadimitriou,
Joy Burchell and Trevor Duhig

Imperial Cancer Research Fund
P O Box 123, Lincoln's Inn Fields
London WC2A 3PX, U.K.

ABSTRACT   Sequencing of partial cDNA clones coding
for the core protein of a human polymorphic
epithelial mucin has shown that a large domain
consists of a highly conserved 60 base pair tandem
repeat. The cDNA clones were originally selected
using three monoclonal antibodies which have now been
shown to react strongly with a synthetic peptide with
an amino acid sequence corresponding to that
predicted by the tandem repeat. The antibodies
recognise epitopes which are differentially exposed
in the mucin produced by normal and malignant breast
indicating that the mucin is processed differently in
breast cancers.

INTRODUCTION

In the last few years it has become apparent that
epithelial mucins represent an important class of tumour
associated antigens, since many antibodies selected for
their reaction with carcinomas are directed to these
complex molecules (1-9). The mucins are characterized by
the presence of a large carbohydrate component, which
consists of oligosaccharides linked to serines and
threonines, via the linkage sugar N-acetylgalactosamine

[1]Parts of this report are the subject of an
International Patent Application, No. PCT/GB88/0011

and by a high content of the amino acids proline, glycine and alanine as well as threonine and serine. Analysis of the primary structure of mucins from various animal species suggest that there is great variety in the structure of the carbohydrate side chains which may be composed of only one type of disaccharide, as in ovine submaxillary mucin, or may be complex, containing several sugars and branched chains as in most gastric mucins. However, the same sugars are used to build up the side chains and similar epitopes may be present on more than one mucin and indeed on other glycoproteins, or even glycolipids. When an antibody reacts with several epithelial tissues and carcinomas or with more than one component on Western blots, it is therefore possible that glycoproteins with different core proteins are being detected. Little is known about the detailed structure of the core protein of mucins, and how variable these are within the same animal species. This question, which relates to the number of genes coding for mucins, and the processing of RNA transcripts of these genes, can best be approached by obtaining some data on the peptide sequence(s) of the mucin core proteins.

A mucin which has received a great deal of attention recently is one produced in abundance by the lactating human mammary gland. Originally purified by Shimizu and Yamauchi (10) and characterized by them as having the properties of a mucin, it was identified as the antigenic component recognized by a range of monoclonal antibodies (1-3). These antibodies, some of which are listed in Table 1, were developed using preparations of either the

TABLE 1
ANTIBODIES REACTIVE WITH THE PEM MUCIN

Antibody	Reaction with PDTR peptide
MAM series (5)	−
M8 (6)	+
MC5 (8)	ND
DF3 (4)	ND
NCRC11 (7)	+
Ca1, Ca2, Ca3 (9)	ND

ND – Not Done

human milk fat globule or human carcinomas. There has
been some confusion in nomenclature with this component
which has been referred to as PAS-0 (10), NPGP (non-
penetrating glycoprotein) (8), as MAM-6 (5) and as EMA
(epithelial membrane antigen) (11). Since this component
exhibits a genetic polymorphism and is produced by many
glandular epithelium, we will refer to it as human
polymorphic epithelial mucin (PEM).

The polymorphism in the PEM glycoprotein is apparent
as a difference in mobilities of antibody-reactive high
molecular weight components in polyacrylamide gels. In
addition, some antibodies detect smaller molecular weight
components in extracts of some tumour cells (1,3). In
order to clarify this complexity we have developed
antibodies reactive with the mucin core protein and have
shown that these do indeed detect both the higher
molecular weight bands showing a size polymorphism and the
lower molecular weight bands which represent precursors
(3). Interestingly, these core protein reactive
antibodies show differential activity with the mucin
produced by normal and malignant breast tissue (see Table
2). In particular, the SM-3 epitope appears to be masked
when the mucin is normally glycosylated but exposed in the
cancer-associated mucin (2), suggesting that the mucin is
differently processed in breast cancers.

To obtain structural information relating to the PEM
core protein we have used the core protein reactive
antibodies to select partial cDNA clones from a λgt11 cDNA
library made from MCF-7 cells (12). Sequencing of these
clones has shown that a large domain of the PEM gene is
made up of a highly conserved 60bp repeating unit which
forms the basis for the polymorphism seen at the
glycoprotein level. We have further been able to show
that a synthetic peptide corresponding to the sequence
predicted from the tandem repeat reacts with the
antibodies used to select the cDNA clones, as well as with
several antibodies developed in other laboratories. This
domain therefore constitutes a highly immunogenic region
of the core protein. Our studies have confirmed that the
mucin is aberrantly processed in breast and other
carcinomas so that epitopes in this region which are
normally masked can be expressed in the cancer associated
mucin.

RESULTS

Sequence of cDNA Clones.

The spectrum of reactivity of the three monoclonal antibodies used to select seven cDNA clones from the MCF-7 cDNA library is indicated in Table 2. Two of these

TABLE 2
REACTIVITY OF ANTIBODIES USED TO SELECT
cDNA CLONES CODING FOR PEM

Antibody	Immunogen	Reactivity
HMFG-1 (1,13)	Extract of human milk fat globule (HMFG)	Reacts well with fully gly-cosylated mucin (FGM) in lactating gland. Less strong reaction with deglycosylated mucin (DGM) and breast cancers
HMFG-2 (1,13)	HMFG and cultured milk epithelial cells	Reacts strongly with DGM and breast cancers. Pos-itive reaction but fewer epitopes on FGM
SM-3 (2)	Deglycosylated milk mucin	Reacts strongly with breast cancers and DGM. No reaction with FGM in lact-ating gland

antibodies, HMFG-1 and -2 were developed several years ago (13) using the immunogens shown in the Table and were, surprisingly, found to react with the deglycosylated mucin (2,12). The third antibody, SM-3, was developed recently against the deglycosylated component and shows a marked selectivity in its reaction with breast and other carcinomas (2). All three antibodies were found to react with the β-galactosidase cDNA encoded fusion proteins produced by all of the clones including the smallest which contained only 73bp. Extensive sequencing of the clones showed that all except the largest clone (pMUC10) were

composed exclusively of a 60bp repeating unit, the
sequence of which is shown in Figure 1. The larger clone
also contains some 3' unique sequence, a stop codon and 3'
untranslated region (14).

(a)

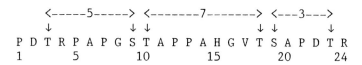

```
    CCG GAC ACC AGG CCG GCC CCG GGC TCC ACC-
    Pro Asp Thr Arg Pro Ala Pro Gly Ser Thr-

    GCC CCC CCA GCC CAC GGT GTC ACC TCG GCC
    Ala Pro Pro Ala His Gly Val Thr Ser Ala
```

(b)

```
      <-----5-----> <--------7--------> <---3--->
           ↓            ↓ ↓               ↓ ↓      ↓
      P D T R P A P G S T A P P A H G V T S A P D T R
      1       5        10        15        20      24
```

FIGURE 1.   (a) Nucleotide and predicted amino acid
sequence of 60bp tandem repeat.   (b) Synthetic peptide
reacting strongly with antibodies HMFG-1, HMFG-2 and SM-3.
Potential sites of glycosylation indicated with arrows.

The tandem repeat is highly GC rich (82%) and the
sequence is remarkably conserved. Each repeat exhibits
the characteristics of a CpG island (15,16) and contains 6
CpGs, 6 GpCs and a GC box. The CpGs at sites within the
tandem repeats appear to be unmethylated as they are
cleaved by restriction enzymes sensitive to methylation as
exemplified by the loss of the identifiable alleles (Fig.
2, Lanes 8-10). This lack of methylation is seen in CpG
islands and would account for the stability of the
sequence among the repeats, since it is the methylated
nucleotide which tends to mutate to TpG and its complement
CpA. The GC richness (60%) continues into the translated
portion 3' to the tandem repeats with 7 CpGs and 9 GpCs
identified, although there are no additional G/C boxes
(14). G/C boxes have been found within the coding
sequences of tissue-specific genes (15,16) and the PEM
gene would fit into this category.
    We have previously shown, using the pMUC10 probe in
Northern blot analysis, that the expression of the mucin

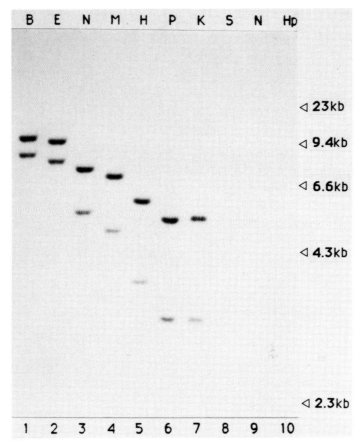

FIGURE 2. Southern blot of MCF-7 genomic DNA
digested with restriction enzymes and hybridized to
pMUC10. Genomic DNA from the breast cancer cell line
MCF-7 was digested by restriction enzymes, seven reveal 2
allelic bands of differing sizes containing the tandem
repeats (lanes 1-7). Lack of methylation at restriction
sites within the tandem repeat is shown by the lack of
bands hybridizing to pMUC10 in DNA cut by enzymes
sensitive to methylation (lanes 8-10) resulting in the
loss of the 2 alleles seen in lanes 1-7. The enzymes used
are designated as follows: B, BamHI; E, EcoRI; N, NcoI;
M, MboI; H, HinfI; P, PstI; K, KpnI; S, SmaI; N, NaeI; and
Hp, HpaII.

mRNA is epithelial specific, and that the polymorphism originally seen in the glycoprotein (1,17) is also apparent in both RNA and DNA (18,19). Since a dominant feature of the mucin gene is the 60bp tandem repeat, it seems likely that the polymorphism is due to different numbers of the repeat being found in the different alleles. That there is only one gene is shown by the presence of only two bands representing the two alleles which hybridize to the mucin probe in digests of DNA prepared with seven restriction enzymes. Figure 2 shows that the smallest fragments (3.3 and 5.3kb) were obtained with KpnI or PstI digestion, and the presence of only 2 allelic bands indicates that the tandem repeat elements are contained within these fragments.

The conservation of sequence within the repeats of the human PEM gene is in striking contrast to the lack of conservation of the sequence in several other mammalian species. The antibodies shown in Table 2 do not react with rodent tissues and accordingly a cross hybridizing gene cannot be detected in Southern blots of rodent DNA digested with restriction enzymes and probed with pMUC10. A similar gene is however detected in primates.

Reaction of Antibodies with a Synthetic Peptide.

The direction of transcription of the repeat was elucidated using synthetic oligonucleotides deduced from each strand of the DNA to probe Northern blots prepared from MCF-7 total RNA, and the coding strand is shown in Figure 1. The correct reading frame (shown in Figure 1) was established by showing a positive reaction of the three antibodies with a synthetic peptide, predicted from a reading frame of the 73bp clone. This peptide contains the 20 amino acid repeat together with 4 amino acids from the adjoining repeat and is referred to as PDTR (see Figure 1b). The positive reactions of antibodies HMFG-1, HMFG-2 and SM-3 with the peptide were demonstrated using a solid phase ELISA assay (Figure 3) and the specificity of the reaction was established by showing that the peptide competed effectively with the deglycosylated milk mucin for binding to the antibodies (data not shown). A range of antibodies developed in other laboratories were tested for their reaction with the PDTR peptide and those showing positive reactions are shown in Table 1.

The reaction of the antibodies with the synthetic

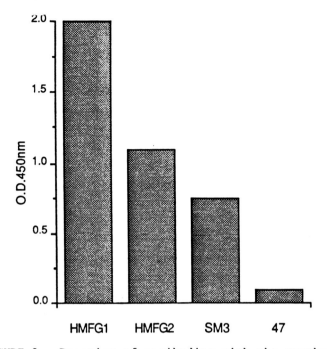

FIGURE 3. Reaction of antibodies with the synthetic
peptide PDTR (see Figure 1). The peptide PDTR was dried
on to wells of a 96 well plate (200 ng/well) and the
plates incubated with antibodies at a concentration of 6
μg/well. Bound antibody was detected in an ELISA assay
using a second antibody labelled with peroxidase (1). (47
is an irrelevant antibody used as a negative control.)
N.B. The fusion protein containing the PDTR sequence was
initially reported to have a negative reaction with HMFG-1
and SM-3 (12) but was later found to be positive when the
level of fusion protein was increased.

peptide PDTR unequivocally establishes the sequence of the
repeating amino acid unit coded for by the 60bp tandem
repeat. The amino acid sequence and composition of the
repeat exhibit features which would be expected for the
core protein of a mucin. There are five potential 0
glycosylation sites represented by serines and threonines
separated by proline-rich stretches of 3,5 and 7 amino
acids (see Figure 1). The prolines would keep the
molecule extended, so that even in the glycosylated
molecule some epitopes on the core protein could be

exposed, and these could be different depending on the pattern of glycosylation.

In a preliminary attempt to identify more precisely the specific epitopes recognized by the three antibodies, portions of the PDTR peptide were synthesized and binding of antibodies to these peptides was tested. The results indicate that the HMFG-1 determinant which is abundantly expressed on the normal mucin produced by the lactating mammary gland is located in the region of the molecule which contains the stretch of 7 amino acids running between the doublets of serine and threonine (see Figure 1). Although the epitopes recognized by SM-3 and HMFG-2 are not identical, both appear to contain the single threonine at position 3 or 23 in the PDTR peptide. Some similarity between these epitopes might be expected since both are expressed abundantly on the breast cancer associated mucin. However they are significantly different since the HMFG-2 determinant is also expressed on the normal mucin (albeit less abundantly than on the cancer mucin), while the SM-3 determinant is not. Further analysis is required to map the epitopes in detail, but the data obtained suggest that the 7 amino acid stretch between the potential sites of glycosylation may be at least in part exposed in the fully processed mucin, and that the one threonine which is not next to a serine (position 3 in the PDTR peptide) may be underglycosylated in tumors.

DISCUSSION

The determination of the sequence of a domain of the PEM mucin has been extremely informative, both in allowing the identification of the region containing the epitopes for several core reactive antibodies, and in defining the basis for the genetic polymorphism previously observed in the PEM glycoprotein. The dominant feature of the nucleotide sequence of the clones isolated from the MCF-7 library is the 60 bp repeating unit, which codes for a repeating peptide unit. In this respect the PEM mucin resembles the structure of a domain of the porcine submaxillary mucin which has recently been sequenced (20) and shown to contain a 243 bp repeating unit. Other proteins found mainly in lower organisms either as surface proteins or extracellular components show a similar motif, which could relate to the protective function that some of these proteins exhibit (for review see 21).

The sequence of the 60bp tandem repeat which makes up
the domain of the mucin described here is unusual in being
highly GC rich (82%) and remarkably conserved. The
conservation of sequence goes beyond that required for
maintaining the amino acid sequence, and results in a
large CpG island being present in the coding sequence of
the gene. Whether there is functional significance in the
sequence apart from coding for the twenty amino acid
repeat unit remains to be seen.

We have previously reported that the PEM gene is
located on chromosome 1 within the region 1q21-24 (22),
where many breaks have been seen in breast carcinomas
(23,24). The large number of tandem repeats in the gene
which have probably led by recombination, duplication or
deletion to the extensive polymorphism seen as restriction
fragment length polymorphism, could mean that the gene is
subjected to modification and/or translocation in cancer.
Initial studies following allele distribution on Southern
blots of digests of DNA from paired samples of blood cells
and tumour tissue from breast cancer patients suggest that
loss or changes in alleles are seen in a relatively high
proportion of patients (unpublished data). Further study
should clarify whether the alterations are functionally
important or are merely monitoring changes occurring at
adjacent sites in the chromosome. In this context it will
be important to identify regulatory sequences in the gene,
since PEM shows tissue specific expression and is
expressed in more than 95% of breast cancers.
Translocation of such sequences could lead to activation
of normally silent genes and conceivably influence the
change to malignancy.

A most important feature of the tandem repeat
structure described here is its immunogenicity. Since
antibodies showing differences in their reaction with
normal and malignant breast tissue recognize epitopes
located in the repeating peptide sequence and react with a
synthetic peptide, it should now be possible, by defining
these epitopes, to determine which portions of the
sequence are exposed in the normally processed mucin, and
in the mucin produced by breast cancer cells. Preliminary
experiments suggest that such an analysis is possible and
should allow a directed approach using synthetic peptides
as immunogens for the production of antibodies with
enhanced specificity for breast and other carcinomas.

REFERENCES

1. Burchell J, Durbin H, Taylor-Papadimitriou J (1983)
    Complexity of expression of antigenic determinants
    recognised by monoclonal antibodies HMFG-1 and HMFG-2
    in normal and malignant human mammary epithelial
    cells. J Immunol 131:508.
2. Burchell J, Gendler S, Taylor-Papadimitriou J, Girling
    A, Lewis A, Millis R, Lamport D (1987) Development and
    characterization of breast cancer reactive monoclonal
    antibodies directed to the core protein of the human
    milk mucin. Can Res 47:5476.
3. Griffiths AB, Burchell J, Gendler S, Lewis A, Blight
    K, Tilly R, Taylor-Papadimitriou J (1987)
    Immunological analysis of mucin molecules expressed by
    normal and malignant mammary epithelial cells. Int J
    Cancer 40:319.
4. Sekine H, Ohno T, Kufe D (1985) Purification and
    characterization of a high molecular weight
    glycoprotein detectable in human milk and breast
    carcinomas. J Immunol 135:3610.
5. Hilkens J, Buijs F, Hilgers J, Hagemann P, Calafat J,
    Sonnenberg A, Van der Valk M (1984) Monoclonal
    antibodies against human milk fat globule membranes
    detecting differentiation antigens of the mammary
    gland and its tumour. Int J Cancer 34:197.
6. Foster C, Edwards PA, Dinsdale EA, Neville AM (1982)
    Monoclonal antibodies to the human mammary gland. I.
    Distribution of determinants in non-neoplastic mammary
    and extra mammary tissues. Virchows Arch (Path Anat)
    394:279.
7. Price M, Edwards S, Owainati A, Bullock JE, Ferry B,
    Robins RA, Baldwin RW (1985) Multiple epitopes on a
    human breast carcinoma associated antigen. Int J
    Cancer 36:567.
8. Ceriani RL, Peterson JA, Lee JY, Moncada R, Blank E
    (1983) Characterization of cell surface antigens of
    human mammary epithelial cells with monoclonal
    antibodies prepared agains human milk fat globule.
    Som Cell Genet 9:415.
9. Bramwell ME, Bhavanandan VP, Wiseman G, Harris H
    (1983) Structure and function of the Ca antigen. Br J
    Cancer 48:177.
10. Shimizu M, Yamauchi K (1982) Isolation and
    characterization of mucin-like glycoproteins in human

milk fat globule membranes. J Biochem 91:515.
11. Ormerod MG, Steele K, Westwood JH, Hazzini MN (1983)
    Epithelial membrane antigen: partial purification
    assay and properties. Br J Cancer 48:533.
12. Gendler SJ, Burchell JM, Duhig T, Lamport D, White R,
    Parker M, Taylor-Papadimitriou J (1987) Cloning of
    partial cDNA encoding differentiation and
    tumour-associated mucin glycoproteins expressed by
    human mammary epithelium. Proc Natl Acad Sci USA
    84:6060.
13. Taylor-Papadimitriou J, Peterson JA, Arklie J,
    Burchell J, Ceriani RL, Bodmer WF (1981) Monoclonal
    antibodies to epithelium-specific components of the
    human milk fat globule membrane: production and
    reaction with cells in culture. Int J Cancer 28:17.
14. Gendler S, Taylor-Papadimitriou J, Duhig T, Rothbard
    J, Burchell J (1988) A highly immunogenic region of a
    human polymorphic epithelial mucin expressed by
    carcinomas is made up of tandem repeats. J Biol Chem
    (submitted).
15. Gardiner-Garden M, Frommer MJ (1987) CpG islands in
    vertebrate genomes. Mol Biol 196:261.
16. Bird AP (1986) CpG-rich island and the function of DNA
    methylation. Nature 321:209.
17. Griffiths B, Gordon A, Burchell J, Bramwell M,
    Griffiths A, Price M, Taylor-Papadimitriou J, Zanin D,
    Swallow D (1988) The tumour-associated epithelial
    mucins and the peanut lectin binding urinary mucins
    appears to be coded by a single highly polymorphic
    gene locus 'PUM'.   1.   Studies on the mammary gland.
    Dis Markers (in press).
18. Gendler S, Burchell J, Girling A, Millis R, Duhig T,
    Taylor-Papadimitriou J (1988) Cloning the polymorphic
    gene for the mammary mucin abnormally glycosylated in
    carcinomas.   In Rich MA, Hager JC, Lopez DM (eds):
    "Breast Cancer: From Research in the Laboratory to
    Control in the Clinic and Community," New York: Kluwer
    Academic Publishers (in press).
19. Swallow D, Gendler S, Griffiths B, Corney G,
    Taylor-Papadimitriou J, Bramwell ME (1987) The human
    tumour-associated epithelial mucins are coded by an
    expressed hypervariable gene locus PUM.   Nature
    328:82.
20. Timpte CS, Eckhardt AE, Abernethy JL, Hill RL (1988)
    Porcine submaxillary gland apomucin contains tandemly
    repeated, identical sequences of 81 residues.   J Biol

Chem 263:1081.
21. Taylor-Papadimitriou J, Gendler S (1988) Molecular aspects of mucins. In Olsson L (ed): "Tumor Associated Antigens on Mucins," (in press).
22. Swallow D, Gendler S, Griffiths B, Kearney A, Povey S, Sheer D, Palmer R, Taylor-Papadimitriou J (1987) The hypervariable gene locus PUM, which codes for the tumour associated epithelial mucins, is located on chromosome 1, within the region 1q21-24. Ann Hum Genet 51:289.
23. Rodgers CS, Hill SM, Hulten MA (1984) Cytogenetic analysis in human breast carcinoma. I. Nine cases in the diploid range investigated using direct preparations. Cancer Genet Cytogenet 13:95.
24. Heim S, Mitelman F (1987) "Cancer Cytogenetics." New York: Alan R Liss Inc.

ISOLATION AND SEQUENCING OF A cDNA CODING FOR THE
HUMAN DF3 BREAST CARCINOMA-ASSOCIATED ANTIGEN

M.Abe, J.Siddiqui, D.Hayes and D.Kufe

Department of Medicine, Dana-Farber Cancer Institute
Boston, MA 02115

ABSTRACT The murine monoclonal antibody (MAb) DF3
reacts with high molecular weight glycoproteins
detectable in human breast carcinomas. The correlation
between DF3 antigen expression and human breast tumor
differentiation, as well as the detection of a cross-
reactive species in human milk has suggested that this
antigen might be useful as a marker of differentiated
mammary epithelium. Other studies have demonstrated
that DF3 antigen circulates at elevated levels in the
plasma of patients with breast cancer. The circulating
MAb DF3-reactive antigens have molecular masses ranging
from approximately 300 to 450 Kd and differ among
individuals. Studies in family members have DF3 antigen
is determined by codominant expression of multiple
alleles at a single locus. We have isolated a cDNA
clone from a λgt11 library prepared from MCF-7 human
breast carcinoma cells by screening with MAb DF3. The
results demonstrated that this 309 bp cDNA, designated
pDF9.3 codes for the DF3 antigen epitope. Southern
blot analysis of EcoRI or PstI digested DNAs from 6
human tumor cell lines with ^{32}P-pDF9.3 have revealed
a restriction fragment length polymorphism (RFLP).
Hybridization of ^{32}P-pDF9.3 with total cellular RNA
from all but one of these cell lines demonstrated
either one or two transcripts. These different sized
transcripts corresponded to RFLPs in EcoRI or PstI
digested DNAs as well as with the polymorphic expression of the DF3 glycoproteins. Nucleotide sequence
analysis of pDF9.3 has revealed a highly conserved
GC-rich tandem repeat.

INTRODUCTION

A human breast carcinoma associated antigen has been
identified by using a murine monoclonal antibody (MAb), designated DF3. MAb DF3 was prepared against a membrane enriched
fraction of a human breast carcinoma metastatic to liver(1).
DF3 antigen is expressed on the apical borders of secretory
mammary epithelial cells and in the cytosol of less differentiated malignant cells(1). DF3 antigen expression also
correlates with the degree of breast tumor differentiation
and estrogen receptor status(2). These findings and the
detection of DF3 antigen in human milk(3), have suggested
that MAb DF3 reacts with a differentiation antigen expressed
in breast carcinoma cells.
       We have examined the characteristics of DF3 antigen
and the genetic mechanisms responsible for the heterogeneity
in antigen expression.

RESULTS

DF3 Antigen

       DF3 antigen has been characterized as a high molecular
weight (MW) glycoprotein(4,5). DF3 antigen in human MCF-7
breast carcinoma cells consists of two distinct glycoproteins
with MWs of 330 & 450 Kd(5). ^{35}S-Methionine or ^{14}C-glucosamine
labeling of DF3 antigen was detectable after immunoprecipitation. Furthermore, N-acetylglucosamine and N-acetylgalactosamine were detected by lectin column analysis(5).
       Figure 1 shows the effects of enzyme treatment on the
antigenicity of DF3 antigen in MCF-7 cells. Two antigens in
Fig.1 correspond to MWs of 330 & 450 Kd. Reactivity of both
MW species with MAb DF3 was almost completely decreased following neuraminidase treatment. Less significant changes were
obtained with chymotrypsin and S.aureus V8 protease. The
higher and lower MW DF3 reactive species were similarly
affected by each of the enzymes. The enzyme digests, however,
failed to yield smaller MW fragments that retained antigenicity. These results suggested that involvement of both
carbohydrate and protein in maintaining antigenicity.
       Although MCF-7 cells express two distinct DF3 antigens
(Fig.1,2), BT-20,an other human breast carcinoma line and
human milk fat globule membrane (HMFGM) have single DF3 antigen with MWs of 310 or 510 Kd, respectively (Fig.2). These
purified DF3 antigens were also detected by other MAs reactive

with breast carcinoma (ref.6). MAb F36/22 was prepared
against MCF-7 cells, MAb 115/D8 against HMFGM and MAb Cal
against HEp-2 human laryngeal carcinoma cells. Competition
assays were performed to determine if these MAbs react with
similar or distinct epitopes on DF3 antigen. MAb F36/22
completely blocks MAb DF3 binding to the DF3 antigen. In
contrast, MAbs 115/D8 and Cal only partially block MAb DF3
reactivity and the extent of this inhibition varies with the
preparation of DF3 antigen (Fig.3). These findings with

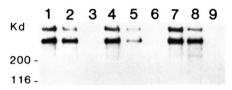

FIGURE 1. Effects of chymotrypsin, neuraminidase and
S.aureus V8 protease on DF3 antigenicity (ref.5). MCF-7
cellular extract was treated with enzymes for 2h at 37°C,
separated by SDS-PAGE, transferred to nitrocellulose paper,
and analyzed for the reactivity with MAb DF3. Lane 1: MCF-7
extract alone; lane 2: MCF-7 extract, chymotrypsin, 6.2u;
lane 3: chymotrypsin alone; lane 4: MCF-7 extract alone;
lane 5: MCF-7 extract, neuraminidase 1.0u; lane 6: neuraminidase alone; lane 7: MCF-7 extract alone; lane 8: MCF-7 extract,
S.aureus V8 protease 57u; lane 9: S.aureus V8 protease alone.

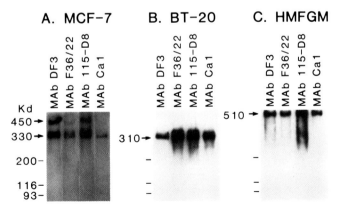

FIGURE 2. Purified DF3 antigens from MCF-7 cells(A),
BT-20 cells(B) and HMFGM(C) were analyzed by SDS-PAGE and
immunoblotting with MAb DF3, F36/22, 115/D8 and Cal, followed
by rabbit anti-mouse Ig and ^{125}I-protein A (ref.6).

28   Abe et al.

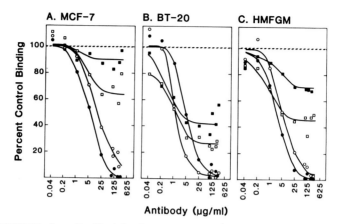

Antibody (μg/ml)

FIGURE 3.   Individual wells were coated with 1.0 U of
purified DF3 antigen from MCF-7(A), BT-20(B) or HMFGM(C) and
incubated with MAb DF3(●), F36/22(○), 115-D8(□) or Cal(■).
Reactivity of MAb DF3-peroxidase was then determined at 490rm.
Percentage of control binding was determined by comparison to
control without MAb (ref.6).

multiple MAbs prepared against a variety of immunogens suggest
the existence of a family of related but not identical high
molecular weight tumor associated glycoproteins.

The Heterogeneity of DF3 Antigen Expression

    MAb DF3 reacts with circulating antigens of different
MWs ranging from 300 to approximately 450 Kd. DF3 antigen is
detectable in plasma from normal subjects and patients with
breast cancer(7). However, levels of circulating DF3 antigen
are significantly higher in patients with breast cancer(7).
Moreover, the electrophoretic mobility patterns of circulating
DF3 antigen differ among individuals (Fig.4).
    Although the level of DF3 antigen varies with clinical
course, the electrophoretic pattern of the reactive moiety
remains the same for each individual(7). Consequently we
studied patterns of DF3 antigen expression in a patient with
metastatic breast cancer and ten of her family members.
Members of this family expressed DF3 antigen with S,I and R
electrophoretic mobilities (Fig.5). The data illustrated in
Fig.5 suggest that DF3 antigen polymorphism are genetically
determined and expressed in an autosomal codominant fashion.
The finding in this single family led us to further examine
the possibility of a genetic basis for the DF3 antigen poly-

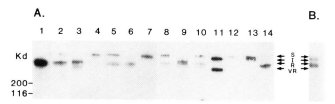

FIGURE 4. Electrophoretic mobilities of DF3 antigen in plasma and tumor (ref.8). (A) Plasma samples (1 μl) from patients with breast cancer were subjected to 3-15% SDS-PAGE, transferred to nitrocellulose paper and analyzed for the reactivity with MAb DF3. (B) Membrane-enriched fraction (0.5 μg) of the breast carcinoma cell line, ZR-75-1 was similarly analyzed. Electrophoretic mobilities are categorized as slow(S), intermediate(I), rapid(R) and vary rapid(VR).

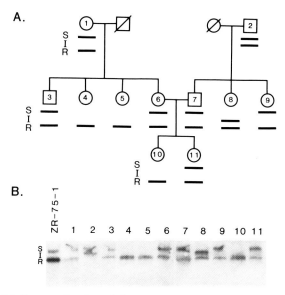

FIGURE 5. Relationship of DF3 antigen electrophoretic mobilities among family members (ref.8). (A) Family pedigree and schematic representation of DF3 antigen mobilities for each member. (B) Actual immunoblot results obtained for plasma samples (6 μl) from the members. Electrophoretic mobilities are categorized as slow(S), intermediate(I) and rapid(R). Lane numbers correspond to subjects designation in family pedigree. Subject 6 is a patient with metastatic breast cancer.

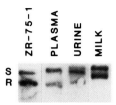

FIGURE 6. Comparison of DF3 antigens in plasma and
other fluid (ref.8). Mobilities of MAb DF3 reactive antigen
in plasma, milk and urine from a lactating woman.

morphisms in 17 additional Caucasian families. The findings
confirm that the DF3 antigens are inherited as codominant
autosomal alleles(8).

Although DF3 antigen polymorphisms are genetically
determined, electrophoretic mobility of the antigen might be
modified by glycosylation. For example, electrophoretic
mobility of DF3 antigen in milk appears to differ from that
in plasma from the same individual (Fig.6). Moreover, the
migration of the urinary R band was slightly slower than that
in plasma (Fig.6). These findings would suggest that separate
alleles code for the core proteins of different sizes and
that heterogeneity with the electrophoretic mobilities might
be related to variation by glycosylation.

cDNA CODING DF3 Antigen Protein Core

MAb DF3 was used to screen a λgt11 library prepared from
MCF-7 cells(9). Screening of 800,000 plaques yielded three
positive clones that were further purified by repeated antibody screening. One 309 bp clone, designated λDF9.3, was
used for further characterization.

Competition assays were performed to confirm that the
epitope expressed by λDF9.3 shares homology with DF3 glycoprotein. A β-galactosidase fusion protein was prepared by
infecting E.coli Y1089 with λDF9.3 phage, applied to SDS-PAGE,
transferred to nitrocellulose sheet. MAb DF3 was preincubated
with purified DF3 glycoprotein before immunoblot analysis with
the sheet to which λDF9.3 fusion protein were bound. Increasing amounts of purified DF3 glycoprotein progressively inhibited the reactivity of the antibody with the fusion protein(10).

Identification of the cDNA was further studied by Southern blot hybridization using ^{32}P-pDF9.3 prepared by subcloning
the insert into the EcoRI site of pUC8. Southern blot analysis of genomic DNAs from the human tumor cell lines digested

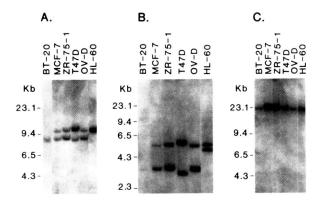

FIGURE 7.   Southern blot analysis of genomic DNA with the
pDF9.3 (ref.10).   DNAs (10 µg) from human tumor cell lines
were digested with EcoRI(A), PstI(B) and HindIII(C), electrophoresed in 0.6% agarose gels, denatured and transferred to
nylon filters.   The filters were hybridized with the ^{32}P-pDF9.3.

with EcoRI, PstI and HindIII are shown in Fig.7. Hybridization
of pDF9.3 with the EcoRI and PstI DNA digests revealed restriction fragment length polycorphisms.   The EcoRI digest
yielded two fragments ranging from 8-11 Kb in size for DNAs
from each of the cell lines except BT-20.   Similar findings
were obtained with the PstI fragments, which ranged in size
from 3.5-6 Kb.   The single EccRI and PstI restriction fragments obtained with BT-20 DNA indicate the presence of two
alleles of identical size or cnly a single allele.   In contrast to these results, digestion of each of the DNA preparations with HindIII revealed only a single fragment of 23Kb.
This finding corresponds to the absence of a HindIII restriction site in the alleles identified by pDF9.3.
     Total cellular RNA was prepared from several human tumor
cell lines and monitored by RNA transfer blot analysis for
transcripts that hybridized to the pDF9.3 probe.   A single
4.7 Kb mRNA was detectable in BT-20 cells (Fig.8).   In contrast, cell lines derived from the other breast and ovarian
carcinomas expressed two transcripts that ranged in size from
approximately 4.1 to 7.1 Kb.   Moreover, HL-60 cells had no
detectable pDF9.3 reactive transcript (Fig.8).
     These findings by RNA transfer blot analysis were com-
pared to DF3 glycoprotein expression obtained by immunoblot
analysis with MAb DF3.   The results indicate concordance in
patterns of expression at the RNA and glycoprotein levels
(Fig.9).   BT-20 cells expressed a single transcript and a

single DF3 glycoprotein, whereas the other epithelial cell lines expressed two transcripts and two DF3 antigens. Moreover, HL60 cells had no detectable RNA and no detectable MAb DF3 reactive species. These findings further suggested that the transcripts detected code for the DF3 core protein and that the size of these transcripts determines the size of the MAb DF3-reactive glycoproteins.

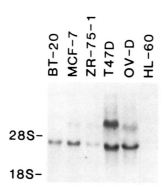

FIGURE 8. RNA transfer blot analysis with pDF9.3 (ref.10). Total cellular RNA (20 µg) from human tumor cell lines was electrophoresed in 1.1% agarose/formaldehyde gels, transferred to nitrocellulose paper and hybridized with the ^{32}P-pDF9.3.

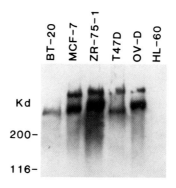

FIGURE 9. DF3 antigen transfer blot analysis (ref.10). Cellular extracts (100 µg protein) of the human tumor cell lines were separated by 3-15% SDS-PAGE, transferred to nitrocellulose paper and analyzed with MAb DF3, rabbit anti-mouse immunoglobulin and ^{125}I-protein A.

```
CGCACGGCTG GGGGGGCGGT GGAGCCCGGG GCCGGCCTGC TCTCCGGGGC CGAGGTGACA   60
.CGTG..... C...C..... .......... .......... .......... ..........  120
.......... .......... .......... ........G .G........ ..........  180
.......... G...G..... .......... .......... .......... ..........  240
.......... .......... .......... .......... .......... ..........  300
.........
```

FIGURE 10.   Nucleotide sequence of the pDF9.3 cDNA
(ref.10).

The reactivity of the fusion protein with MAb DF3 indicated that the cDNA insert (pDF9.3) contained the open reading frame that codes for the DF3 epitope. The nucleotide
sequence of pDF9.3 was found to be highly GC-rich (85%), 309
bp (Fig.10). Moreover, the sequence was found to consist
entirely of 60 bp tandem repeat. These repeats were nearly
identical with the exception of some transversions (Fig.10).

DISCUSSION

MAb DF3 reacts with a family of high molecular weight
glycoproteins. The reactivity of MAb DF3 with fusion protein
from λgt11 expression library suggests that this antibody
reacts with the core protein of DF3 antigen(10). However,
DF3 antigenicity has also been shown to be sensitive to
neuraminidase besides protease(4,5,Fig.1). Thus, MAb DF3
binding to the protein may be enhanced by the adhered
carbohydrate structure.

Southern blot analysis of EcoRI, PstI digested DNAs from
6 human tumor cell lines with ^{32}P-pDF9.3 have revealed a restriction fragment length polymorphism (10, Fig.7). The variation in allele size corresponded with the presence of differently sized transcripts. Furthermore, these patterns coin-
cided with the electrophoretic mobilities of DF3 antigen from
the same lines(10, Fig.7-9). Taken together, these findings
support our previous findings that the heterogeneity of DF3
antigen production is controlled by multiple alleles at a
single locus expressed in an autosomal codominant fashion(8).
Additionally, the electrophoretic mobility of DF3 antigen
could be modified by differences in glycosylation(8,Fig.6).

The observation that the pDF9.3 contains a 60 bp tandem
repeat suggests that the variation in the size of alleles
coding for the polymorphic DF3 glycoprotein may represent
differences in the numbers of repeats. The presence of

closely related repeats may also explain the existence of multiple antigen determinant sites on a DF3 antigen molecule(7).

REFERENCES

1. Kufe D, Inghirami G, Abe M, Hayes D, Justi-Wheeler H, Schlom J (1984). Differential reactivity of a novel monoclonal antibody (DF3) with human malignant versus benign breast tumor. Hybridoma 3:223.
2. Lundy J, Thor A, Maenza R, Schlom J, Forouhar F, Testa M, Kufe D (1985). Monoclonal antibody DF3 correlates with tumor differentiation and hormone receptor status in breast cancer patients. Breast Cancer Res Treat 5:269.
3. Abe M, Kufe D (1984). Sodium butyrate induction of milk-related antigens in human MCF-7 breast carcinoma cells. Cancer Res 44:4574.
4. Sekine H, Ohno T, Kufe D (1985). Purification and characterization of a high molecular weight glycoprotein detectable in human milk and breast carcinomas. J Immunol 135:3610.
5. Abe M, Kufe D (1986). Effects of maturational agents on expression and secretion of two partially characterized high molecular weight milk-related glycoproteins in MCF-7 breast carcinoma cell. J Cell Physiol 126:126.
6. Abe M, Kufe DW (1987). Identification of a family of high molecular weight tumor-associated glycoproteins. J Immunol 139:257.
7. Hayes D, Sekine H, Ohno T, Abe M, Keefe K, Kufe D (1985). Use of a murine monoclonal antibody for detection of circulating plasma DF3 antigen levels in breast cancer patients. J Clin Inves 75:1671.
8. Hayes DF, Sekine H, Marcus D, Alper CA, Kufe DW (1988). Genetically determined polymorphism of the circulating human breast cancer-associated DF3 antigen. Blood 71:436.
9. Walter P, Green S, Greene GM, Krunst A, Bornert JM, Heltsch JM, Staub A, Jensen E, Scrace G, Waterfield M, Chambon P (1985). Cloning of the human estrogen receptor cDNA. Proc Natl Acad Sci USA 82:7889.
10. Siddiqui J, Abe M, Hayes D, Shani E, Yunis E, Kufe D (1988). Isolation and sequencing of a cDNA coding for the human DF3 breast carcinoma-associated antigen. Proc Natl Acad Sci USA 85:2320.

Human Tumor Antigens and Specific Tumor Therapy, pages 35–44
© 1989 Alan R. Liss, Inc.

SELECTIVE COAMPLIFICATION LEADS TO INCREASED REPRESENTATION
OF INTERSPECIFICALLY TRANSFECTED HUMAN GENES ENCODING
THE 100K AND THE 96K MELANOMA-ASSOCIATED ANTIGENS[1]

Lloyd H. Graf, Jr.[2,3], Mark C. Fagan[2], Soldano Ferrone[4],
Karen A. Kozlowski[2], Valeria Mancino[2],
Charles D. Rosenberg[5], and James P. Schrementi[2]

ABSTRACT   In order to derive recombinant probes to
investigate the tissue distribution and the regulation of
expression of human tumor-associated antigens (TAA), we
initiated transfer of genes encoding TAA identified by
mouse monoclonal antibodies (MoAb). Use of highly
competent mouse B16 melanoma recipient cell clone B78H1,
and of an indirect red cell rosetting assay resulted in
total human DNA-mediated primary (1°) transfer of genes
encoding 4 glycoprotein TAA, including 3 membrane-bound
melanoma-associated antigens (MAA). This communication
describes cell DNA-mediated transfers and selective
coamplification in the mouse host cell background of
human genes encoding 2 of the 3 MAA, "100K MAA," identified by MoAb CL376.96, and "96K MAA," identified by MoAb
CL203.4. These MAA exhibit distinctive, severely limited
patterns of expression by normal tissues, characteristic
distributions on tumors of diverse embryological origins,
and specific responses to treatments with lymphokines.
B78H1 transfectant cells were shown by immunochemical
criteria to express surface molecules closely resembling
the 100K MAA or 96K MAA synthesized by human melanoma

[1]This work was supported by NIH grants CA44107 and
CA37959.
[2]Center for Research in Periodontal Diseases and Oral
Molecular Biology, University of Illinois at Chicago,
Chicago, IL 60612.
[3]Department of Physiology and Biophysics, University of
Illinois at Chicago, Chicago, IL 60612.
[4]Department of Microbiology and Immunology, New York
Medical College, Valhalla, NY 10595.
[5]Cornell University Graduate School of Medical Sciences,
New York, NY 10021.

cells. After 2° or 3° transfers by transfectant cell
DNAs, specific MAA gene-associated human alu family
repeat sequence (h-alu)-positive restriction fragments
are present in mouse host cell genomes. An indirect
dihydrofolate reductase (dhfr) gene vector-targeted
selective coamplification procedure applied to 100K MAA
and to 96K MAA gene transfectant cells led to increases
in the copy numbers of all assayable donor DNA sequences,
including the h-alu's, in the host cell DNAs. Dhfr gene
transcript levels, DHFR enzyme activities, and synthesis
and cell surface expression of the transfected MAA were
highly elevated following stepwise selections with up to
100µM methotrexate (MTX). The increased copy number
representation of active 96K MAA and 100K MAA-encoding
genes in the MTX-coamplified transfectant cells is
potentially useful for isolation of recombinant genomic
and cDNA clones specific for the 2 MAA.

INTRODUCTION

Human TAA defined by MoAbs are of interest as cell
surface molecules involved in the onset or progression of
malignancy, as markers for developmental lineages or for
stages of differentiation, as products of genes responsive to
lymphokines and other modulators, and as possible targets for
immunodiagnostic or immunotherapeutic approaches to malignant
diseases.
    Inasmuch as these aspects of antigen biology will be most
effectively addressed by the use of recombinant probes and
vectors for genes encoding the protein domains of TAA, experiments aimed at isolating such recombinants were performed. A
genetic approach based on interspecific human-cell DNA-
mediated transfer of active genes coding for TAA was employed.
A highly competent mouse melanoma cell line, B78H1, was used
as DNA recipient, and TAA$^+$ colonies were detected by a red
cell immunorosetting assay.
    Transfections in which panels of screening MoAbs against
various TAA were used led to identification of independent
transfectant colonies expressing each of 4 glycoprotein cell
surface antigens: gp130 (1), 100K MAA (2), and 96K MAA (3),
and the widely-distributed antigen "VCA-2" defined on renal
carcinoma cells (4). Each of the transfected TAA exhibits
restricted tissue distribution, a potential role in cell
recognition and adhesion, or regulated expression in response
to physiological modulators.
    We report results from use of a multistep genetic proce-
dure aimed at isolation of the transfected human genes

encoding the 100K MAA and the 96K MAA. One element of this
procedure, selective coamplification designed to increase the
dosages of transferred MAA-specific genes, and thus to sim-
plify their genomic cloning, is considered in genetic, biochemical, and immunological terms.

MATERIALS AND METHODS

Cell Lines

     B78H1 mouse melanoma cells, transfectants derived from
B78H1, Colo 38 and SK-MEL-37 human melanoma cells, and cells
of malignant mouse fibroblast line LMTK⁻ were obtained and
cultured as described (3).

Monoclonal Antibodies and Antisera

     Anti-96K MAA MoAb CL203.4 and anti-100K MAA MoAb 376.96
were derived as described (5, 6). Purified rabbit antimouse
Ig antibodies, purchased from Cappell-Worthington, a division
of Cooper Biomedical, Malvern, PA, were radiolabeled with ^{125}I
NaI as described (7).

Origin and Preparation of DNAs, DNA-mediated Gene Transfer,
and Selective Coamplification of Introduced DNA Sequences

     Aminoglycoside phosphotransferase (neo) gene vector
pGCcos3neo, dihydrofolate reductase (dhfr) gene vector pFD11,
and plasmid pBlur8, which contains an h-alu sequence, were
obtained as described (3). Purifications of cell and plasmid
DNAs, gene transfers using calcium phosphate coprecipitated
DNAs, and primary Geneticin (G418) selections for transfectant
cells expressing neo gene vector were as described (3).
Cotransfections with 1° or 2° transfectant cell DNAs mixed
with dhfr and neo gene vectors, followed by stepwise MTX
selections were as described (3).

Serological, Immunochemical, and Enzymological Assays

     The indirect binding assay involving sequential incuba-
tion of cells with MoAb CL203.4 or MoAb 376.96, followed by
^{125}I-labeled antimouse Ig xenoantibodies, was performed as
described (3). Surface radioiodination of viable cells,
indirect immunoprecipitation, and sodium dodecylsulphate
polyacrylamide gel electrophoresis (SDS-PAGE) were as
described (3). The protein-level assay for DHFR, involving
the binding of ^{3}H MTX was performed as described (8).

Nucleic Acid Electrophoresis, Southern and Northern Hybridization Analyses, and Dot Blot Analyses

DNAs were digested with restriction endonucleases EcoR1
or BamH1 as recommended by the manufacturer (International
Biotechnologies, Inc., New Haven, CT) and were electrophoresed
in 0.8% agarose gels and transferred to nitrocellulose as
described (9). For DNA dot blotting, cell DNAs were sheared,
denatured, and transferred to nitrocellulose by published
procedures (10). Total cell RNAs were isolated (11) and were
enriched, where indicated, for the polyA$^+$ fraction by standard
methods (11, 12). Formaldehyde-agarose electrophoresis and
transfer to nitrocellulose were as described (13). Filter-
bound nucleic acids were hybridized (11) to the indicated
probes which were radiolabeled as described (14).

RESULTS

Transfer of Genes Encoding 96K and 100K MAA

Primary (1°) human melanoma cell DNA-mediated transfers
of the 100K MAA$^+$ and of the 96K MAA$^+$ phenotypes into B78H1
mouse melanoma cells were human DNA dependent and occurred at
frequencies of $4x10^{-6}$ and $7x10^{-7}$ MAA$^+$ colonies/host cell
plated, respectively, as previously described (2, 3). Subsequent 2° and 3° transfections were similarly dependent on DNAs
from 1° or 2° transfectant cells.

Coamplification of Transfected 100K and 96K MAA Genes

A selective procedure involving cotransfection and
coamplification was used in order to increase the dosages of
transferred MAA gene sequences in transfectant cell genomes
and thus in recombinant transfectant cell libraries in lieu of
direct biochemical selection for overproduction of MAA (2, 3).
Efficacy of the procedure depended on the validity for
MAA$^+$ dhfr$^+$ B78H1 cotransfectants of several reported characteristics of exogenous DNA sequences in transfected rodent
cells: (i) most introduced DNA fragments which associate
heritably with the host cell genome are joined together in a
single (or a low number of) larger multigenic entities (15);
(ii) transferred genes encoding an amplifiable product, e.g.,
dhfr gene vector pFD11, respond more readily than the homologous chromosomal dhfr genes of the host cells to biochemical
selection (MTX) for gene amplification (15); and (iii) a large
block of foreign DNA encompassing most of the transferred DNA,
and thus including the MAA genes, increases in dosage under

selective pressure for amplification of the transferred dhfr
gene component (15). The following results suggest that transferred DNA
sequences including the intact 100K and 96K MAA genes did
respond in this hypothesized manner to MTX selection.

Dosage of Transfected Plasmid DNA Sequences in MTX-Amplified
Transfectant Cells

Dot blot hybridization analyses of cell DNAs (not shown)
revealed that the dosages of human DNA-associated h-alu
repeats, dhfr sequences and plasmid domains of transfecting
vectors increased in parallel with stringency of MTX selection
of 3° 96K and of 2° 100K MAA gene transfectants.
Southern hybridizations showed that specific h-alu$^+$ DNA
fragments heritably present in 2° or 3° MAA gene transfectant
cells respond to MTX selection by copy number amplification.
These include EcoRl fragments of 13kb, 11kb, and 9kb from 2°
100K MAA transfectant cells (2) and a BamHl fragment of 19kb
and EcoRl fragments of 5.8, 4.1 and 1.2kb from 3° 96K MAA
transfectant cells (3).

Dhfr Gene Transcripts and DHFR Enzyme Activities in MTX-
Coamplified Transfectant Cells

Northern Blot analyses of total cell and polyadenylated
RNAs demonstrated that MTX-selected MAA gene amplificants
produce large amounts of a dhfr gene probe-homologous species
of 1.4-1.6kb, and lesser amounts of a larger (2-2.5kb) probe-
hybridizable RNA (not shown). Levels of active DHFR protein
increased progressively to maximum levels 100-200 times
greater than that in unamplified transfectant cells in
response to increasingly stringent MTX selections of 100K MAA
or 96K MAA gene transfectant cells (results not shown).

Effects of Selective Amplification of Transfected DNA
Sequences on B78H1 Host Cell Expression of 100K and 96K MAA

Serological and immunochemical assays showed that MTX-
driven amplification of transfected gene(s) led to B78H1 host
cell overexpression of 100K MAA and 96K MAA from transferred
genes. Table 1 summarizes effects of a 5-step selective
coamplification sequence on mouse transfectant cell binding of
MoAbs CL376.96 or CL203.4, as estimated by binding assays with
radiolabeled anti-mouse IgG antibodies.

TABLE 1
CELL SURFACE EXPRESSION OF MOLECULES
RECOGNIZED BY MoAbs 376.96 OR CL203.4

| | CPM ^{125}I Second Antibody Bound (Actual/Normalized) | |
| | MoAb Added | |
Cell Lines	376.96	203.4
Human melanoma[a]	45,026/1	38,482/1
B78H1 Mouse melanoma	14,660/0	18,654/0
MAA[+] mouse melanoma transfectant/G418[b]	47,756/1.1	43,231/1.2
MAA[+] mouse melanoma transfectant/MTX[c]	549,455/17.6	115,908/4.7

Reactivities of intact cells with MoAb 376.96 or MoAb 203.4 in
the indirect binding assay are tabulated as averages of direct
CPM from duplicate incubations and as relative values derived
by normalization against CPM bound to human melanoma cells.
Prior to normalizations, a negative control consisting of CPM
adhering to B78H1 cells that had been treated with the
indicated MoAb was subtracted. Results of one representative
experiment for each MoAb are presented.
[a]SK-MEL-37 and Colo 38 human melanoma cells were used in
experiments with MoAbs 376.96 and CL203.4 respectively.
[b,c]Transfectant B78H1 cells expressing either 100K MAA
(left column) or 96K MAA (right), as selected in G418 medium
(b) and after 5-step MTX selections that reached a maximum
concentration of 100μM (c).

    SDS-PAGE analysis confirmed overproduction of the anti-
genic structures immunoprecipitated by MoAb 376.96 and by MoAb
CL203.4 from extracts of radiolabeled coamplified 100K MAA and
96K MAA gene transfectant cells. Representative results shown
in figure 1 illustrate ≥20x overproduction of MoAb 376.96-
reactive antigen by coamplified 2° 100K MAA transfectant mouse
melanoma cells. The species immunoprecipitated from 2°
transfectant mouse cells is not electrophoretically separated

from that immunoprecipitated from Colo 38 human melanoma cells
at the ambient level of resolution (lanes 1-3).

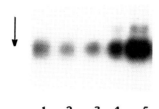

1   2   3   4   5

FIGURE 1.   MoAb 376.96 reactive cell surface molecules
overproduced by coamplified mouse transfectant cells.   Components immunoprecipitated by MoAb 376.96 from extracts of
^{125}I labeled cells were adjusted to a common concentration of
$\approx3-4\times10^4$ cell equivalents/µl and were analyzed by SDS-PAGE:
Colo 38 human melanoma cells, 40µl (lane 1); a mixture of 2°
100K MAA B78H1 mouse melanoma transfectant clone A,
nonamplified, 14µl, with human melanoma Colo 38, 20µl (lane
2); 2° transfectant A, 27µl (lane 3); 2° B78H1 transfectant
clone B, MTX (100µM) amplified, 2 µl (lane 4), and 4µl (lane
5).   Electrophoresis was run under reducing conditions in a
7.5% polyacrylamide gel.   Molecular weight markers (not shown)
indicate a mass of 90-100kDa for the precipitated species.

Efficiency of DNAs from Coamplified Transfectants for Transfer
of MAA Genes into B78H1 Cells and into Mouse Fibroblasts

The frequencies with which the DNAs from maximally
MTX-coamplified 2° 100K MAA$^+$ or 3° 96K MAA$^+$ transfectant cells
transferred the respective MAA genes into B78H1 cells,
$4-5\times10^{-4}$ and 3×10^{-4}, represented a ≥100x increase relative to
1° transfer frequencies indicating marked MTX-mediated
increases in the dosages of biologically active genes encoding
the MAA.   Comparative tests of host cell capabilities to
express foreign MAA genes, made feasible by the high donor
efficiency of coamplified transfectant cell DNAs, demonstrated
that the highly competent mouse fibroblast cell line LMTK$^-$ is
specifically deficient in transgenomic expression of the 96K
MAA gene in transfections in which other dishes of LMTK$^-$ cells
tested in parallel efficiently express the introduced 100K MAA
genes (3).

DISCUSSION

A sequence of genetic steps involving serial gene transfers and selective coamplification appears to provide a useful
approach for cloning of transfected genomic genes encoding TAA
or other transfectable products. By adding donor human DNAs
to mouse melanoma host cells and screening by red cell
immunorosetting with mouse MoAbs that define a number of
different TAA, transfectant colonies have been detected which
stably express any of 4 human cell surface glycoprotein
antigens: 100K MAA, 96K MAA, MAA gp130, and CVA-2. A
selective coamplification procedure applied to transfectant
cells expressing each of the former 2 MAA genes led to marked,
stepwise increases in copy numbers both of gene-associated
h-alu DNA fragments and of MTX-selected dhfr gene and
PGCcos3neo sequences. DHFR enzymatic specific activity and
serologically assayed 100K MAA or 96K MAA increased in
parallel with gene dosages, indicating that the genes were
amplified in a functionally intact form.

The maximum MTX-selected gene and gene product amplification attained for each of the MAA is in the range of 50-100
times the levels in nonamplified, G418-selected transfectant
cells, as estimated by a number of criteria including relative
intensities of h-alu DNA hybridizations, quantities of components immunoprecipitated from radiolabeled transfectant cell
extracts, and donor efficiencies of coamplified cell DNAs for
transfer of the MAA genes. On the other hand, coamplifi-
cation-mediated increases in densities of 96K MAA and of 100K
MAA molecules on transfectant cell surfaces were 5-20-fold, as
compared to densities of the MAA on human melanoma cells and
on nonamplified transfectant cells.

Recent results of in situ chromosomal hybridizations
suggest localization of transferred coamplified h-alu and
vector sequences to ≥2 chromosomes each from coamplified 100K
MAA[+] and from coamplified 96K MAA[+] transfectants. The as yet
unidentified transgenome-positive chromosomes include one
bicentric marker chromosome in the case of 100K MAA gene
transfectant cells. No localization of transferred sequences
to "double minute" subchromosomal elements (16) was detected.

The demonstration of a specific defect in transgenomic
expression of 96K MAA, as opposed to 100K MAA, by the mouse
fibroblast cell line LMTK⁻ is a prototype for studies in which
the high efficiency of MAA gene donation by DNAs of coamplified transfectant cells is utilized in comparative transfection experiments. Such studies will make possible assessment
of the relative capacities of murine host cells representing
diverse developmental lineages or stages of malignancy to
express either of the 2 MAA.

Recombinant clones that contain h-alu elements having presumed association with the 100K MAA and 96K MAA genes have recently been isolated from bacteriophage libraries containing chromosomal DNA fragments from coamplified transfectant cells. The frequencies, ≈10^{-3}, at which these 2 sets of h-alu$^+$ clones were identified were approximately 2 orders of magnitude higher than the frequencies that would be expected in the absence of gene amplification. The relation of the h-alu$^+$ clones to the active 100K MAA and 96K MAA genes is currently being analyzed.

Probes and vectors derived through the application of genomic and/or cDNA cloning methods in combination with gene transfer and coamplification will be useful for analyzing the cellular distribution patterns and the physiological regulation of the 100K MAA and the 96K MAA.

ACKNOWLEDGEMENTS

The authors thank Dr. Lawrence A. Chasin, Columbia University, NY, and his associates for assaying DHFR activities and John Schuchert and Deborah Solomon for preparation of the manuscript.

REFERENCES

1. Albino AP, Graf LH Jr, McLean WJ, Kantor RRS, Silagi S, Old LJ (1985). DNA-mediated transfer of a human melanoma cell surface glycoprotein gp130: identification of transfectants by erythrocyte rosetting. Molec Cell Biol 5:692.
2. Graf LH Jr, Ferrone S, Rosenberg CD (1986). Interspecific DNA-mediated transfer and selective coamplification of a gene for a melanoma surface antigen. J Cell Biol 103:51a.
3. Graf LH Jr, Rosenberg CD, Mancino V, Ferrone S (1988). Transfer and coamplification of a gene encoding a 96 kilodalton immune interferon induced human melanoma-associated antigen: preferential expression by mouse melanoma host cells. J Immunol in press.
4. Kantor RRS, Bander NH, Graf LH Jr, Old LJ, Albino AP (1987). DNA-mediated gene transfer of a human cell surface 170-kilodalton glycoprotein: evidence for association with an endogenous murine protein. J Biol Chem 262:15166.

5. Imai K, Wilson BS, Bigotti A, Natali PG, Ferrone S (1982). A 94,000 dalton glycoprotein expressed by human melanoma and carcinoma cells. J Natl Cancer Inst 68:761.

6. Matsui M, Temponi M, Ferrone S (1987). Characterization of a monoclonal antibody-defined human melanoma-associated antigen susceptible to induction by immune interferon. J Immunol 139:2083.

7. Fraker PS, Speck JC Jr (1978). Protein and cell membrane iodinations with a sparingly soluble chloroamide, 1, 3, 4, 6-tetrachloro-3α, 6α-phenyl glycouril. Biochem Biophys Res Comm 80:849.

8. Urlaub G, Chasin LA (1980). Isolation of Chinese hamster cell mutants deficient in dihydrofolate reductase activity. Proc Natl Acad Sci USA 77:4216.

9. Graf LH Jr, Chasin LA (1982). Direct demonstration of genetic alterations at the dihydrofolate reductase locus after gamma irradiation. Molec Cell Biol 2:93.

10. Cirullo RE, Dana S, Wasmuth JJ (1983). Efficient procedure for transferring specific human genes into Chinese hamster cell mutants: interspecific transfer of the human genes encoding leucyl- and asparaginyl-tRNA synthetases. Mol Cell Biol 3:892

11. Chirgwin JM, Przybala AE, McDonald RJ, Rutter WJ (1979). Isolation of biologically active ribonucleic acid from sources enriched in ribonuclease. Biochemistry 24:5294.

12. Jacobson A (1987). Purification and fractionation of polyA$^+$ RNA. In Berger SL, Kimmel AR (eds): "Guide to Molecular Cloning Techniques," Methods in Enzymology, vol. 152, New York: Academic Press, p. 202.

13. Maniatis T, Fritsch EF, Sambrook J (1982). "Molecular Cloning." Cold Spring Harbor, NY: Cold Spring Harbor Press, p. 202.

14. Feinberg AP, Vogelstein B (1984). A technique for radiolabeling DNA restriction endonuclease fragments to a high specific activity. Anal Biochem 137:206.

15. Perucho M, Hanahan D, Wigler M (1980). Genetic and physical linkage of exogenous sequences in transformed cells. Cell 22:309.

16. Kaufman RJ, Brown PC, Schimke RJ (1979). Amplified dihydrofolate reductase genes in unstably methotrexate-resistant cells are associated with double minute chromosomes. Proc Natl Acad Sci USA 76:5669.

Human Tumor Antigens and Specific Tumor Therapy, pages 45–52
© 1989 Alan R. Liss, Inc.

cDNA CLONING OF TWO CLOSELY RELATED MELANOMA GLYCOPROTEINS: MUC18 A MARKER FOR TUMOR PROGRESSION AND MUC18rep A NEW MEMBER OF THE IMMUNOGLOBULIN SUPERFAMILY[1]

Jürgen M.Lehmann, Christine Sers, Gert Riethmüller and Judith P.Johnson

Institute of Immunology, University of Munich, D8000 Munich 2, Federal Republic of Germany

ABSTRACT   MUC18 is a 113,000 dalton surface glycoprotein whose expression is correlated with tumor progression in human malignant melanoma. MUC18, or at least the epitope defined by MoAb MUC18, has not yet been detected on benign melanocytic nevi or other types of tumors and in normal tissue its expression is limited to smooth muscle cells. cDNA cloning resulted in the isolation of two different gene products which were cross-reactive at both the protein and nucleic acid levels. While both genes are expressed in melanomas, transfection into COS-7 cells indicated that only one encodes the MUC18 antigen. The deduced amino acid sequence of the MUC18 related protein predicts an integral membrane glycoprotein with 3 extracellular immunoglobulin like domains.

INTRODUCTION

The pigmented nature of melanocytes and their epidermal location allow identification of and easy access to a large variety of benign and malignant melanocytic lesions and make human melanoma a good model system in which to identify molecular changes occurring during tumor progression.

[1]This work was supported by the Deutsche Krebshilfe, Mildred Scheel Stiftung

Using monoclonal antibodies (MoAb) which discriminate between benign melanocytic nevi and malignant melanoma, 5 groups of melanocytic lesions could be distinguished by antigenic profile (1). These groups could be ranked in relation to each other on the basis of sequential acquisition or loss of antigens. A scheme of stepwise antigenic changes is therefore proposed to accompany the histopathological and clinical alterations observed during the transformation of normal skin melanocytes into highly metastatic melanoma cells. One of these progression steps is characterized by the appearance of the antigen defined by MoAb MUC18 (2).

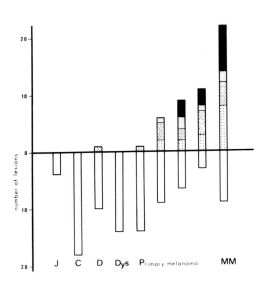

Figure 1. Reaction pattern of MoAb MUC18 with various melanocytic lesions. J: junctional nevus, C: compound nevus, D: dermal nevus, DYS: dysplastic nevus. Primary melanomas are divided according Breslow index (≤0.75mm, 0.76-1.5mm, 1.51-3.0mm, ≥3.0mm). M: metastatic melanoma. The percent positive cells per lesion were divided into 5 intensity groups (☐ :no reactivity, ☐ :≤5, ∷ :5-25, ▦ :26-50, ▨ :51-75, ■ :76-100)

REACTIVITY OF MoAB MUC18 WITH NORMAL TISSUES, BENIGN LESIONS AND MALIGNANT TUMORS OF VARIOUS ORIGINS

Figure 1 shows the reaction pattern of MoAb MUC18 (IgG2a) on various melanocytic lesions as tested by immunoperoxidase staining on frozen tissue sections. With the exception of a single nevus cell nest in one compound nevus, no reactivity was seen with melanocytic nevi. Nevi are benign melanocytic tumors with activated and proliferative characteristics. In addition no reactivity of MoAb MUC18 was seen on dysplastic nevi which are postulated to be premalignant lesions (3). Among primary melanomas expression of MUC18 is correlated with tumor thickness. MUC18 is not seen on the very early (i.e.,thin) tumors but appears when tumors reach a thickness of 1 mm. The frequency of positive lesions as well as the number of positive tumor cells per lesion increases with increasing tumor thickness. Because tumor thickness (i.e. Breslow index; 4) is the most predictive parameter of poor prognosis and the eventual incidence of metastatic disease, MUC18 may play a role in tumor progression, endowing cells with a selective advantage which contributes to the successful formation of metastasis. Outside the melanocytic lineage no reactivity has yet been observed with any other tumor tested and in normal tissue, antigen expression seems to be limited to hair follicles and smooth muscle cells (Table 1). Using the Western blotting reactive antibody MUCBA18.1 (see below), the MUC18 antigen could be immunoprecipitated from a smooth muscle cell lysate. Therefore MoAb MUC18 reactivity is not due to a cross reactive epitope but indicates that the MUC18 antigen itself is a normal component of smooth muscle cells.

BIOCHEMICAL CHARACTERIZATION OF MUC18

Immunoprecipitation from radiolabelled melanoma cells revealed that MUC18 is a heavily sialylated surface glycoprotein of M_r of 113,000 daltons,with a protein backbone of M_r of 67,000 daltons. The reduction to a M_r of 98,000 daltons under reducing conditions suggests that the antigen is a single polypeptide chain with intrachain disulfide bonds.

Table 1: Reactivity of MoAb MUC18 with normal tissues, benign lesions and malignant tumors of various origins

---

Tissues with positive reactivity	Tissues scored as negative[a]	Carcinomas scored as negative
Smooth muscle cells	Skin epidermis	Colorectal Ca (9)[b]
Hair follicles	Sweat gland	Gastric Ca (8)
	Sebaceous gland	Breast Ca (10)
	Lung (3)	Ovarian Ca (3)
	Spleen (1)	Renal cell Ca (4)
	Thymus (2)	Bronchial Ca (1)
	Lymph node (3)	Thyroid Ca (1)
	Kidney (3)	Adrenal Ca (1)
	Liver (4)	Vaginal Ca (1)
	Bile duct	Chorion Ca (1)
	Stomach (4)	Retinoblastoma(1)
	Intestinal	Basal cell Ca (1)
	Metaplasia (2)	Glioma (2)
	Colon (10)	Neuroblastoma (1)
	Small intestine	EBV transformed
	Gall bladder (1)	B-LCL (16)[c] [d]
	Pancreas (1)	T-cell Leukemia(3)
	Thyroid gland	
	Goiter (2)	
	Mammary gland	
	Mastopathia (2)	
	Brain Cerebrum	
	Cerebellum (1)	
	Peripheral nerves	
	Skeletal muscle of	
	colon and stomach	
	Bone Marrow (2)	
	Blood cells	
	PMC (5)[e]	
	PHA stimulated PMC (5)	

---

[a] Tissue were scored as negative only if no reactive cell could be detected. Isotype control was UPC10 (IgG2a, Sigma, St.Louis,MO)
[b] Numbers in parentheses, number of tissues tested
[c] EBV transformed B-LCL, Epstein-Barr virus transformed B-lymphoblastoid cell line
[d] T-cell lines: Molt4; CEM; and Jurkat
[e] PMC, peripheral mononuclear cell; PHA, phytohemagglutinin

MOLECULAR CLONING OF MUC18 AND A MUC18 RELATED PROTEIN

To obtain a probe that can be used to screen a human melanoma cDNA library in the lambda gt11 and lambda zap expression vector systems, 5 MoAbs reactive with the denatured MUC18 antigen were isolated. All 5 MoAbs showed strong reactivity with melanoma on tissue sections. On other tissues a slightly broader reactivity pattern was observed as compared to that of MoAb MUC18 but this was not characterized in more detail. One of these Western blotting antibodies reacts as well with unfixed cells in immunofluoresence staining. Therefore the 5 MoAbs include antibodies directed against at least two different epitopes on MUC18.

Screening of 750,000 lambda plaques yielded 10 cDNA clones positive in immunoblotting. These clones could be divided into three non cross-hybridizing groups. Because of an expression pattern in Northern blot analyses similar to that of MUC18 antigen expression (data not shown), one group was chosen for further analyses. This group contained four cross-hybridizing cDNA clones encoding two different but apparently closely related gene products. Transfection experiments, using the CDM8 vector into COS-7 cells (5), showed that the product encoded by cDNA clones drop1 and drop6 is recognized by MoAb MUC18 (data not shown). The COS-7 product encoded by the cDNA clones drop4 and zapy reacted weakly with 3 out of 5 Western blotting antibodies but did not react with MoAb MUC18. cDNA cloning has therefore identified 2 melanoma proteins: MUC18 whose expression is correlated with tumor progression and a MUC18 related protein (MUC18rep) with an expression pattern in Northern blot analyses similar to that of MUC18 antigen expression. cDNA clones encoding MUC18rep contain sequence information for approximately 2,900bp and identified a single mRNA band of 3,300bp in melanoma cells. The restriction pattern in Southern blot analyses is consistent with a single copy gene as only a single hybridization fragment was obtained with several different restriction endonucleases. Comparison of restriction patterns in autologous B-LCL and melanoma cells provides no indication that the gene is rearranged in melanoma.

Suitable restriction fragments were subcloned into pUC18 and the double stranded cDNA inserts were sequenced by the dideoxy chain termination method (6). The cDNA of MUC18rep includes a single open reading frame of at least 1,160 bp and a 1,450bp 3'non-coding region, which includes the consensus polyadenylation signal (AATAAA). Sequencing of the 5'prime region is not yet completed but in the carboxyl terminal region the predicted amino acid sequence contains a 24 residue hydrophobic putative transmembrane domain followed by 21 residues of basic and hydrophilic amino acids comprising the cytoplasmic domain. The sequence contains 8 potential extracellular N-linked glycosylation sites (Arg-X-Thr/Ser) and at least 2 sites for potential O-linked glycosylation (acidic residue-X-Ser-Gly).

MUC18rep IS A MEMBER OF THE IMMUNOGLOBULIN SUPERFAMILY

Inspection of the MUC18rep sequence revealed three extracellular repeats with internal homology (9 residues are conserved) fulfilling the criteria of a typical C2-SET sequence as proposed for members of the immunoglobulin superfamily (7). This family of immunoglobulin related structures is proposed on the basis of sequence similarities. The characteristic feature of C2-SET sequences is a folded sandwich structure of 7 anti-parallel beta sheets stabilized by a disulfide bond. Moreover several additional residues highly characteristic for the immunoglobulin domain structure are conserved in the MUC18rep sequence. Among the immunoglobulin related molecules, the myelin-associated glycoprotein (MAG) (8) (26% identity over 159 residues) showed the greatest similarity to the MUC18rep sequence. However the T-cell surface glycoprotein CD8 (22% identity over 50 residues) and the T-cell receptor alpha (38% identity over 39 residues) and beta (35% identity over 31 residues) subunits showed great similarity to MUC18rep sequence. Outside the immunoglobulin superfamily, searches of protein sequence data bases using the FASTP program detected only weak similarities over a small number of residues.

CONCLUSION

During the course of tumor progression, tumor cells acquire many new properties normally not expressed by their progenitor cells. In order to initiate secondary growth at distant sites, tumor cells have to invade the host stroma, penetrate vascular/lymphatic systems, attach in the capillary beds of distant organs and finally penetrate into organ parenchyma. During this process tumor cells must resist destruction from mechanical stress as well as from

```
                              ....S......................................S....
                                  :                                      :
MUC18  (I)   TEKVWLEVEPVGMLKEGDRVFIRCLADGNPPPHFSISKQN--------PSTREAFEETTNDNGVLVLEPARKEHSGRYECQAWNLDTMISLLSEPQELLVN
MUC18 (II)   YVSDVRVSPAAPERQEGSSLTLTCEAESSQD--LE--FQWLREETDQVLERGPVL----------LQLHDLKREAGGGYRCVA---SVPSTPGLNRTQLVKL
MUC18 (III)  GPPWMAFKERKVWVKENMVLNLSCEASGHPRPTISWNVNGTASEQDQDPQRVLST----------LNVLVTPELLEGTVECTA---SNDLGKNTSTLFLELV

MAG   (III)  YPPVIVEMNSSVEAIEGSHVSLLCGADSNPPPLLTWMRDG--------MVLREAVAESLY----LDLEEVTPAEDGIYACLA---ENAYGQDNRTVELSVM
MAG   (IV)   YAPWKPTVNGTVVAVEGETVSTLCSTQSNPDPILTIFKEKQILATVIYESQLQ-----------LELPAVTPEDDGEYWCVA---ENQYGQRATAFNLSVE
```

Figure 2. Internal homology between repeated domains in MUC18rep and relationship to the immunoglobulin superfamily. Rows 1,2, and 3 contain the contiguous 270 amino acid sequence of MUC18rep, and rows 4 and 5 the contiguous amino acid sequence of MAG (residues 237-410), aligned to show greatest similarity. Amino acids (237-410) form the third and fourth immunoglobulin related domains of MAG.

the immune system. The expression pattern of MUC18 on melanocytic lesions strongly suggests that this molecule, a normal component of smooth muscle cells, is involved in some aspect of this process. Northern analyses indicate that the closely related MUC18rep also appears to be melanoma restricted. MUC18rep membership in the immunoglobulin superfamily suggests that it may function as a receptor for soluble or cell bound factors controlling movement or differentiation.

REFERENCES

1. Holzmann B, Bröcker EB, Lehmann JM, Ruiter DJ, Riethmüller G, Johnson JP (1987). Tumor progression in human malignant melanoma: Five stages defined by their antigenic phenotypes. Int J Cancer 39:466.
2. Lehmann JM, Holzmann B, Breitbart EW, Schmiegelow P, Riethmüller G, Johnson JP (1987). Discrimination between benign and malignant cells of melanocytic lineage by two novel antigens, a glycoprotein with a molecular weight of 113,000 and a protein with a molecular weight of 76,000. Cancer Research 47:841
3. Clark WH, Elder DE, Guerry D, Epstein MV, Greene MH, van Horn M (1985). A study of tumor progression. The precursor lesions of superficial spreading and nodular melanoma. Hum Pathol 15:1147
4. Breslow A (1970). Thickness, cross-sectional areas and depth of invasion in the prognosis cutaneous melanoma. Ann Surg 172:902
5. Aruffo A, Seed B (1987). Molecular cloning of a CD28 cDNA by a high-efficiency COS cell expression system. Proc.Natl.Acad.Sci.USA 84:8573
6. Sanger F, Nicklen S, Coulson AR (1977). DNA sequencing with chain termination inhibitors. Proc.Natl.Acad.Sci.USA 74:5463
7. Williams AF (1987). A year in the life of the immuno- globulin superfamily. Immun Today 8:298
8. Arquint M, Roder J, Chia L-S, Down J, Wilkinson D, Bayley H, Braun P, Dunn R (1987) Molecular cloning and primary structure of myelin-associated glycoprotein. Proc.Natl.Acad.Sci.USA 84:600

Human Tumor Antigens and Specific Tumor Therapy, pages 53–62
© 1989 Alan R. Liss, Inc.

MONOCLONAL ANTIBODIES FOR DETECTION OF NORMAL AND ONCOGENIC RAS P21

Walter P. Carney, Peter J. Hamer, Joyce LaVecchio, Simon Ng, Debra Petit, Thaddeus G. Pullano and Kevin L. Trimpe

Medical Products Dept., E. I. Dupont, North Billerica, MA 01862

ABSTRACT   The ras gene family is composed of the Harvey, Kirsten and N ras genes which encode immunologically related proteins of approximately 21,000 daltons that are collectively referred to as p21. Several reports have implicated the overexpression of normal p21 in breast and colon carcinomas; other studies have led to the discovery of oncogenic ras genes in a wide variety of cancers. These oncogenic ras genes encode activated proteins with amino acid substitutions at positions 12, 13 or 61.

In this report, we describe monoclonal antibodies (Mab) designated   Ras 10 and Ras 11 that detect both normal and activated forms of p21 as well as the three families of the Harvey, Kirsten and N-ras p21. We also describe Mab R256, DWP and E184 that detect only activated p21 with amino acid substitutions at position 12. Monoclonal antibodies specific for normal and activated p21 will be valuable for assessing the role of ras proteins in the initiation and progression of cancer.

INTRODUCTION

The ras family includes the Harvey (H), Kirsten (Ki) and N ras genes which encode 21,000 dalton proteins that bind guanine nucleotides, have GTPase activity and are associated with the inner face of the plasma membrane (1). The ras genes have been highly conserved in eukaryotic organisms (2) and have been implicated in cell proliferation (3) and terminal differentiation (4). Since ras proteins have functional and biochemical properties similar to the G proteins, they have been implicated in the transduction of signals across the cell membrane (5).

Previous studies have proposed that ras proteins contribute to the neoplastic process by either overexpression of the p21 or by an alteration in the amino acid structure of the p21. For example, reports by Spandidos, et al., utilized nucleic acid hybridization procedures to demonstrate the presence of elevated levels of ras specific RNA in breast and colon carcinomas (6, 7). Reports such as these have led to the hypothesis that overexpression of ras p21 may be important in the development of cancer.

Transfection studies using NIH3T3 cells as recipients of human tumor cell DNA have led to the discovery of activated ras genes that encode proteins with amino acid substitutions at positions 12, 13 and 61. Activated p21s have been discovered in a variety of human and animal cancers including solid tumors and leukemias. Recent reports have shown the presence of activated p21 in 40% of human colorectal cancers and in preneoplastic lesions of the colon (8, 9). Similarly, activated p21s with amino acid substitutions at position 12 (10) or 13 have been discovered in acute myelogenous leukemias (11) as well as in preleukemic syndromes (12). Since activated p21s have not been detected in normal cells, they may be considered specific cancer markers and their detection may be of diagnostic and prognostic significance.

In this report, we describe Mab Ras 10 and Ras 11 that specifically detect the normal and activated forms of p21 as well as the H, Ki and N forms of the ras protein. These monoclonal antibodies will be valuable in a variety of assays for assessing the overall level of cellular p21 and for understanding the role of ras proteins in the neoplastic process.

We also describe Mab R256, DWP and E184 which are valuable reagents in the Western blot format for detecting activated ras proteins with arginine, valine or glutamic acid, respectively at position 12.

MATERIALS AND METHODS

Immunization, Hybridoma Selection and Mab Characterization

To produce Mab that react with both normal and activated p21, we immunized Balb/c X C57Bl/6 mice with a recombinant protein representing the human Harvey p21 (r-p21) mixed with Complete Freund's Adjuvant.

To generate Mab that could discriminate between activated and normal p21, we immunized mice with synthetic peptides corresponding to positions 5-16 of activated ras proteins. The peptides used for immunization contained amino acid substitutions that corresponded to activated p21, i.e. with arginine

(Arg-12), valine (Val-12) or glutamic acid (Glu-12) at position 12 instead of the normal amino acid glycine (Gly-12). To enhance immunogenicity, the peptides were coupled to carrier proteins Keyhole Limpet Hemocyanin or Bovine Thyroglobulin using the glutaraldehyde method of Kagan and Glick (13).

The production of hybridomas, ascites fluid and purified immunoglobulins were as described previously (14).

The detection of antibodies in hybridoma supernatants and the characterization of purified Mab was performed using ELISA, immunoprecipitation and Western blot procedures as previously described (14).

Cell Culture

To characterize Mab Ras 10 and Ras 11 the following cell lines were kindly provided by Dr. G.M. Cooper, Dana Farber Cancer Institute: NIH3T3 cells, NIH3T3 cells transformed by overexpression of the normal cellular H-ras (designated 3T3-H), NIH3T3 cells transformed by an activated human cellular Ki-ras gene (designated 3T3-Ki) and NIH3T3 cells transformed by an activated human cellular N-ras gene. Cell lines used to characterize the specificity of Mab R256, DWP and E184 were described previously (14).

RESULTS

Mab for the Detection of Normal and Activated p21

ELISA

To generate Mab that would detect both normal and activated p21, sera from mice immunized with r-p21 were tested by ELISA. Mice that exhibited serum reactivity with r-p21 of greater than 1:50,000 were selected for hybridoma production.

To select hybridomas secreting anti-p21 antibodies, cell supernatants were analyzed by ELISA and immuno-precipitation procedures for reactivity with normal and activated r-p21. From several hundred wells tested, hybridomas designated Ras 10 and Ras 11 were selected and purified for subsequent studies. Subclass analysis of the purified monoclonal antibodies demonstrated that Ras 10 was an IgG2a whereas Mab Ras 11 was an IgG2b.

Purified Ras 10 or Ras 11 were evaluated by ELISA for the ability to react with the various r-p21 coated onto microtiter wells. Results demonstrated that Ras 10 or Ras 11 could detect the normal r-p21 and a variety of recombinant ras proteins activated by amino acid substitutions at positions 12 or 61. ELISA results also demonstrated that Ras 10 or Ras 11 could react with r-p21 representing the human H, Ki and N ras proteins.

In the next series of ELISA experiments, we compared Ras 10, Ras 11 and the rat Mab Y13-259 (15) for the ability to react with the various forms of r-p21. Results clearly demonstrated the strong reactivity of Ras 10 or Ras 11 with the normal and activated forms of r-p21 whereas Y13-259 consistently showed very weak reactivity with the recombinant ras proteins.

Biochemical Evaluation of Ras 10

We next evaluated the ability of Ras 10 to specifically immunoprecipitate ras p21 from cells overexpressing normal H-p21 (3T3-H) or cells with activated Ki-ras p21 (3T3-Ki) or activated N-ras p21 (3T3-N). Fig 1 illustrates the results in which cell lysates were incubated with Ras 10 or a class matched negative control antibody to immunoprecipitate ras p21. To visualize the p21 we employed Ras 10 in a Western blot format. Results in panel A show that Ras 10 was able to immunoprecipitate normal p21 from the 3T3-H cell lysate (lane 1) as well as the activated Ki-p21 (lane 2) or the activated N-p21 (lane 3). Panel B shows that the negative control antibody did not immunoprecipitate p21 from any of the cell lines. These studies demonstrate that Ras 10 is capable of detecting both normal and activated cellular p21 as well as the three families of H, Ki and N ras. Similar results were obtained with Mab Ras 11 (data not shown). Therefore, Mab Ras 10 or Ras 11 can be used to immunoprecipitate p21 as well as to visualize ras proteins by the Western blot procedure.

Numerous reports have evaluated human tumor cell lines and human tumors for the presence and level of ras p21 using Mab Y13-259. Since our ELISA data demonstrated that Y13-259 was far less reactive with r-p21 than Ras 10 or Ras 11, it suggested that Y13-259 might also be less reactive than Ras 10 in detecting p21 by Western blot.

To test this hypothesis, we evaluated a variety of human and animal tumor cell lines as well as human tumors for reactivity with Ras 10, Ras 11 or Y13-259. In the majority (>90%) of samples tested, the Mab Y13-259 was far less reactive with cellular p21 than Ras 10 or Ras 11. In many samples, the p21 was not detected at all with Y13-259. Variations in the concentration of Y13-259 as well as in the reagents to detect the rat Mab did not improve results significantly.

These observations suggest that previous studies with rat Mab Y13-259 may be inaccurate in the assessment of the presence, absence or overall level of ras expression.

ras10

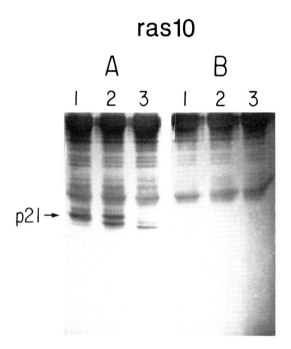

FIG 1. Immunoprecipitation of p21 with Ras 10
Cell lysates 3T3-H (1), 3T3-Ki (2) and 3T3-N (3). Lysates were incubated with Ras 10 (A) or a negative control antibody (B) and the immunoprecipitation and Western blot procedures completed as described.

Mab for Detection of Activated P21

To generate Mab that would react specifically with activated p21 we immunized mice with synthetic peptides corresponding to amino acids 5-16 of activated p21 containing Arg-12, Val-12 or Glu-12 as described in Materials and Methods.

To select anti-peptide Mab, hybridoma supernatants were screened by ELISA for reactivity with peptides containing Arg-12, Val-12, Glu-12 or the normal Gly-12. Hybridomas secreting antibodies which reacted specifically with the immunizing peptide and that did not react with peptides containing Gly-12 were selected for further analysis.

Mab R256 was derived from a mouse immunized with the peptide containing Arg-12, Mab DWP was derived from a mouse immunized with a peptide containing Val-12 and Mab E184 was isolated from a mouse immunized with peptide Glu-12. Mabs R256 and E184 did not react with peptides containing serine, cysteine, alanine, aspartic acid or glycine at position 12. Mab DWP did not react with peptides containing serine, alanine, aspartic acid or glycine, however, DWP did show some cross reactivity with the peptide containing cysteine (14).

To determine whether anti-peptide Mab R256, DWP and E184 would react specifically with activated cellular p21, we performed the following analysis. Cell lysates containing normal p21 or p21 activated by various mutations at position 12 were applied to a 12.5% polyacrylamide gel and proteins were separated using SDS-PAGE.

The proteins were electrophoretically transferred to nitrocellulose filters and the remaining steps of the Western blot were carried out as described in Materials and Methods. Fig. 2 illustrates Western blot results whereby lysates from four cell lines containing either normal (panel A) or activated p21 (B, C & D) were tested for reactivity with anti-p21 Mab Ras 11 (lane 1), R256 (lane 2), DWP (lane 3) or E184 (lane 4). Panel A represents a cell lysate containing normal p21 with Gly-12; lysate in panel B contains activated p21 with Arg-12, lysate in panel C contains activated p21 with Val-12 and lysate in panel D contains activated p21 with Glu-12.

Results illustrated in lane 1 of panels A, B, C and D show that the positive control, anti-p21 Mab Ras 11 was reactive with both normal and activated p21. However, panel A also shows that R256 (lane 2), DWP (lane 3) and E184 (lane 4) were not reactive with normal cellular p21. Panel B shows the specificity of Mab R256 for activated p21 with Arg-12 (lane 2), panel C shows the specificity of Mab DWP for activated cellular p21 with Val-12 (lane 3) and panel D shows the specificity of Mab E184 for activated cellular p21 containing Glu-12 (lane 4). Additional studies demonstrated that R256, DWP and E184 did not crossreact with p21 activated by position 12 substitutions of serine, cysteine or aspartic acid. Similarly, these Mab did not crossreact with p21 activated by aspartic acid at position 13 or cellular p21 activated by histidine, lysine, leucine or arginine at position 61.

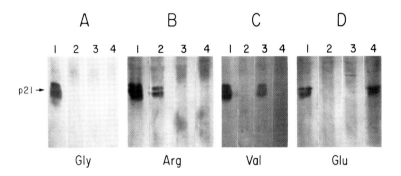

Fig 2. Western blot of Activated p21
Cell lysates containing normal p21 (Gly-12) (A), or p21s activated by Arg-12 (B), Val-12 (C) or Glu-12 (D). Cell proteins were separated by electrophoresis in a 12.5% SDS-PAGE and transferred to nitrocellulose filters. Filters were incubated with the anti-p21 Mab Ras 11 (lane 1), R256 (lane 2),   DWP (lane 3) or E184 (lane 4).   The monoclonal antibodies were detected with goat anti-mouse IgG-HRP and the Western blot completed as previously described.

DISCUSSION

Although ras proteins are normal cellular constituents, their overexpression or activation has been proposed as possible mechanisms by which normal cells are transformed to cancer cells. To better understand the role of ras proteins in neoplastic progression and to help elucidate mechanisms by which p21s contribute to the transformation process, we raised a series of Mab to normal and activated p21.

Mab Ras 10 or Ras 11 were raised against recombinant p21 and were subsequently shown to react specifically with recombinant and cellular p21 using procedures such as ELISA, immunoprecipitation and Western blot. We have demonstrated in these assays that Ras 10 or Ras 11 can detect both normal and activated p21 as well as the H, Ki and N forms of the p21. Comparative biochemical studies of human tumors and human tumor cell lines have revealed that Ras 10 and Ras 11 are significantly more reactive with p21 than the rat Mab Y13-259. Therefore, Ras 10 and Ras 11 are valuable reagents for establishing accurate levels of ras p21 in normal and neoplastic cells.

Flow cytometry studies (data not shown) showed that tumor cells known to overexpress the ras p21 stained more intensely than cells expressing normal levels of p21. We are currently using Ras 10 in flow cytometry to address the issue of whether level of ras expression in leukemic cells has any diagnostic or prognostic significance.

Preliminary immunoperoxidase studies (data not shown) demonstrated that Ras 10 and Ras 11 could specifically detect p21 in tumor cells that had been fixed in formalin and embedded in paraffin. Competitive inhibition studies revealed that Ras 10 or Ras 11 immunoreactivities could be inhibited by the preincubation of the Mabs with r-p21. Immunohisto-chemistry studies also demonstrated that the differential expression of ras p21 detected by flow cytometry and Western blot could also be visualized at the cellular level using the immunoperoxidase technique.

In summary, our results demonstrate that Mab Ras 10 and Ras 11 are valuable reagents for the biochemical, flow cytometric and immunohistochemical analysis of ras expression in normal, hyperplastic and neoplastic cells.

Activated ras p21 with amino acid substitutions at position 12, 13 or 61 have been detected in a variety of neoplastic and preneoplastic cells. In this report, we describe a series of Mab raised against synthetic peptides with amino acid substitutions at position 12 of the p21. We demonstrated the ability of these anti-peptide Mab to detect activated cellular p21. Western blot studies of ras transformed NIH cells indicated that Mab R256 specifically reacted with lysates containing activated p21 with Arg-12, Mab DWP specifically reacted with lysates containing activated p21 with Val-12 and E184 specifically reacted with activated p21 containing Glu-12. Mab R256, DWP, E184 and additional monoclonal antibodies with specificity for activated p21 may be useful in detecting the presence and determining the frequency of activated p21 in preneoplastic and neoplastic cells.

REFERENCES

1. Barbacid M, (1987). Ras Genes.   Ann. Rev. Biochem, 56:779.

2. Shilo BZ, Weinberg RA, (1987).   DNA sequences homologous to vertebrate oncogenes are conserved in Drosphila melanogaster.   PNAS USA 78:6789.

3. Mulcahy LS, Smith MR, Stacey DW, (1985).   Requirement for ras proto-oncogene function during serum stimulated growth of NIH 3T3 cells.   Nature (London) 313:241.

4. Bar-Sagi D, Feramisco JR, (1985).   Microinjection of the ras oncogene protein into PC12 cells induces morphological differentiation.   Cell 42:841.

5. Koin LJ, Siebel CW, McCormick F, Roth RA, (1987).   Ras p21 as a potential mediator of insulin action in Xenopus ocytes.   Science 236:840.

6. Spandidos DA, Agnantis NJ.   (1984) Human malignant tumors of the breast, as compared to their respective normal tissue, have elevated expression of the Harvey ras oncogene.   Anticancer Research 4:269.

7. Spandidos DA, Kerr IB, (1984).   Elevated expression of the human ras oncogene family in premalignant and malignant tumors of the colorectum.   Br. J. Cancer 49:681.

8. Bos JL, Fearon ER, Hamilton SR, Verlaan-deVries M, Van Boom JH, van der Eb AJ, Volgelstein B.   (1987) Prevalence of ras gene mutations in human cancers.   Nature 327:293.

9. Forrester K, Almoguera C, Han K, Grizzle WE, Perucho M.   (1987)   Detection of high incidence of K-ras oncogenes during human colon tumorigenesis.   Nature 327:299.

10 Farr CJ, Saiki RK, Erlich HA, McCormick F, Marshall C.   (1988) Analysis of ras gene mutations in acute myeloid leukemia by polymerase chain reaction and oligonucleotide probes.   PNAS 85:1629.

11 Bos JL, Toksoz D, Marshall CJ, Verlaan-de Vries M, Veeneman GH, van der Eb AJ, VanBoom JH, Janssen JWG, Steenvoorden ACM.   (1985) Amino acid substitutions at codon 13 of the N ras oncogene in human acute myeloid leukemia.   Nature 315:726

12 Liu E, Hjelle B, Morgan R, Hecht F, Bishop MJ (1987). Mutations of the Kirsten-ras proto-oncogene in human preleukemia. Nature 330:186.

13 Kagan A, Glick SM, (1979). Methods of Hormone Radioimmunoassay. 2nd Ed. Academic Press, Inc. 327-339.

14 Carney WP, Petit D, Hamer PJ, Der CJ, Finkel T, Cooper GM, Lefebvre M, Mobtaker H, DeLellis R., Tischler AS, Dayal Y, Wolfe H, Rabin H. (1986) Monoclonal antibody specific for an activated Ras Protein . PNAS USA 83:7485.

15 Furth ME, Davis LJ, Fleurdelys B, Scolnick E. (1982) Monoclonal Antibodies to the p21 Product of the Tranforming Gene of Harvey Murine Sarcoma Virus and of the Cellular ras Gene Family. J. of Virol. 43(1):294.

Human Tumor Antigens and Specific Tumor Therapy, pages 63–71
© 1989 Alan R. Liss, Inc.

Gp96 MOLECULES : RECOGNITION ELEMENTS IN TUMOR IMMUNITY[1]

Pramod K Srivastava[2] and Lloyd J Old

Samuel Freeman Laboratory
Memorial Sloan-Kettering Cancer Center
New York, NY 10021

ABSTRACT Cell surface molecules of 96,000 d (gp96)
mediate   the individually distinct antigenicity of
chemically   induced   tumors of inbred mice.   This
claim rests on the following observations : (a) the
unique immunogenicity of BALB/c sarcomas Meth A and
CMS5 copurifies with gp96 molecules from these tumors
through several independent purification steps. (b) the
cross   reactive immunogenicity of BALB/c sarcomas Meth
A   and and   CMS13 also   copurifies   with   gp96
molecules   from   these   tumors.   (c)   specific
immunogenicity is removed from antigen extracts by
immunoaffinity chromatography through rabbit anti-gp96
columns. (d) lymphocytes from mice immunized with Meth
A gp96 preparations can passively transfer resistance
to Meth A sarcoma. Gp96 molecules (detected by rabbit
anti-gp96 antiserum) are ubiquitous in the tumors and
normal tissues tested; however, immunization with gp96
from BALB/c liver did not elicit resistance to   Meth
A or CMS5 sarcomas. Comparison of sequences of gp96
cDNAs from   Meth A and spleen   shows a structural
divergence. The relationship of this difference to the
individually distinct tumor antigenicity remains to be
elucidated.

[1] This work was supported by a First   Independent
Research Support and Transition Award of the NIH to P.K.S.
(CA-44786) and National Cancer Institute grant CA-08748 and
the Samuel Freeman Trust.
[2] To whom correspondence should be addressed.

INTRODUCTION

Immunogenicity of chemically induced tumors in syngeneic and autologous rodents provided the initial conceptual framework for contemporary tumor immunology and remains the prototypical example of immunity against syngeneic tumors (1). Studies with tumors induced by a variety of chemical carcinogens have demonstrated the generality of these antigens and their two fundamental properties : (a) they elicit immunity in syngeneic hosts and (b) they are highly polymorphic. These tumors have been criticized as being inappropriate models in tumor immunology because they are artificially induced and highly immunogenic – thus their study may not be applicable to human tumors, which are 'spontaneous' and presumably non-immunogenic (2). Clearly, it is not evident whether human tumors are infact 'spontaneous' or non-immunogenic nor is it clear what the appropriate models for human cancers should be. The significance of experimental cancer immunology lies not so much in the hope that its results will be immediately relevant to human cancer, as in the likelihood that these studies will permit a glimpse into the immunological mechanisms that go into tumor immunity. In particular, the precise structure of antigens eliciting immunity to experimental tumors needs to be determined, if cancer immunology is to achieve the status of an objective science rather than an empirical art. Studies with these tumors have already elucidated some general principles, which could not have emerged without them : to wit, the significance of cellular immunity in tumor resistance, role of immunological suppression in abrogation of tumor immunity, adoptive immunotherapy of tumor bearing hosts and the demonstration that immunity can be generated against apparently non-immunogenic tumors (3-5).

Our work on the molecular definition of the individually distinct immunogenic antigens of these tumors has led us to propose (6) that these tumor rejection antigens (TRAs) belong to a family of cell surface glycoproteins of 96,000 d , which are distinct from previously described antigens . In the present communication, we describe further evidence that the gp96 molecules are indeed the recognition elements in tumor immunity and we discuss the current status of studies with respect to the structural basis of polymorphism of gp96 molecules.

METHODS

Inbred BALB/c mice were obtained from our mouse colonies. BALB/c sarcomas used in the present study have been described earlier (7).

Gp96 antigens were purified from cytosol of Meth A, and plasma membranes of CMS5 and CMS13 sarcomas, as earlier described (6,8). For purification of gp96 from BALB/c liver, purified plasma membranes were used as the starting material and gp96 molecules were monitored with rabbit anti-gp96 antiserum.

Tumor rejection assays have also been described (6). For adoptive transfer of immunity, mice were immunized once, twice or three times with gp96 preparations; one week after the last immunization, spleen of immunized mice were removed and a lymphocyte suspension was prepared. Lymphocytes obtained from one spleen were injected (intravenous) into one mouse challenged with 250,000 live Meth A cells four days earlier. The kinetics of tumor growth was monitored at weekly intervals.

cDNA libraries were generated and screened with probes described by Srivastava et al. (9). One Meth A cDNA library was generously provided by Dr. Varda Rotter of Weisman Institute, Rehovot, Israel. DNA sequencing was carried out by the dideoxynucleotide chain terminator method of Sanger et al. (10). DNA and protein sequence analysis, homology search and hydropathicity plots were carried out using computer programs of BIONET (Palo Alto, CA).

RESULTS

Gp96 Molecules from Non Cross Reactive Tumors Elicit Non Cross Reactive Immunity.

BALB/c sarcomas Meth A and CMS5 are antigenically distinct in that they elicit tumor specific immunity. Components of the murine leukemia viruses or polyoma virus are not involved in their immunogenicity (6,11). Gp96 preparations from the two tumors also elicit the same pattern of immunity as obtained by immunization with whole irradiated tumor cells. Mice immunuzed with Meth A gp96 resist challenge with Meth A but not CMS5 cells; conversely, mice immunized with CMS5 gp96 preparations elicit immunity specifically against CMS5 (Fig.1).

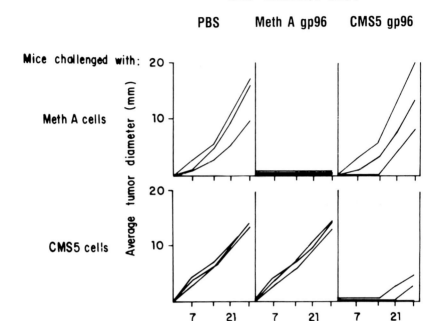

FIGURE 1. Growth of Meth A and CMS5 in BALB/c female mice after immunization with Meth A gp96 or CMS5 gp96. Lines represent tumor growth in mice challenged with 125,000 Meth A cells or 75,000 CMS5 cells.

Gp96 Molecules from Cross Reactive Tumors Elicit Cross Reactive Immunity.

    In contrast to the tumor specific immunity elicited by Meth A and CMS5, Meth A and another chemically induced BALB/c sarcoma CMS13 show a partially cross-reactive pattern of immunity (8). Immunization with irradiated Meth A cells elicits complete immunity against Meth A challenge, no immunity against CMS5 challenge and partial protection against CMS13 challenge. Similiarly, immunization with irradiated CMS13 trocar fragments offers complete protection against CMS13, no protection against CMS5 and

TABLE 1
INDUCTION OF IMMUNITY AGAINST METH A, CMS5 AND CMS13 SARCOMAS BY GP96 PREPARATIONS DERIVED FROM THEM

| | % Inhibition of growth of tumor challenge[b] | | |
Immunization with	Meth A	CMS13	CMS5
Meth A gp96[a]	>90 (0/3)[d]	59 (2/3)[e]	<10 (3/3)[f]
CMS13 gp96[a]	65 (3/3)	>90 (3/3)[c]	<10 (3/3)[f]
CMS5 gp96[a]	<10 (3/3)	<10 (3/3)[f]	80 (2/3)[c]

[a] Meth A gp96 was purified to apparent homogeneity as judged by silver staining. CMS5 and CMS13 gp96 preparations contained >90% gp96 but were not homogeneous.
[b] Percentage of tumor growth based on average tumor diameter 14 days after tumor challenge.
[c] P<0.001.
[d] Numbers in parantheses represent number of tumor-bearing mice over total number of mice.
[e] P<0.05.
[f] P not significant.

partial protection against Meth A. Immunization with gp96 preparations from these tumors elicits the same pattern of immunity (Table 1).

Gp96 Molecules from Normal Liver Do Not Protect Against Meth A or CMS5 Sarcomas.

Our earlier studies have shown that gp96 molecules detected by rabbit antisera are expressed on normal tissues also (6). Because of this, immunogenicity of BALB/c liver gp96 to Meth A and CMS5 sarcomas was tested in tumor rejection assays. Immunization with liver gp96 did not render mice immune to challenges with either tumor (results not shown).

Lymphocytes from Mice Immunized with Gp96 Can Mediate Partial Regression of Pre-Existing Tumors.

Mice were immunized with one, two or three injections of Meth A gp96 preparations at weekly intervals. Spleens from immunized mice were adoptively transferred to Meth A bearing mice as described in Methods. Spleens from unimmunized mice were also transferred to tumor bearing mice in control experiments. The kinetics of tumor growth shows that lymphocytes of mice immunized two or three times with gp96 preparations were able to effect inhibition of tumor growth in mice with pre-existing tumors (P.K.Srivastava, N.Ohta, H.F.Oettgen and L.J.Old : unpublished observations). Lymphocytes from normal mice and mice immunized only once with gp96 preparations were unable to mediate inhibition of tumor growth (data not shown).

Sequencing of Gp96 Genes from Normal Spleen and Meth A Sarcoma : Structural Diversity.

Isolation and sequencing of gp96 encoding cDNA clones from normal BALB/c spleen, Meth A and CMS5 sarcomas was initiated in order to explore the structural basis of polymorphism of gp96. 5' structural analysis of gp96 genes

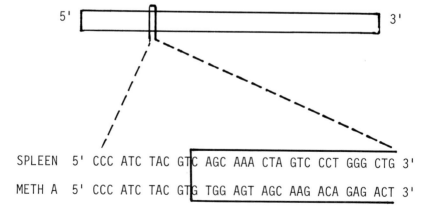

SPLEEN   5' CCC ATC TAC GTC AGC AAA CTA GTC CCT GGG CTG 3'

METH A   5' CCC ATC TAC GTG TGG AGT AGC AAG ACA GAG ACT 3'

FIGURE 2. Schematic representation of a gp96 encoding cDNA molecule and the observed divergence between spleen and Meth A gp96 cDNA. Boxed sequences represent the beginning of the region of divergence.

from Meth A, CMS5 and spleen did not reveal any sequence differences or gross alterations (9). However, comparison of internal regions of Meth A and spleen cDNA clones shows that while the sequences are identical from the initiation ATG codon to basepair 842, they begin to diverge after that point (Fig.2; unpublished observations). Junctional fragments spanning regions of identity as well as regions of divergence are being used to probe Southern blots of spleen and Meth A genomic DNA and in ribonuclease protection experiments with Meth A and spleen RNA in order to characterize this divergence.

DISCUSSION

The evidence that gp96 molecules are the tumor rejection antigens of chemically induced sarcomas comes from the following results : (a) The individually distinct immunogenicity of BALB/c sarcomas Meth A and CMS5 copurified with gp96 through several biochemical separation methods based on independent criteria (b) cross-reactive immunogenicity of Meth A and CMS13 sarcomas also copurifies with gp96 molecules derived from these tumors. (c) specific immunogenicity is removed from antigen extracts by immunoaffinity chromatography through rabbit anti-gp96 sera. (d) Lymphocytes from mice immunized with Meth A gp96 preparations can passively transfer immunity to Meth A sarcoma. These observations indicate that gp96 molecules do indeed mediate the tumor specific immunogenicity of chemically induced tumors. Studies with expressed products of gp96 genes or with defined gp96 synthetic peptides will be needed to substantiate this proposal.

Dr. Michael Green from St.Louis University has very recently brought to our attention the striking similarity between the 5' ends of genes of gp96 and an endoplasmic reticulum protein Erp99, isolated by his group (12). Further structural analysis of gp96 encoding genes has extended this homology. The gp96 and Erp99 genes also show significant homology with a glucose regulated protein (13) and heat shock proteins (14). These observations suggest that gp96 encoding genes belong to an 'extended family' of genes.

The structural basis for the polymorphism of individually specific tumor rejection antigens is still unclear. 5' structural analysis of genes encoding gp96 molecules (9) or their chromosomal localization (15) provide no clues to it. While internal 3' sequence data reported here show diversity between spleen and Meth A gp96 cDNAs, the relationship of this to the antigenic polymorphism remains to be elucidated. Furthermore, the possibility that gp96 antigens are related to tumor antigens of similar sizes and molecular properties reported in rats (16) and humans (17) remains to be explored.

With the isolation of a purified antigen which induces tumor immunity, it will now be interesting to explore active immunization strategies that will cause inhibition of established tumors. Another approach will expand on our observation that T cells from animals immunized with purified tumor antigen can adoptively transfer immunity; attempts are now being made to in vitro sensitize lymphocytes with purified tumor antigen alone or in combination with relevant H-2 antigens on liposomes. In addition, a precise dissection of the cellular and humoral immune response to a purified tumor antigen can be initiated.

REFERENCES

1. Srivastava PK, Old LJ (1988) Individually distinct transplantation antigens of chemically induced mouse tumors. Immunology Today 9 : 78-83.
2. Hewitt HB, Blake ER, Walder AS (1976) A critique of the evidence for active host defense against cancer based on personal studies of 27 murine tumors of spontaneous origin. British J Cancer 33 : 241-259.
3. Boon T (1983) Antigenic tumor cell variants obtained with mutagenesis. Adv Cancer Research 39 : 121-152.
4. North R (1983) Down-regulation of anti-tumor immune response. Adv Cancer Research 45 : 1-43.
5. Rosenberg SA, Terry WD (1977) Passive immunotherapy of cancer in animal and man. Adv Cancer Research 25 : 323-388.
6. Srivastava PK, DeLeo AB, Old LJ (1986) Tumor rejection antigens of chemically induced sarcomas of inbred mice. Proc Natl Acad Sci USA 83 : 3407-3411.
7. DeLeo AB, Shiku H, Takahashi T, John M, Old LJ (1977) Cell surface antigens of chemically induced sarcomas of the mouse. I. Murine leukemia virus related antigen alloantigens on cultured fibroblasts and sarcomas; description of a unique antigen on BALB/c Meth A sarcoma. J exp Med 146 : 720-734.

8. Palladino MA, Srivastava PK, Oettgen HF, DeLeo AB (1987) Expression of a shared Tumor-specific antigen by two chemically induced BALB/c sarcomas. Cancer Research 47 : 5074-5079.
9. Srivastava PK, Chen YT, Old LJ (1987) 5'Structural analysis of genes encoding polymorphic antigens of chemically induced tumors. Proc Natl Acad Sci USA 84 : 3807-3811.
10. Sanger F, Nicklen S, Coulson AR (1977) DNA sequencing with chain-terminating inhibitors. Proc Natl Acad Sci USA 74 : 5463-5467.
11. DeLeo AB, Srivastava PK (1985) Cell surface antigens of chemically induced sarcomas of murine origin. Cancer Surveys 4 : 21-34.
12. Mazzarella RA, Green M (1987) ERp99, an abundant conserved glycoprotein of the endoplasmic reticulum is homologous to the 90 kDa heat shock protein (hsp90) and the 94 kDa glucose regulated protein (GRP94). J Biol Chem 262 : 8875-8883.
13. Sorger PK, Pelham HRB (1987) The glucose regulated protein grp94 is related to heat shock protein hsp90. J Mol Biol 194 : 341-344.
14. Farrelly FW, Finkelstein DB (1984) Complete sequence of the heat shock - inducible HSP90 gene of Saccharomyces cerevisiae. J Biol Chem 259 : 5745-5751.
15. Srivastava PK, Kozak CA, Old LJ (1988) Chromosomal assignment of the gene encoding murine tumor rejection antigen gp96. Immunogenetics (In press).
16. Srivastava PK, Das MR (1984) Serologically unique cell surface antigen of Zajdela ascitic hepatoma is also its tumor associated transplantation antigen. Int J Cancer 33 : 417-422.
17. Real FX, Furukawa K, Mattes MJ, Gusik, SA, Cordon-Cardo C, Oettgen HF, Old LJ (1988) Class 1 (unique) tumor antigens of human melanoma : Identification of unique and common epitopes on a Mr 90,000 glycoprotein. Proc Natl Acad Sci USA (In press).

Human Tumor Antigens and Specific Tumor Therapy, pages 73–82
© 1989 Alan R. Liss, Inc.

CDNA CLONING OF THE PROGRESSION ASSOCIATED MELANOMA ANTIGEN P3.58: IDENTITY TO ICAM-1, A LEUKOCYTE INTERCELLULAR ADHESION MOLECULE[1]

Barbara G. Stade, Bernhard Holzmann[2], Gert Riethmüller and Judith P. Johnson

Institute for Immunology, University of Munich, 8000 Munich 2, West Germany

ABSTRACT   The 89kd cell surface glycoprotein, P3.58, is expressed on advanced human melanomas in situ but not on benign melanocytes or early melanomas indicating that the expression of this molecule is associated with tumor progression. cDNA cloning of P3.58 from melanoma cells revealed identity with the intercellular adhesion molecule-1 (ICAM-1). Northern and southern analyses indicated that no qualitative differences in mRNA species or gene organization could be seen in the P3.58/ICAM-1 molecule between melanoma cells and hematopoietic cells. The acquisition of a new cell adhesion molecule during the process of tumor progression is speculated to contribute to the development of metastasis in melanoma.

INTRODUCTION

The progression of a malignant tumor to metastatic disease is a dynamic process during which tumor cells acquire invasive and locomotory behavior and become capable of autochthonous growth (1). In human melanoma the

[1]This work was supported by the Deutsche Krebshilfe, Mildred Scheel Stiftung, and the Deutsche Forschungs gemeinschaft SFB 217 (A3)
[2]Present address: Stanford University School of Medicine, Department of Pathology, 300 Pasteur Drive, Stanford CA 94305

isolation of monoclonal antibodies (mabs) which distinguish
distinct stages in tumor progression has led to the
identification of several molecules which may be directly
involved in the development of metastasis (2-4). One of
these molecules is P3.58, a 89kD cell surface glycoprotein
defined by two monoclonal antibodies (mabs P3.58[a], P3.58[b])
which were selected to discriminate between benign
melanocytic nevi and malignant melanoma in situ (2).

P3.58 EXPRESSION IS AN EARLY EVENT IN MELANOMA PROGRESSION

P3.58 is not detectable on quiescent melanocytes and is
only rarely found on benign melanocytic lesions (Fig 1).
Expression of P3.58 on primary melanomas depends on the
vertical thickness of the tumor. Thin tumors (≤ 0.75 mm) re-
semble benign nevi while 60-70% of all tumors 1mm or greater

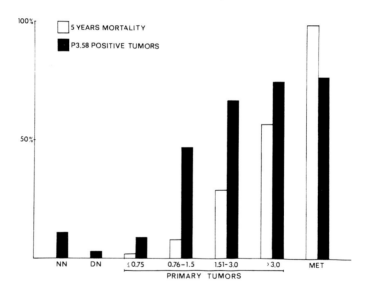

FIGURE 1. P3.58 expression on melanocytic lesions.
Reactivity was determined by immunoperoxidase staining of
frozen tissue sections. NN: nevocellular nevi; DN:
dysplastic nevi; MET: metastases. Primary tumors are grouped
according to their thickness (mm). Mortality rates are from
reference 5.

in thickness express P3.58. Expression is heterogeneous, ranging from 5 to 90 per cent of the cells and increases slightly with increasing tumor thickness. The vertical thickness of primary tumors is a measure of progression in melanoma and is directly correlated with the probability of metastatic disease (5,6; Fig 1). The association between P3.58 expression and tumor thickness suggests that the appearance of this molecule reflects a change in the tumor cells which may contribute directly to the development of metastatic capacity. The appearance of P3.58 on tumors which still have a good prognosis indicates that this is one of the earliest events in melanoma progression.

P3.58 IS A NORMAL COMPONENT OF THE IMMUNE SYSTEM

Expression of P3.58 in normal tissues in situ is limited to blood vessel endothelia, cells in germinal centers of lymphoid follicles and macrophage populations. It is strongly expressed on adherent monocytes in vitro, is found on Epstein Barr Virus transformed B cell lines and can be induced on many different cell types by interferon-γ and TNFα (4,7). These observations suggest that P3.58 is normally involved in the development of immune reactivity. Studies in vitro support this, revealing that antibodies directed to P3.58 partially inhibit antigen specific and anti CD3 induced T cell proliferation and completely block antigen independent monocyte-lymphocyte clustering (8).

P3.58 IS BIOCHEMICALLY AND IMMUNOLOGICALLY DISTINCT IN DIFFERENT CELL TYPES

The P3.58 antigen precipitated from radiolabelled melanoma cell lines is a 89kD glycoprotein and comparison of its migration under reducing and nonreducing conditions indicates that it is a single polypeptide chain with intramolecular disulfide bonds (2). Analysis of the antigen precipitated from various hematopoietic cells lines reveals a cell type specific migration pattern (7; Fig 2). B cell P3.58 migrates as a broad smear around 83kD and monocyte P3.58 as a sharp band at 95kD. These differences appear to be due to variations in N-linked glycosylation since P3.58 precipitated from tunicamycin treated cells of all types migrates as a sharp band with an apparent molecular weight of 53kD. Differences between the P3.58 antigens in different cell types

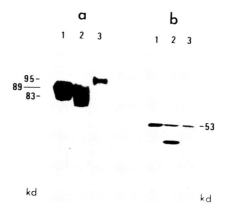

FIGURE 2. Biochemical analyis of radiolabelled P3.58 antigen isolated from various cell lines and separated on SDS-polyacrylamide gels under reducing conditions. a, Immunoprecipitation of P3.58 from ^{125}I-surface-labelled cells, using mab P3.58[b]. Lane 1: L89 (P3.58[+] L cell transfectant) lane 2: Ramos (Burkitt's lymphoma), lane 3: U937 (monoblast like cell line). b, Immunoprecipitation of P3.58 from tunicamycin treated ^{35}S-methionine-labelled cells, using mab P3.58[b]. Lane 1: L89 ; lane 2: Ramos; lane 3: U937.

are also seen in terms of antibody defined epitopes. Mabs P3.58[a] and P3.58[b] consistently fail to bind antigen specific T cell lines and clones although most other antibodies reacting with the melanoma P3.58 antigen (mabs gp89-1,2,3,7F7) clearly bind (9; unpublished observations). It is not yet known whether this variation affects P3.58 function although differences in glycosylation have been shown to regulate function of the neural cell adhesion molecule NCAM (10).

MOLECULAR CLONING OF P3.58 : IDENTITY TO ICAM-1

To isolate P3.58 encoding cDNA, a lambda expression library was produced from interferon-γ stimulated Mel JuSo melanoma cells. The library was screened with a pool of monoclonal antibodies produced against denatured P3.58

immunoprecipitates isolated from 3 x 10⁹ melanoma cells. All mabs also reacted with the native P3.58 antigen and precipitated only this molecule from radiolabelled melanoma cells. A single clone, λ89-1, containing a 2.7kb insert and encoding a product reactive with six mabs was isolated. Two additional clones isolated by hybridization (λ89-48, λ89-49) showed identical restriction maps to λ89-1. To confirm that these clones contained P3.58 cDNA, they were hybridized to DNA and RNA isolated from L89, a P3.58 expressing L cell transfectant (7; Fig 3). Identical genomic fragments and

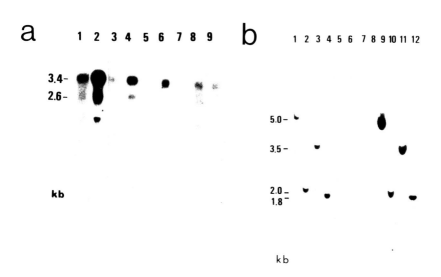

FIGURE 3. a, Northern analysis of P3.58/ICAM-1 mRNA . 20ug total RNA (11) was hybridized with the clone λ89-1. lane 1: Mel Wei (melanoma cell); lane 2: SkMel28 (melanoma cell); lane 3: Mel JuSo (melanoma cell); lane 4: L89 (P3.58⁺ L cell transfectant); lane 5: Ltk⁻ cells; lane 6: interferon-γ stimulated A375 (melanoma cell); lane 7: unstimulated A375; lane 8: U937 (monoblast like cells); lane 9: Daudi (Burkitt's lymphoma). b, Southern analysis of the P3.58/ICAM-1 gene. 15ug genomic DNA (11) was hybridized with a 700bp PstI-subclone from the coding region of λ89-1. Lanes 1-4: L89; lanes 5-6: Ltk⁻; lanes 7-8: Mel JuSo. Restriction enzymes: lanes 1,5,9: EcoRI; lanes 2,6,10: TaqI; lanes 3,7,11: PvuII; lanes 4,8,12: BglII.

mRNA species were observed in L89 and Mel JuSo and no
hybridization was seen with DNA or RNA isolated from the
untransfected Ltk⁻ cells. In the melanoma cell line A375
where the P3.58 antigen is seen only following exposure to
interferon-ɣ (4), hybridizing mRNA was also detectable only
after stimulation.

Subfragments of λ89-1, λ89-48 and λ89-49 were cloned
into puc18 and the double stranded DNA sequenced using the
dideoxy method (12). The sequence obtained was identical to
the recently published sequence of ICAM-1 (intercellular
adhesion molecule 1) isolated from myeloid and endothelial
cells (13,14;Fig 4).

Northern blotting analyses showed no quantitative differences in the P3.58/ICAM-1 mRNAs between melanoma cells
and hematopoietic cells. In both cell types, 2 species of
mRNA (3.4 kb, 2.6kb) were found (Fig 3). Southern analyses
revealed one major band with four difference restriction endonucleases, results consistent with a single copy gene. No
evidence was obtained for rearrangement of the P3.58/ICAM-1
gene in melanomas as identical fragments were observed in
DNA from melanomas, EBV transformed B cells and peripheral
blood mononuclear cells (Fig 3).

THE ROLE OF P3.58/ICAM-1 IN MELANOMA TUMOR PROGRESSION

One of the earliest events in metastasis is the separation of individual cells from the primary tumor. In carcinomas this is often associated with a reduction in the expression of a family of epithelial intercellular adhesion molecules, the cadherins (15). We speculate that in melanomas
this event may be associated with the acquisition of a new
cell adhesion molecule. ICAM-1 has been shown to be a ligand
of the lymphocyte function associated molecule 1 (LFA-1;16)
and to mediate LFA-1 dependent leukocyte adhesion in a
variety of systems (17,18). The expression of P3.58/ICAM-1
may encourage melanoma cells to preferentially interact with
LFA-1 bearing hematopoietic cells comprising the tumor infiltrate. This would effectively reduce intercellular adhesion between melanoma cells and at the same time allow the
tumor cells to interact with cells which are naturally mig-
ratory and invasive, characteristics which would clearly
contribute to the dissemination of the tumor cells.

The expression of P3.58/ICAM-1 can be induced by lymphokines in vitro and the observation of a correlation bet-

FIGURE 4: Continued on following page.

A: AlaGlnLysGlyThrProMetLysProAsnThrGlnAlaThrProPro*** 505
B: GCCCAAAAAGGGACCCCCATGAAACCGAACACAACAGCCACGCCTCCTGAACCTATCCC 1665
C: GCCCAAAAAGGGACCCCCATGAAACCGAACACAACAGCCACGCCTCCTGAACCTATCCC

B: GGGACAGGGCCTCTTCCTCCGGCCTTCCCATATTGGTGGCAGTGGTGCCACCTGAACAGA 1725
C: GGGACAGGGCCTCTTCCTCCGGCCTTCCCATATTGGTGGCAGTGGTGCCACCTGAACAGA

B: GTGGAAGACATATGCCATGCAGCTACACCTACCGGCCCTGGGACGCCGGAGGACAGGGCA 1785
C: GTGGAAGACATATGCCATGCAGCTACACCTACCGGCCCTGGGACGCCGGAGGACAGGGCA

B: TTGTCCTCAGTCAGATACAACAGCATTTGGGGCCATGGTACCTGCACACCTAAAACACTA 1845
C: TTGTCCTCAGTCAGATACAACAGCATTTGGGGCC

B: GGCCACGCATCTGATCTGTAGTCACATGCATTAGCCAAGAGGAAGGAGCAAGACTCAAGA 1905
C: CATCTGATCTGTAGTCACATGCATTAGCCAAGAGGAAGGAGCAAGACTCAAGA

B: CATGATTGATGGATGTTAAAGTCTAGCCTGATGAGAGGGGAAGTGGTGGGGGAGACATAG 1965
C: CATGATTGATGGATGTTAAAGTCTAGCCTGATGAGAGGGGAAGTGGTGGGGGAGACATAG

B: CCCCACCATGAGGACATACAACTGGGAAATACTGAAACTTGCTGCCTATTGGGTATGCTG 2025
C: CCCCACCATGAGGACATACAACTGGGAAATACTGAAACTTGCTGCCTATTGGGTATGCTG

B: AGGCCCAGACTTACGAGAGAAGTGGCCCTCCCATGACATGTGTAGCACAAAAACACAA 2085
C: AGGCCCAGACTTACGAGAGAAGTGGCC   T CATAGACAT
        C

B: AGGCCCAACTTCCGGACGGATGGCACTGCTGTCTACTGACCCCAACCCTT 2145
C: A CCAGCT GCACTGCTGTCTACTGACCCCA CCC T

B: GATGATATGTATTTATTCATTGTATTTACCAGCTATTTATTGAGTGTCTTTTATGTA 2205
C: GATGATATGTATTTATTCATTGTATTTACCAGCTATTTATTGAGTGTCTTTTATGTA

B: GGCTAAATGACATAGGTCTGTGGCCTCACGGAGCTCCCATGTCCATTCAATTCAAGGT 2265
C: GGCTAAATGACATAGGTCTGTGGCCTCA GGAGCTCCCAGTCC   TCACATTCAAGGT

B: CACCAGGTACAGTTGTACAGGTGTGCACTGACGAGGAGTGCCTGGCAAAAAGATCAAAT 2325
C: CACCAGGTACAGTTGTACAGGTGT CTGCAGGAGAGTGCCTGGCAAAAAGATCA AT

B: GGGGCTGGGGACTTCCATTGGCCAACCTGCCTTTCCCCAGAAGGAGTGATTTTTCTATCG 2385
C: GGGGCTGGGACTTCCATTGGCCAACCTGCCTTTCCCCAGAAGGAGTGATTTTTCTATCG

B: GCACAAAAGCACTATATGACTGGTAATGGTTCACAGGTTCAGAGATTACCCAGTGAGGC 2445
C: GCACAAAAGCACTATATGACTGGTAATGGTT ACAGGTTCAGAGATTACCCAGTGAGGC

B: CTTATTCTCCCTTCCCCCAAAACTGACACCTTGTTAGCCACCTCCCCACCCCACCATAC 2505
C: CTTATTCTCCCCTTCCCCCAAAACTGACACCTTGTTAGCCACCTCCCCACCCACCATAC
                                                           G

B: ATTTTCTGCCAGTGTTCAAATGACACTCAGCGGTCATGTCTGGACATGAGTGCCCAGGGA 2565
C: ATTTTCTGCCAGTGTTCACAA ACACTCAGCGGTCATGTCTGGACATGAGTGCCCAGGGA

B: ATATGCCCAAGCTATGCCTTGTCTCCTTGTCTCCTGTTTGCATTTCACTGGGAGCTTGCACT 2625
C: ATATGCCCAAGCTATGCCTTGTCTCCTTGTCTCCTGTTTGCATTTCACTGGGAGCTTGCACT

B: ATTTGCAGCTCCAGTTTCCTGCAGTGATCAGGGTCCCGCAAGCAGTGGGGAAGGGGGCCAA 2685
C: AT GCAGCTCCAGTTTCCTGCAGTGATCAGGGTCCCGCAAGCAGTGGGGAAGGGGGCCAA

B: GGTATTGGAGGACTCCCTCCCAGCTTTGGAAGGGTCATCCGGCGTGTGTGTGTGTGTAT 2745
C: GGTATTGGAGGACTCCCTCCCAGCTTTGGAAG TCATCCGGCGTGTGTGTGTGTGTAT

B: GTGTAGACAAGCTCTCGCTCGTGTCACCCAGGCTGGAGTGCAGTGGTGCAATCATGGTTCA 2805
C: GTGTAGACAAGCTCTCGCTCGTGTCACCCAGGCTGGAGTG GTGGTGCAATCATGGTTCA

B: CTGCAGTCTTGACCTTTGGCCTCAAGTGATCCTCCCACCTCAGCCTCCTGAGTAGCTGG 2865
C: CTGCAGTCTTGACCTTTGGCCTCAAGTGATCCTCCCACCTCAGCCTCCTGAGTAGCTGG

B: GACCATAGGCTCACAACACCACCTGGCAAATTGATTTTTTTTTTTTTTTTCAGAGAC 2925
C: GACCATAGGCTCACAACACCACCTGG AAATTGATTTTTTTTTTTTTT CAGAGAC

B: GGGGTCTCGCACAATTGGCCCAGACTTCCTTGTGTAGTTAATAAAGCTTTCTCAACTGC 2985
C: GGGGTCTCGCCACAATTGGCCCAGACTTCCTTGTGTAGTTAATAAAGCTTTCTCAACTGC

B: CAAAAAAAAAAAAAAAAAAAAAAAAAAAAAAAAAAAA 3' 3024

FIGURE 4. Comparison of the cDNA sequences of P3.58 and ICAM-1. A: Predicted protein sequence; amino acid numbering is at right. B: Nucleotide sequence of ICAM-1 cDNA (14); nucleotide numbering is at right. C: Sequence of cDNA clone λ89-1. Gaps indicate regions still not sequenced. Nucleotides below line C were detected only in P3.58 cDNA. Potential N-linked glycosylation sites are boxed and lines denote the putative hydrophobic signal peptide and the transmembrane sequences (line above) and the polyadenylation signal AATAAA (line below).

ween P3.58 expression and the presence of interferon-γ, in situ suggests that this may also occur in vivo (19). Thus it appears that the mononuclear cellular infiltrate, by regulating tumor cell gene expression, may directly participate in the acquisition of characteristics required for metastasis. These observations underscore the complexity of the interactions which occur between tumor cells and the host microenvironment and suggest that at least in human melanoma, metastasis may result from interactions occurring between the tumor cell and the immune system.

REFERENCES

1. Fidler IJ, Hart IR (1982). Biological diversity in metastatic neoplasms: origins and implications. Science 217:998.

2. Holzmann B, Johnson JP, Kaudewitz P, Riethmüller G (1985) In situ analysis of antigens on malignant and benign cells of the melanocyte lineage. Differential expression of two surface molecules gp75 and p89. J. Exp. Med. 161:366.

3. Lehmann JM, Holzmann B, Breitbart EW, Schmiegelow P, Riethmüller G, Johnson JP (1987) Discrimination between benign and malignant cells of melanocytic lineage by two novel antigens, a glycoprotein with a molecular weight of 113,000 and a protein with a molecular weight of 76,000. Cancer Res 47:841.

4. Holzmann B, Bröcker EB, Lehmann JM, Ruiter DJ, Sorg C, Riethmüller G, Johnson JP (1987) Tumor progression in human malignant melanoma:five stages defined by their antigenic phenotypes. Int. J. Cancer 39:466.

5. Sober AJ (1984) Prognostic factors for cutaneous melanoma. In Ruiter DJ, Welvaart K, Ferrone S (eds): "Cutaneous Melanoma and Precursor Lesions," Dordrecht: Martin Nijhoff Publishers, p 126.

6. Breslow A (1970). Thickness, cross-sectional areas and depth of invasion in the prognosis of cutaneous melanoma. Ann. Surg. 172:902.

7. Holzmann B, Lehmann JM, Ziegler-Heitbrock L, Funke I, Riethmüller G, Johnson JP (1988) Glycoprotein P3.58, associated with tumor progression in malignant melanoma, is a novel leukocyte activation antigen. Int J. Cancer 41:542.

8. Johnson JP, Lehmann JM, Riethmüller G (1988) Metastasis in human melanoma correlates with the

expression of two distinct immune function molecules. Submitted.

9. Schulz TF, Vogetseder W, Mitterer M, Böck G, Johnson JP Dierich MP (1988) Individual epitopes of an 85 Kd membrane adherence molecule are variably expressed on cells of different lineage. Submitted.

10. Edelman GM (1986) Cell adhesion molecules in the regulation of animal form and tissue pattern. Ann.Rev.Cell.Biol. 2:81.

11. Maniatis T, Fritsch EF, Sambrook J (1982). "Molecular Cloning: A Laboratory Manual." Cold Spring Harbor: Cold Spring Harbor Laboratory.

12. Sanger F, Nicklen S, Coulson AR (1977) DNA sequencing with chain termination inhibitors. Proc. Natl. Acad. Sci. 74:5463.

13. Simmons D, Makgoba MW, Seed B (1988) ICAM, an adhesion ligand of LFA-1, is homologous to the neural cell adhesion molecule NCAM. Nature 331:624.

14. Staunton DE, Marlin SD, Stratowa C, Dustin ML, Springer TA (1988) Primary structure of ICAM-1 demonstrates interaction between members of the immunoglobulin and integrin supergene families. Cell 52:925.

15. Behrens J, Mareel MM, Van Roy FM, Birchmeier W (1988) Essential steps in tumor cell invasion: epithelial cells acquire invasive properties following the loss of uvomorulin-mediated cell-cell adhesion. Cell in press.

16. Marlin SD, Springer T (1987) Purified intercellular adhesion molecule-1 (ICAM-1) is a ligand for lymphocyte function-associated antigen (LFA-1). Cell 51:813.

17. Dustin ML, Rothlein R, Bhan AK, Dinarello CA, Springer TA (1986) Induction by IL-1 and interferon, tissue distribution, biochemistry and function of a natural adherence molecule (ICAM-1). J. Immunol. 137:245.

18. Dustin ML, Singer KH, Tuck DT, Springer TA (1988) Adhesion of T lymphoblasts to epidermal keratinocytes is regulated by interferon gamma and is mediated by intercellular adhesion molecule-1 (ICAM-1). J. Exp Med. 167:1323.

19. Bröcker EB, Zwaldo G, Holzmann B, Macher E, and Sorg C (1988) Inflammatory cell infiltrates in human melanoma of different stages of tumor progression. Int.J.Canc. 41:562.

Human Tumor Antigens and Specific Tumor Therapy, pages 83–92
© 1989 Alan R. Liss, Inc.

DIFFERENT FINE BINDING SPECIFICITIES OF MONOCLONAL ANTIBODIES TO GANGLIOSIDE GD2[1]

Tadashi Tai[*], Ikuo Kawashima[*], Nobuhiko Tada[**], and Takao Fujimori[***]

[*]Department of Oncology, Tokyo Metropolitan Institute of Medical Science, Bunkyo-ku, Tokyo 113, [**]Department of Pathology, Tokai University School of Medicine, Isehara, Kanagawa 250-11, and [***]Meiji Institute of Health Science, Odawara, Kanagawa 250, Japan

ABSTRACT The fine structural specificities of six monoclonal antibodies (MAbs) to ganglioside GD2 were studied. These MAbs were produced by hybridomas obtained from A/J mice immunized with EL4 (C57BL/6 derived-T lymphoma). The binding specificities of these MAbs were found to differ from each other by virtue of their binding to structurally related authentic standard glycosphingolipids as revealed by three different assay systems. The MAbs examined could be divided into three binding types. Three MAbs A1-201, A1-410, and A1-425 bound specifically to ganglioside GD2 and none of the other gangliosides tested. Two other MAbs A1-245 and A1-267 reacted not only with GD2, but also several other gangliosides. In addition, these MAbs were found to distinguish between different N-acetyl- and N-glycolylneuraminic acid derivatives of ganglioside GD3. The last MAb A1-287 reacted with several other gangliosides but with lower avidity than A1-245 and A1-267. These six MAbs, furthermore, reacted with ganglioside GD2 lactones. The reactivities of these antibodies to various ganglioside lactones also differed from each other.

[1]This work was supported in part by a grant from the Science and Technology Agency of Japan and a Grant-in-aid for scientific research from the Ministry of Education, Science and Culture of Japan.

INTRODUCTION

Many tissue-specific and tumor-specific mouse and human monoclonal antibodies (MAbs) have been described that recognize carbohydrate determinants of glycolipids, glycoproteins or mucins (1-4). The antibodies that react preferentially with tumors of neuroectodermal origin such as melanoma, neuroblastoma, and glioma, but not with normal cells have been shown to be directed to gangliosides. It is of importance to study the fine binding specificity of an MAb. If the precise epitope specificity of the MAb has not been determined, there is no way to judge whether the antibody binds to the authentic antigen or to structurally related substances. There have been few reports on precise binding specificities of MAbs to gangliosides. We recently produced six MAbs to ganglioside GD2 by immunizing mice with a mouse T-cell lymphoma (5). In the present report we determined fine binding specificities of the MAbs by several assay systems. These MAbs also reacted with ganglioside GD2 lactones which are inner esters formed between carboxyl group of sialic acid and hydroxyl group of ganglioside.

RESULTS

Immunostaining on TLC of Brain Gangliosides and Various Authentic Gangliosides with the Six MAbs.

Using six MAbs, we have found that mouse and human T lymphoma-associated antigen is ganglioside GD2. We tested the binding reactivities of the MAbs to bovine brain gangliosides. The results of the enzyme-immunostaining on TLC are shown in Fig. 1. MAb A1-201 reacted with only GD2 of brain gangliosides (Fig. 1B). The reactivities of the other three antibodies (A1-287, A1-410, and A1-425) were identical. In contrast, MAb A1-245 reacted with a variety of gangliosides which have the same chromatographic mobility as standards GD3, GD2, and GD1b on TLC (Fig. 1C). These findings were confirmed by the observation that MAb A1-245 reacts with authentic gangliosides GD3, GD2, and GD1b (Fig. 1C). Authentic ganglioside GT1b was faintly stained, although GT1b of brain gangliosides appeared to be negative. Similar results were obtained with MAb A1-267. Thus, we concluded that the two MAbs have a broad binding specificity for GD3 and the other three gangliosides. The results of

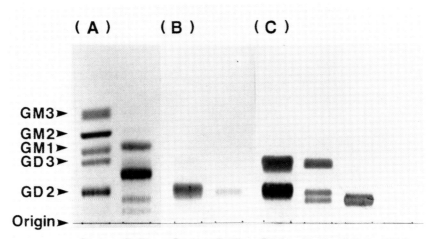

(A)   (B)   (C)

GM3►
GM2►
GM1►
GD3►

GD2►

Origin►

Stds B.B.   Stds B.B.   Stds B.B. GD1b GT1b

FIGURE 1. TLC immunostaining of brain gangliosides with six MAbs. (A), ganglioside fraction (total 10 nmol) from bovine brain and the same amount of standard gangliosides were chromatographed with chloroform/methanol/0.22% $CaCl_2$ in water (55/45/10, v/v) and visualized with resorcinol. Stds, mixture of standard gangliosides GM3, GM2, GM1, GD3, and GD2; B.B., gangliosides of bovine brain. (B) and (C), the same ganglioside fraction (total 1 nmol/lane), the same amount of standard gangliosides, GD1b and GT1b were also developed similarly and immunostained with MAbs A1-201 and A1-245, respectively. The enzyme-immunostaining on TLC plates were performed as previously described(6). The reactivities of the other three MAbs A1-287, A1-410, and A1-425 were similar to that of A1-201. The reactivity of A1-267 was similar to that of A1-245.

enzyme immunostainings on TLC of various authentic di-, tri- and tetra-sialosylgangliosides and all other glycolipids tested are summarized in Table 1. Monosialogangliosides (GM4, GM3, GM2, and GM1) and neutral glycolipids (GlcCer, LacCer, $GbOs_3Cer$, $GbOs_4Cer$, $GgOs_3Cer$, and $GgOs_4Cer$) were negative (data not shown). The MAbs were classified into at least three binding types according to their cross-reactivities with some authentic gangliosides.

TABLE 1

SUMMARY OF ENZYME IMMUNOSTAINING ON TLC OF VARIOUS AUTHENTIC GANGLIOSIDES WITH SIX MONOCLONAL ANTIBODIES[a]

Ganglioside[b]	A1-201[c]	A1-245[d]	A1-287
GD3	-[e]	++	-
GD2	+++	+++	+++
GD1a	-	-	-
GD1b	-	++	-
GT1a	-	++	++
GT1b	-	+	-
GQ1b	-	++	++
GT3	-	-	-
GT2	-	-	-

[a]Two MAbs, A1-201 and A1-245, are of the IgM (k) class. The other four MAbs, A1-267, A1-287, A1-410, and A1-425 are of the IgG3 (k) class. [b]Gangliosides were prepared as previously described (7, 8). All of the gangliosides used contain NeuAc as a sialic acid moiety. None of neutral glycolipids (GlcCer, LacCer, $GbOs_3Cer$, $GbOs_4Cer$, $GgOs_3Cer$ and $GgOs_4Cer$) or monosialogangliosides (GM4, GM3, GM2 and GM1) tested were detected. [c]The reactivities of A1-410 and A1-425 were similar to that of A1-201. [d]The reactivity of A1-267 was similar to that of A1-245. [e]+++ , strong; ++ , moderate; + , weak or trace; - , negative.

TLC Immunostaining of Four Ganglioside GD3 Isomers.

Since various standard gangliosides having NeuAc and /or NeuGc are not available, four ganglioside GD3 variants including (NeuAc-NeuAc-)GD3, (NeuGc-NeuAc-)GD3, (NeuAc-NeuGc-)GD3, and (NeuGc-NeuGc-)GD3 were tested with the six MAbs (Fig. 2). As would be predicted from the results in Table 1, only MAbs of the second type reacted with some of these GD3. MAbs of the first and the third types did not react with any GD3 isomers (data not shown). The second type reacted with (NeuAc-NeuAc-)GD3 and (NeuGc-NeuAc-)GD3, but not with (NeuAc-NeuGc-)GD3 or (NeuGc-NeuGc-)GD3. These results clearly indicate that the inner sialic acid of GD3 must be a NeuAc residue and it is very crucial for the reactivity with the MAbs, and that the requirement of NeuAc

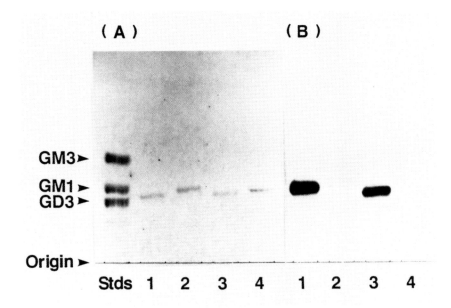

FIGURE 2. TLC immunostaining of four isomers of
ganglioside GD3 with six MAbs. (A), four kinds of
ganglioside GD3 (5 nmol of ganglioside/lane) and standard
gangliosides (total 10 nmol) were chromatographed as
described in Fig. 1 and visualized with resorcinol. Stds,
mixture of GM3, GM1, and GD3; 1, (NeuAc-NeuAc-)GD3; 2,
(NeuAc-NeuGc-)GD3; 3, (NeuGc-NeuAc-)GD3; 4, (NeuGc-NeuGc-)
GD3. (B), the same ganglioside isomers (1 nmol/lane) were
developed similarly and immunostained with MAb A1-245. The
reactivity of A1-267 was identical to that of A1-245.

for the terminal sialic acid residue seems to be less
important, because ganglioside GD3 with external NeuGc was
also reactive. Whether the other two types of MAbs can
distingush sialic acid derivatives of GD2 molecule still
remains to be determined, since GD2 isomers were not
available.

Enzyme-Linked Immunosorbent Assay (ELISA) with Various
Authentic Glycolipids.

The solid-phase ELISA was performed as previously
described (9). The ELISA results using these MAbs agreed

well with those obtained by immunostaining of gangliosides
and neutral glycolipids (data not shown). However, several
discrepancies were found between them. For example,
although neither (NeuAc-NeuAc-)GD3 nor (NeuGc-NeuAc-)GD3
reacted with the third type MAb in the TLC immunostaining,
both of them reacted in the ELISA. These findings suggest
that ELISA may be more sensitive than immunostaining.

Reactivities of MAbs with Various Authentic Glycolipids by
Immune Adherent (IA) Inhibition Assay.

   IA inhibition assay was performed as previously
described (10). The results were similar to those of the
TLC immunostaining (data not shown).

TLC Immunostaining of Ganglioside GD2 lactones with the
MAbs.

   Purified GD2 showed one clear band, while GD2 lactones
revealed several bands (Fig 3A). A major component (90
mol%) migrated in the region between GM2 and GM1 on the TLC.
After the GD2 lactones were treated with base, they changed
their chromatographic behaviors and migrated exatctly as the
purified GD2, indicating that these components are simply
lactones of GD2. TLC immunostaining showed that MAb A1-201
reacted with GD2 lactones as well as the purified GD2 (Fig.
3B). GD2 lactones revealed several bands, probably due to
the potential for lactone formation in either or both of the
two sialic acids. Reactivity of the major ganglioside GD2
lactone appeared to be similar to that of the purified GD2.
None of other ganglioside lactones tested were detected by
MAb A1-201. The pattern using the other three MAbs (A1-410,
A1-425, and A1-287) was identical to that of A1-201.
   In contrast, MAb A1-245 reacted with three gangliosides
lactones (GD2, GD1b, and GT1b), but not with the other three
(GD3, GT1a, and GQ1b) among the six gangliosides tested
(data not shown). The major components of the three
ganglioside lactones (GD2, GD1b, and GT1b) appeared to
retain their reactivities compared to these purified
gangliosides, while those of the other three ganglioside
lactones (GD3, GT1a, and GQ1b) lost their binding activities
completely. Identical reactivities were obtained by A1-267.
Effects of sialidase on major components of ganglioside
lactones were tested. None of the major components of
ganglioside lactones prepared from the six gangliosides were

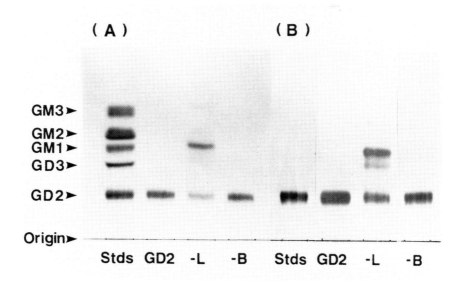

FIGURE 3. TLC immunostaining of ganglioside GD2 lactones. (A), Ganglioside GD2 lactones (Total 10 nmol as sialic acid content) and the same amount of standard ganglioside were chromatographed as described in Fig. 1 and visualized with resorcinol. Stds, mixture of standard gangliosides GM3, GM2, GM1, GD3, and GD2; GD2, purified GD2; -L, GD2 lactones; -B, GD2 after base treatment of the GD2 lactones. (B), the same fraction as in (A), total 1 nmol/lane was developed similarly and immunostained with MAb A1-201. Lactones were prepared from purified ganglioside as previously described (11). The reactivities of the other five MAbs were identical to that of A1-201.

sensitive with the sialidase, while all of these purified gangliosides were sensitive, demonstrating that at least the outer sialic acid moietiies of these gangliosides were involved in lactone formation (11).

DISCUSSION

The reactivities of the MAbs to ganglioside GD2 with GD3 isomers and ganglioside lactones have not been studied yet. None of these studies investigated the involvement of

REFERENCES

1. Hakomori S (1984). Tumor-associated carbohydrate antigens. Annu Rev Immunol 2: 103.
2. Marcus D (1984). A review of the immunogenic and immunomodulatory properties of glycosphingolipids. Mol Immunol 21: 1083.
3. Feizi T (1985). Demonstration by monoclonal antibodies that carbohydrate structures of glycoproteins and glycolipids are oncodevelopmental antigens. Nature (London) 314: 53.
4. Reisfeld RA, Cheresh DA (1987). Human tumor antigens. Adv Immunol 40: 323.
5. Kawashima I, Tada N, Ikegami S, Nakamura S, Ueda R, Tai T (1988). Mouse monoclonal antibodies detecting disialogangliosides on mouse and human T-lymphomas. Int J Cancer 41:267.
6. Tai T, Sze L, Kawashima I, Saxton RE, Irie RF (1987). Monoclonal antibody detects monosialogangliosides having a sialic acidα2-3galactosyl residue. J Biol Chem 262: 6803.
7. Tai T, Kawashima I, Tada N, Dairiki K (1988). Different fine binding specificities of monoclonal antibodies to disialosylganglioside GD2. J Biochem (Tokyo) 103: 313.
8. Tai T, Kawashima I, Furukawa K, Lloyd KO (1988). Monoclonal antibody R24 distinguishes between different N-acetyl- and N-glycolylneuraminic acid derivatives of ganglioside GD3. Arch Biochem Biophys 260: 51.
9. Tai T, Cahan LD, Paulson JC, Saxton RE, Irie RF (1984). Human monoclonal antibody against ganglioside GD2: Use in development of enzyme-linked immunosorbent assay for the monitoring of anti-GD2 in cancer patients. J Natl Cancer Inst 73: 627.
10. Tai T, Paulson JC, Cahan LD, Irie RF (1983). Ganglioside GM2 as a human tumor antigen (OFA-I-1). Proc Natl Acad Sci USA 80: 5392.
11. Tai T, Kawashima I, Tada N, Ikegami S (1988). Different reactivities of monoclonal antibodies to ganglioside lactones. Biochim Biophys Acta 958: 134.
12. Acquotti D, Fronza G, Riboni L, Sonnino S, Tettamanti G (1987). Ganglioside lactones: H-NMR determination of the inner ester position of GD1b-ganglioside lactone naturally occuring in human brain or produced by chemical synthesis. Glycoconjugate J 4: 119.

Human Tumor Antigens and Specific Tumor Therapy, pages 93–103
© 1989 Alan R. Liss, Inc.

TUMOR INFILTRATING LYMPHOCYTES IN COLORECTAL CANCER ARE MAINLY CYTOTOXIC T CELLS: EVIDENCE FOR AN ONGOING IMMUNE RESPONSE ?

M.Slaoui,[1][x] C.Bruyns,[1] K.Thielemans,[2] M.Marechal[2], T.Schuurs[3], and J.Urbain[1].

From ULB, Brussels[1], AZ-VUB, Jette Hospital[2], Brussels and Organon International, Oss, the Netherlands[3].

ABSTRACT We have designed experiments aimed at identifying the nature of the spontaneous anti-tumor response in patients bearing colon carcinomas. The T cell response was analyzed by producing T cell clones from the proximal or distal lymph node T cells, or tumor infiltrating lymphocytes (TIL). Interestingly, all T cell clones derived from the TIL population had a cytolytic phenotype (OKT8[+] OKT4[-] OKT3[+]) and were able to lyse a Fc receptor + target cell in the presence of OKT3 mAbs. In contrast, only 1 out of 7 T cell clones derived from the draining lymph nodes belonged to the cytotoxic compartment. This strongly suggests a preferential infiltration of the tumor burden by cytolytic T cells. The specificity of the CTL clones was analyzed in a direct ^{51}Cr release assay. 2 out of 5 TIL derived clones demonstrated a significant specific lysis of the autologous tumor cells.

---

[1][x]Present address:Laboratoire de Physiologie animale,ULB,67,rue des Chevaux,1640 Rhode-st-Genèse Belgium.

INTRODUCTION

Many human solid tumors are infiltrated with mononuclear cells (1). In some instances, the extent of lymphocyte infiltration was demonstrated to be an important parameter in prognosis and survival of the cancer patients (2).

The analysis of T lymphocytes infiltrating tumor tissues may provide major clues toward developing an efficient strategy for immunotherapy. In many instances, TIL cell populations have been expanded and their lytic activity against autologous or unrelated tumor targets tested (3),(4), (5),(6). Depending on the concentrations of IL-2 used for T cell stimulation (ranging from 10 U/ml to 150.000 U/ml), on the presence or absence of autologous tumor cells during T cell expansion and on the nature of the neoplasms analyzed, the data yielded conflicting results as to the nature and the specificity of the TIL cells (NK,LAK, tumor specific CTL).

T cell cloning is a powerful tool for analysing many important questions such as the extent, the nature and the specificity of cellular immune responses. Thus, in order to carefully analyze the contribution of the different cytolytic phenotypes in the host anti-tumor response, one should analyse the cellular response at the clonal level. In human tumors, the tumor targets can rarely be adapted to in vitro growth, regardless of the fact that they may change their antigenic expression after adapting to in vitro growth. Thus, for T cell cloning, one has to rely on small cryopreserved tumor fragments. The amount of tumor cells usually recovered from these fragments does not allow long term cloning, maintenance or testing for receptor stability of the T cell clones.

The aim of the present study was to develop a general approach that allows the cloning,maintenance and functional analysis of tumor infiltrating lymphocytes with a minimal use of autologous tumor target cells. Because, T cell stimulation, through CD3 is the one that most closely mimicks a physiological stimulation (7), we have maintained and functionally characterized T cell clones using a Fc receptor[+] cell line and OKT3 antibodies, in the

absence of the nominal antigen, instead of the
usual T cell cloning and characterization technics.
This approach was used to evaluate, in a colon
carcinoma patient, the autologous tumor specific
cytotoxic activity of T cell clones derived from
the PBL, proximal lymph nodes, distal lymph nodes
or TIL populations. Interestingly, all clones
derived from the TIL population had a cytolytic-
suppressor phenotype (OKT8$^+$ OKT4$^-$ OKT3$^+$) and were
able to lyse a Fc receptor$^+$ target cell in the
presence of OKT3 antibodies. In contrast, only
14 % of the T cell clones derived from the proximal draining lymph nodes demonstrated a cytolytic
effector function. Furthermore, 2 out of 5 TIL
derived T cell clones tested, proved to be specific for the autologous tumor cells without significant lysis of autologous normal lymphocytes.
The implications of these data in terms of cloning
of tumor specific T cells, and in terms of the
host spontaneous tumor specific T cell response
are discussed.

MATERIALS AND METHODS

Tumor : a surgically resected specimen of malignant colon carcinoma was obtained from a 69-year-
old female patient.
Tumor separation : the processing of the tumor
specimen was carried out as described (3),(4).
Briefly, the tumor specimen was minced, and the
fragments suspended in an enzyme mixture of collagenase, hyaluronidase and DNAse. The fragments
were digested for 4 to 16 hours at 37°C. The cells
were then harvested by centrifugation, washed and
incubated in complete medium for 12 to 18H to allow
maximal reexpression of surface antigens. Aliquots
of the single cell suspension, containing both
tumor cells and infiltrating lymphocytes (TILs)
were either cryopreserved for later use, or irradiated and used as stimulators for autologous PBL
and lymph-node derived lymphocytes or directly
incubated in the presence of r-IL-2 and condition-
ned medium for TIL expansion.

Experimental design : Ficoll-Hypaque separated
lymphocytes from the peripheral blood (PBL) or
from the proximal or distal draining lymph-nodes
(P.LN or D.LN) were extensively washed and 10^7
cells stimulated with 10^3 irradiated (6000 rads)
autologous tumor cells, in complete medium supplemented with 10 U/ml r-IL-2 and 10 % supernatant
from PHA stimulated PBL cells (conditioned medium).
The cells were fed every 3 days. After 1 week,
live cells were harvested and restimulated according to the same protocol. One week later, live
cells were plated under limiting conditions and
stimulated with 10^3 irradiated tumor cells and
10^5 irradiated heterologous feeder cells in conditioned medium. Proliferating clones were expanded,
recloned and maintained as described below.
    For the TIL population, a fraction of the
single cell suspension of the tumor was incubated
for 2 weeks, with occasional feedings, in conditioned medium. Growing T lymphocytes were then
expanded, cloned and maintained for over 7 months
as described below.
Maintenance of the T cell clones : all clones that
scored positive in our retargeting assay (see
below) were restimulated at weekly intervals with
conditioned medium in the presence of heterologous
irradiated PBL as feeder cells, or in the presence
of 10^5 mouse Fc receptor[+] B cell hybridoma cells
(TA3 (8)) and 10 % OKT3 supernatant. The cytolytic
effector function of the clones was routinely
tested as well as their specificity towards the
autologous colon carcinoma tumor cells.
Chromium release assays : in order to test the
cytolytic effector function of the growing T cell
clones, regardless of their specificity, we have
used a retargeting assay (7), (9), based on the
fact that T cells can be activated to perform
their effector function through the cross-linking
of their T cell receptor complex (TcR and the CD3
complex). Thus the incubation of CTL clones with
a chromium labeled Fc receptor[+] cell line (acts as
a cross-linking agent) and anti-CD3 antibodies
(recognize a monomorphic determinant on all TcR[+]
T cells) will induce a retargetted lysis of the Fc
receptor[+] cells.
    For specificity testing, autologous and hete-

rologous tumor cells were thawed and incubated overnight in complete medium before ^{51}Cr incorporation. The K 562 myeloid leukemia cell line (NK sensitive targets) and TA3 mouse B cell hybridoma cells (the retargeting cell) were maintained in complete medium. All targets were labeled with 500 μCi Na$_2$^{51}CrO$_4$ according to standard procedures. 100 μl of ^{251}Cr-labeled target cells (5x10^3) and 100 μl of effector cells were assigned at different effector to target ratios (E:T) to wells of round-bottomed microtiter plates for 4 hrs at 37°C. The percentage of cytotoxicity was determined using the formula : (experimental cpm-spontaneous cpm)/ (maximum cpm-spontaneous cpm) x 100 = % cytotoxicity.

Phenotypic analysis : cell surface expression of CD3, CD4 and CD8 markers was monitored respectively with the monoclonal antibodies OKT3, OKT4 and OKT8. Staining was visualized with FITC-conjugated rabbit anti-mouse antibody and analyzed with an orthocytofluorograph.

RESULTS AND DISCUSSION

Production of T cell clones from a colon carcinoma patient.
        In order to investigate the putative presence of a spontaneous, tumor specific immune response in cancer patients, we have analyzed T cells from different origins for a possible tumor-specific activity.
PBL, P.LN and D.LN cells were cocultured with irradiated (6000 rads) autologous tumor cells (10^3 cells/well) in 24 well culture trays, in the presence of irradiated heterologous PBL as feeders (10^5 cells/well) in complete conditioned medium (10 % supernatant from PHA activated PBL and 10 U/ml r-IL-2). After two rounds of stimulation, the blast cells were harvested on a density gradient and cloned under limiting dilution conditions. 12 clones of PBL origin, 7 clones of P.LN and 8 clones of D.LN origin, scored positive for cell growth after two cloning procedures. Of these clones, one from PBL origin, 2 of D.LN origin and all 7 of P.LN origin were succesfully maintained

for further characterization.
    TIL derived T cell clones were obtained as
described in Materials and Methods;briefly, surgically resected tumor tissue was enzymatically
dissociated and a fraction of the single cell
suspension was cultured for 2 weeks in complete
conditioned medium. After that period, a sizable
population of lymphocytes could be harvested
$(1.5 \ 10^6)$, and was cloned. A very large number of
clones was recovered among which 9 clones were
randomly selected for further growth and characterization.
Since all the clones analyzed were positive for
CD3 expression, they were maintained and restimulated weekly in the absence of the autologous
tumor cell target, but in the presence of irradiated (6000 rads) Fc receptor[+] TA3 mouse hybridoma
cell line and 10 % OKT3 hybridoma supernatant
as described in Materials and Methods.
Functional and phenotypic characterization of
the T cell clones : in order to analyze the effector function of our T cell clones, we have used
the retargeting assay as described in Materials
and Methods.

TABLE 1

	TARGETS			TARGETS	
CLONES	TA3	TA3+ OKT3	CLONES	TA3	TA3+ OKT3
TIL1	8,3%	68,4%	D.LN1	15,8%	57,1%
TIL2	8,0%	52,0%	P.LN1	10,2%	9,5%
TIL3	4,2%	60,0%	P.LN2	2,9%	9,5%
TIL4	4,4%	59,1%	P.LN3	26,6%	64,1%
TIL5	6,9%	45,3%	P.LN4	8,1%	10,0%
TIL6	15,5%	62,7%	P.LN5	7,0%	15,0%
TIL7	10,9%	66,1%	P.LN6	1,5%	7,0%
TIL8	12,2%	63,8%	P.LN7	1,0%	4,0%
TIL10	13,7%	66,5%	PBL.1	8,0%	11,0%

Legend to TABLE 1 : the T cell clones were functionally characterized using a retargeting assay as described. The data
are presented as % lysis of the Fc receptor[+]cell TA3,in the
presence or absence of the retargeting antibody OKT3 and
were obtained at an E:T ratio of 10:1.

The data presented in Table 1 show the cytolytic effector function of the T cell clones tested.
Very interestingly, all T cell clones derived
from the TIL population (9 out of 9) demonstrate
a cytolytic effector function, in sharp contrast
with the clones derived from the proximal lymph
nodes, where only one out of 7 clones proved to
be a cytolytic effector T cell. It is important to
stress here that our T cell clones are maintained
in low concentrations of r-IL-2 (10 U/ml),such
that the cytolytic functions observed are more
likely to reflect the actual effector phenotype
of the cells tested, rather than a lymphokine induced cytotoxic phenotype as observed with high
concentrations of r-IL-2 (10) (LAK cells). Furthermore, the retargeting assay with OKT3 antibodies, that triggers T cells through their T cell
receptor complex, demonstrate that it is a receptor mediated function and suggest that these T
cell clones, unlike LAK or NK cells, use a lytic
machinery that is characteristic of typical cytotoxic T cells.
The data obtained with the PBL and D.LN derived
lymphocytes cannot be taken into account because
of the small numbers of clones analyzed.
The expression of surface membrane CD3, CD4 and
CD8 molecules on the T cell clones was analyzed
by cytofluorometry. All TIL derived clones proved
to be $CD3^+$ $CD4^-$ and $CD8^+$(data not shown).
    Thus, our data demonstrate that, in the ana-
lyzed colorectal carcinoma patient, the tumor
infiltrating lymphocytes are exclusively of the
cytolytic effector phenotype, in contrast with the
T cell clones derived from the proximal draining
lymph nodes. Since the normal CD4/CD8 ratio in the
PBL or lymph nodes is around 2 to 1, there clearly
is a bias toward the cytolytic phenotype in the
TIL population and a converse bias in the proximal
lymph nodes. We believe that this bias in the TIL
population is a strong suggestion of an ongoing
host cytotoxic response against the tumor burden.
Whether such a bias correlates with a good prognosis of the disease will have to be determined in
a larger scale study. Furthermore, the depression
of effector cytolytic lymphocytes from the proximal draining lymph nodes may reflect the presence

of an active, tumor induced, immune suppression
mechanism, as suggested by several authors (11-12).
Test for the fine specificity of the TIL derived
T cell clone.
     As hypothesized above, if the bias for cytoly-
tic function in the TIL population is the reflect
of a spontaneous host immune response, then, it
is important to define the specificity of such a
response. To do so, we have analyzed our TIL derived clones for cytotoxicity, in a standard 4hr
^{51}Cr release assay, against labeled autologous
tumor cells, heterologous fresh tumor cells, autologous PBL and the NK sensitive K562 cell line.
The data presented in Table 2 clearly show that 2
out of 5 TIL derived cell clones are specifically
cytotoxic when tested against the autologous tumor cells and demonstrate no significant lysis of
normal autologous lymphoblasts, heterologous
fresh colon carcinoma tumor cells, nor against the
NK sensitive K562 cell line. These clones were not
tested for LAK activity since they were maintained
in very low concentrations of r-IL-2. Such cytolytic assays were repeated several times over a 7
months period, with the T cell clones restimulated
in the absence of the autologous tumor cells as
described in Materials and Methods.

TABLE   2

TARGETS

Effector	AUTOLOGOUS TUMOR	AUTOLOGOUS PBL	HETEROLOGOUS TUMOR	K562
TIL2	17%	1%	1%	2%
TIL3	8%	2%	ND	ND
TIL7	1%	1%	1%	3%
TIL8	30%	8%	1%	2%

Legend to Table 2 : 5 TIL derived T cell clones were tested
in a direct ^{51}Cr release assay, for autologous tumor specificity. The data are presented as % specific lysis and were
obtained at an E:T ratio of 1:1.

Thus, our data clearly demonstrate a preferential localization of effector cytolytic T lymphocyte precursors within the tumor site. A large fraction of these lymphocytes behave as conventional cytotoxic T cells in terms of their lymphokine requirements, T cell receptor mediated lysis and restricted specificity for the autologous infiltrated tumor target. We believe that this is the reflect of a spontaneous host tumor specific cellular immune response. Our cloning procedure, as well as the phenotypic characterization of our T cell clones using the retargeting assay, allows us to analyze an ongoing, presumably weak immune response in terms of the functional phenotype of the cells involved and also, importantly, in terms of the changes in the normal balances of the different T cell effector types. Such analysis should now be extended to a larger number of colorectal carcinoma patients to confirm our observation and to test whether a correlation can be made between the change in the balance of cytotoxic effector cells and the prognosis of the disease.

For the last several years, the general trend in human tumor immunotherapy has largely focused on what may be called "non-specific approaches", in which attempts have been made to generate large numbers of NK or LAK cells and test for their ability to reject or slow down the progression of the tumor target. The recent observation of the much higher efficiency of TIL derived lymphocytes in reducing the tumor burden (13), the observed side effects of the inoculation of large quantities of r-IL-2 in vivo and the preferential homing of in vitro grown T lymphocytes to the lung has made it more appealing to look for a preexisting, spontaneous tumor specific immune response. Our approach relies on such a preexisting response. Recent reports are now suggesting the oligoclonality of the TIL lymphocytes in terms of TcR rearrangements (14). This suggests that cloning may not be necessary to derive a largely tumor specific cytolytic T cell population from TIL and use it for immunotherapy. One can, for instance, inject such cells to the patient in case of a reapparance of a metastatic tumor after surgery. One may also design original

approaches that could allow the definition of the
tumor associated antigen(s) that is (are) the
target(s) of such an immune response.

REFERENCES

1. Bennet SH, Futre JW, Roth JA, Hoy ERC,
    Ketcham AS (1971). Prognostic significance of
    histological host response in cancer of the
    larynx or hypopharynx. Cancer 28:1255.
2. Lander I, Ahern EW (1985). The significance
    of lymphocytic infiltration and prognosis in
    colorectal carcinoma. Br J Cancer 49:375.
3. Heo DS, Whiteside TL, Johnson JT, Chen K,
    Barnes EL, Herberman RB (1987). Long term
    interleukin 2-dependent growth and cytotoxic
    activity of tumor-infiltrating lymphocytes
    from human squanous cell carcinomas of the
    head and neck. Cancer Res 47:6353.
4. Belldegnm A, Muul LM, Rosenberg SA (1988).
    Interleukin 2 expanded tumor-infiltrating
    lymphocytes in human renal cell cancer :
    isolation, characterization and antitumor
    activity. Cancer Res 48:206.
5. Topalian SL, Muul LM, Solomon D, Rosenberg SA
    (1987). Expansion of human tumor infiltrating
    lymphocytes for use in immunotherapy trials.
    J of Immunol Methods 102:127.
6. Rabinowich H., Cohen R., Bpuderman I, Steiner
    Z, Klajman A (1987). Functional analysis of
    mononuclear cells infiltrating into tumors:
    lysis of autologous human tumor cells by
    cultured infiltrating lymphocytes. Cencer Res
    47:173.
7. Hoffman RW, Bluestone JA, Leo O, Shaw S (1985).
    Lysis of anti-T3 bearing murine hybridoma cells
    by human allospecific cytotoxic T cell clones
    and inhibition of that lysis by anti-T3 and
    anti-LFA-1 antibodies. J Immunol 135:5.
8. Glimcher LH, Sharrow SO, Paul WE (1983).
    Serologic and functional characterization of
    a panel of antigen presenting cell lines ex-
    pressing mutant I-A class II molecules. J
    Exp Med 158:1573.

9. Spits H, Yssel J, Leeuwenberg J, De Vries JE
(1985). Antigen-specific cytotoxic T cell and
antigen-specific proliferating T cell clones
can be induced to cytolytic activity by monoclonal antibodies against T3. Eur J Immunol
15:88.
10. Rosenberg SA (1985). Lymphokine-activated
killer cells. A new approach to immunotherapy
of cancer. J. Natl Cancer Inst 75:595.
11. Hoon DSB, Bowker RJ, Cochran AJ (1987).
Suppressor cell activity in melanoma draining
lymph nodes. Cancer Res 47:1529.
12. Catalona WJ, Ratliff TL, Mc Cool RE (1979).
Concanavalin-A inducible suppressor cells in
regional lymph nodes of cancer patients.
Cancer Res 39:4372.
13. Rosenberg SA, Spiess P, Lafrenière R (1986).
A new approach to the adoptive immunotherapy
of cancer with tumor-infiltrating lymphocytes.
Science 233:1318.
14. Flatow J, Wood N, Dobrzanska E, Iverson S,
Ko JL, Snider ME (1988). T lymphocytes from
lung tumors : phenotype, function and antigen
receptor analysis. Abstract. The FASEB J1
72nd annual meeting : A.898.

Human Tumor Antigens and Specific Tumor Therapy, pages 105–114
© 1989 Alan R. Liss, Inc.

HUMAN MONOCLONAL ANTIBODIES[1]

June Kan-Mitchell

Department of Microbiology
University of Southern California
Los Angeles, California 90033

ABSTRACT   The spectra of reactivity of 2 human IgG
monoclonal antibodies (MAbs), 2-139-1 and 14-31-10,
are presented to illustrate that MAbs of human origin
may be useful to study novel tumor-associated
antigens (TAAs). Because these MAbs were generated
from lymphocytes sensitized in vivo in the cancer
patients, the TAAs detected are by definition
immunogenic to man. The MAb 2-139-1, derived from a
melanoma patient, was reactive against all melanomas
tested. It, however, also stained colon and several
other types of carcinomas that are not
embryologically related to melanoma. No reactivity
was detected against banal nevus cells as well as
adult and fetal melanocytes. Thus, the antibody does
not identify a differentiation antigen of neural
crest cells. In contrast, limited reactivity was
detected in preneoplastic melanocytic lesions. The
MAb 14-31-10, derived from a patient with colon
carcinoma, was selected for its noncrossreactivity to
melanoma. While it stained colon carcinomas, little
reactivity was noted in normal or inflammatory
colonic epithelia. However, some reactivity was also
noted in preneoplastic lesions. Thus, a parallel
exists for the spectra of reactivities of these two
antibodies. Both discriminated between normal and
malignant cells, with limited reactivities against
preneoplastic lesions.   Their target antigens differ
from others previously identified by mouse MAbs and
may be involved in neoplastic transformation.

[1]This work was supported by USPHS Grants CA 43220 and
CA 26233.

INTRODUCTION

The advent of mouse monoclonal antibodies (MAbs) has revolutionized the study of human tumor-associated antigens (TAAs). Because of this success, recent attention has turned to the generation of MAbs of human origin. Human MAbs potentially offer several advantages. For therapeutic purposes, the usefulness of mouse MAbs is severely limited by a strong antimouse immunoglobulin antibody response induced in the patients (1). One possible method to circumvent this immune response is to produce human-mouse chimeric antibodies of various isotypes (2). Indeed, several directed against human cancer cells have been described (3,4,5,6). The utility of such genetically engineered immunoglobulins is still limited by the difficulty of producing large amounts of purified antibody. A more direct approach, however, is to produce MAbs of human origin, which should also be less immunogenic.

Indeed, human MAbs may identify novel TAAs. In the case of human malignant melanoma, which is perhaps the most well studied immunologically, the same TAAs were independently identified by mouse MAbs produced in different laboratories despite the use of a variety of immunization schedules and antigenic preparations. While this might reflect the inability of the mouse to recognize other human tumor antigens (7), it is more likely that without specialized immunization procedures, reactivity was always directed to the same immunodominant antigens.

On the other hand, human MAbs may identify TAAs that are not readily immunogenic to other animals. In some situations, human antibodies exhibit a higher degree of discrimination than xenoantibodies (7). The precedence for this exists in tissue typing, where human antibodies have a wider range of specificities against allotypic determinants of HLA than antibodies of xenogeneic origin.

Lastly, only human MAbs can identify TAAs that are immunogenic to man. In fact, several of the human melanoma-associated antigens defined by mouse MAbs did not induce a detectable humoral response in man and other animals (8). On the other hand, three gangliosides (the monosialoganglioside GM2 and the disialogangliosides GD2 and GD3) associated with cells of neuroectodermal origin have been detected both by mouse MAbs (9,10,11) as well as human sera and human MAbs (12,13,14). One human MAb,

HJM1, identified an epitope common to GD3, GD2, GD1b and GM3 (14). This type of discrimination in the ganglioside antigens has not been described in mouse antibodies raised against GD2 or GD3.

PRODUCTION OF PURIFIED HUMAN MABs

There are two major technological obstacles for the production of human MAbs; namely, the generation of specifically immunized human B lymphocytes and their immortalization into antibody-producing cell lines (15,16). To overcome these difficulties, we made human-mouse heterohybridomas by fusing lymphocytes (LNLs) from regional lymph nodes of melanoma patients with a nonsecreting mouse myeloma cell line.

We chose to use LNLs because they are better fusion partners than circulating lymphocytes and more available than splenic lymphocytes (17). Since human MAbs produced from LNLs of patients with breast carcinomas were reactive to their homologous tumors (18), we used draining LNLs from melanoma patients without further immunization.

To identify TAAs that are spontaneously antigenic to the patients, we decided not to perform a large number of fusions and to screen for predetermined reactivities as have been the approach of other laboratories (19). Instead, we concentrated on solving the technical problem of producing sufficient quantities of purified human MAbs for careful evaluation of their reactivities.

To favor detection of T cell-dependent antigens by our human MAbs, we studied only those of the IgG class. IgG antibodies, as contrast to IgM, are more likely to reflect active specific humoral response to the tumor antigens.

A total of 6 stable hybridoma cell lines were cloned from different LNLs from three melanoma patients (19). By early cloning and freezing of early passages, we have maintained these heterohybridomas for more than 4 years. These cell lines grew readily in an ascitic form in pristane-primed nude mice, producing up to 25 mg of antibody from each mouse. A procedure was developed to purify the human MAbs from the ascitic fluids by ammonium sulfate precipitation and hydroxyapatite chromatography. An important step (termed "affinity depletion") was included for the complete removal of mouse Ig from the ascites by an affinity column of sheep antimouse IgG with no crossreactivity to human IgG (20).

Purified preparations of the 3 classes (IgG, IgM and IgA) of human MAbs were found to be greater than 80% homogeneous by SDS-polyacrylamide gel electrophoresis (20). Estimations of the molecular weights of their heavy and light chains proved that these human MAbs were intact immunoglobulins. Furthermore, no contaminating mouse IgG were detected in the prepartions of IgM and IgA human MAbs, confirming the efficacy of the affinity depletion column and that the human IgG MAbs were indeed human in origin.

ALTERED ANTIGENICITY OF HUMAN MABs MOLECULES

When a standard enzyme immunoassay was used to determine the concentrations of these human IgG MAbs, their titration curves were found to reach maximal plateau values that were much lower than that for the polyclonal control (20). By comparing the concentrations of purified preparations of human MAbs determined by protein determination with that predicted by the immunoassay, it was discovered that the human MAbs were antigenically distinct from their polyclonal counterparts. In particular, the human IgG MAbs were not well recognized by a goat antibody raised against human polyclonal IgG. This artefact in the immunoassay has an important practical corollary in subsequent studies of the reactivities of human MAbs. Corrective measures must be included when xenoantibodies to polyclonal human immunoglobulins are used to study human MAbs, particularly those of the IgG class. For this reason, we used a direct binding assays to study the reactivities of our human MAbs. After the human MAbs were purified, they were conjugated to biotin. Binding was visualized by the avidin-biotin-peroxidase complex.

IMMUNOREACTIVITIES OF THE HUMAN MAB 2-139-1

One of the IgG human MAb (2-139-1) generated from a melanoma patient was studied in the greatest detail. When tested against cell lines, 2-139-1 was found to identify a cytoplasmic antigen in all melanoma cells tested, including both short-term and continuous cultures derived from metastases of cutaneous melanoma and primary lesions

of ocular melanoma.   In contrast to many mouse MAbs raised
against human melanoma, no reactivity was detected against
neuroectodermal tumors.   Reactivity was also not detected
against lymphomas, leukemias and lymphoblastoid cell lines
or sarcoma cell lines.   On the other hand, 2-139-1 reacted
aginst 12 of the 16 carcinoma cell lines tested, staining
in particular, all those of colon origin with an intensity
equal to that of melanoma.
    The reactivity of 2-139-1 against cell lines were
further confirmed by immunohistochemistry.   The antibody
stained frozen sections of melanoma with moderate to high
intensity without detectable reactivity against normal
colon, stomach, breast, skin and lung under identical
conditions.   To characterize the reactivity of 2-139-1
against the broadest possible spectrum of tissues,
formalin-fixed and paraffin-embedded sections of human
tissues were also studied.

          TABLE 1: 2-139-1 AGAINST SKIN TUMORS

    Malignant melanoma
            Primary   20/20 (3-4+)
            Metastatic   17/17 (3-4+)
            Ocular   7/7 (2-4+)
            Lentigo maligna   1/5 (2+)
    Basal cell carcinoma   0/2
    Squamous cell carcinoma   0/2

    The antibody reacted against all the fixed sections
of melanoma specimens tested, including both primary and
metastatic lesions and ocular melanomas (Table 1).
Reactivity was also observed in 1 of the 5 cases of
lentigo maligna, a low grade form of melanoma.   On the
other hand, reactivity was not detected in basal cell and
squamous cell carcinoma of the skin.   Of interest, 2-139-1
did not stained adult and fetal skin melanocytes.   No
reactivity was detected in a variety of nonpigmented
normal tissues, such as normal skin, liver, lung and
colon, or a variety of benign tumors, such as mammary
fibroadenoma and benign prostate hypertrophy.
    The most interesting and unique aspect of the
reactivity of 2-139-1 is its ability to distinguish
cutaneous melanoma from benign nevi in fixed sections
(21).   All 22 specimens of banal nevi representing a

spectrum of histologic types were not stained (Table 2), with the exception of 2 cases of dysplastic nevi, where 40% of the melanocytic cells were reactive. These are putatively premalignant lesions.

TABLE 2: 2-139-1 AGAINST NEVUS CELLS AND MELANOCYTES

Nevi:	Blue	0/2
	Compound	0/3
	Congenital	0/2
	Intradermal	0/2
	Junctional	0/1
	Epithelioid (Spitz)	0/7
	Halo	0/2
	Dysplastic	2/5
Skin melanocytes:		0/15

As suggested by the immunocytochemical results, the antibody exhibited strong crossreactivity against adeno-carcinomas of the colon, prostate, rectum and pancreas. However, not all carcinoma were stained. Excluding the cases of colon and prostate cacinomas, reactivity was observed only against 13 of the 23 specimens of carcinoma studied, including only borderline reactivity against squamous cell carcinoma of the lung and transitional cell carcinoma of the bladder. No reactivity was detected in 5 specimens of sarcomas and other miscellaneous tumors.

IMMUNOREACTIVITIES OF THE HUMAN MAB 14-31-10

The striking crossreactivity of 2-139-1 to colon carcinomas suggested that human MAbs thus generated might recognize only a limited number of target antigens. To test this hypothesis, we developed a series of human MAbs from regional LNLs of colon carcinoma patients (22). Immunohistochemical characterization of 4 MAbs with a panel of 19 tumor xenografts revealed reactivities in the cytoplasm of the tumor cells, however, that only 1 of the 4 antibodies reacted with both colon tumors and melanomas. Three MAbs reacted only to colon carcinoma and not melanoma.
The noncrossreacting IgG MAb, 14-31-10, was selected for further characterization against fixed sections of

human tissues. The reactivity of the MAb was more
restricted than that of 2-139-1. Although 15 of the 18
cases of colon carcinoma were stained, reactivity was
observed only in 4 of 16 breast adenocarcinomas. No
reactivity was detected in 18 adenocarcinomas, 4 squamous
cell carcinomas, 1 transitional cell carcinoma, 12
melanomas, 7 sarcomas, 3 carcinoids and 10 tumors of a
variety of histopathology.

No reactivity was found in 10 sections of normal
adult colon, 4 of normal fetal colon as well as a variety
of other normal tissues such as skin, liver stomach,
pancreas, kidney and lung.

In parallel with studies of 2-139-1 in melanoma, the
human MAb 14-31-10 was tested against inflammatory and
preneoplastic lesions of the colon (23). The antibody was
found not to be reactive against diverticulosis, regional
enteritis, amebic colitis, colitis cytstica profunda and
acute appendicitis. In contrast, 6 of the 38
preneoplastic lesions were reactive to a moderate degree.
These included one of 5 benign polyps, 3 of 9 villous
adenomas and adenomatous polyps, 1 of 5 cases of
ulcerative colitis and 1 of 19 cases of familial
polyposis.

SUMMARY

Our results illustrate that human MAbs can add a new
dimension to the identification of TAAs. The human MAbs
described were derived from regional LNLs of patients with
melanoma and colon carcinoma spontaneously sensitized in
vivo. Immunocytochemical and immunohistochemical studies
defined apparently novel cytoplasmic TAAs that are
preferentially expressed by neoplastic cells. While
absolute discrimination may be impossible with any MAb,
the spectrum of reactivity of these human MAbs are
sufficiently restricted and distinct from those previously
described using mouse MAbs to warrant additional studies.
Indeed some of these may have applications in pathological
and serological diagnosis.

In these studies, we have only used LNLs from
patients as a source of specifically sensitized cells.
This approach has resulted in identifying mostly
cytoplasmic antigens. Because human MAbs reactive to cell
surface antigens would be more desirable for therapeutic

applications, we will use lymphocytes from patients that
have been immunized with an allogeneic melanoma cell
preparation for our future fusions.

REFERENCES

1. Sears, HF, Bagli, DJ, Herlyn, D, DeFreitas, E,
    Suzuki, H, Steele, G and Koprowski, H (1987). Human
    immune response to monoclonal antibody administration
    is dose-dependent. Arch Surg 122:1384.
2. Bruggemann, M, Williams, GT, Bindon, CI, Clark, MR,
    Walker, MR, Jefferis, R, Waldmann, H and Neuberger,
    MS (1987). Comparison of the effector functions of
    human immunoglobulins using a matched set of chimeric
    antibodies. J Exp Med 166:1351.
3. Sahagan, BG, Dorai, H, Saltzgaber-Muller, J,
    Toneguzzo, F, Guindon, CA, Lilly, SP, McDonald, KW,
    Morrissey, DV, Stone, A, Davis, GL, McIntosh, PK and
    Moore, GP (1986). A genetically-engineered
    murine/human chimeric antibody retains specificity
    for human tumor-associated antigens. J Immunol
    137:1066.
4. Sun, LK, Curtis, P, Rakowicz-Szulczynska, E, Ghrayeb,
    J, Morrison, SL, Chang, N and Koprowski, H (1986).
    Chimeric antibodies with 17-1A-derived variable
    regions and human constant regions. Hybridoma 5:S17.
5. Liu, SY, Robinson, RA, Hellstrom, KE, Murray, ED,
    Chang, CP and Hellstrom, I (1987). Chimeric mouse-
    human IgG1 antibody that can mediate lysis of cancer
    cells. Proc Natl Acad Sci USA 84:3439.
6. Brown BA, Davis GL, Saltzgaber-Muller J, Simon P, Ho
    M-K, Shaw PS, Stone BA, Sands H and Moore GP (1987).
    Tumor-specific genetically engineered murine/human
    chimeric monoclonal antibody. Cancer Res 47:3577.
7. Kaplan HS, Olsson L (1982). Human-human hybridomas
    in diagnosis and treatment. In Mitchell MS, Oettgen
    HF (eds): "Hybridomas in Cancer Diagnosis and
    Treatment, Vol. 21 of Progress in Cancer Research and
    Therapy," New York: Raven Press, p 113.
8. Hamby CV, Liao S-K, Ferrone, S (1987).
    Immunogenicity of human melanoma-associated antigens
    defined by murine monoclonal antibodies in allogeneic
    and xenogeneic hosts. Cancer Res 47:5284.

9. Natoli EJ, Livingston PO, Pukel CS, Lloyd KO, Wiegandt H, Szalay J, Oettgen HF, Old LJ (1986). A murine monoclonal antibody detecting N-acetyl- and N-glycolyl-GM2: Characterization of cell surface reactivity. Cancer Res 46:4116.
10. Cheung N-KV, Saarinen UM, Neely JE, Landmeier B, Donovan D, Coccia PF (1985). Monoclonal antibodies to a glycolipid antigen on human neuroblastoma cells. Cancer Res 45:2642.
11. Cheresh DA, Harper JR, Schulz G, Reisfeld RA (1984). Localization of the gangliosides GD3 and GD2 in adhesion plaques and on the surface of human melanoma cells. Proc Natl Acad Sci USA 81:5767.
12. Tai T, Paulson JC, Cahan LD, Irie RF (1983). Ganglioside GM2 as a human tumor antigen (OFA-I-1). Proc Natl Acad Sci USA 80:5392.
13. Watanabe T, Pukel CS, Takeyama H, Lloyd KO, Shiku H, Li LTC, Travassos LR, Oettgen HF, Old LJ (1982). Human melanoma antigen AH is an autoantigenic ganglioside related to GD2. J Exp Med 156:1884.
14. Yamaguchi H, Furukawa K, Fortunato SR, Livingston PO, Lloyd KO, Oettgen HF, Old LJ (1987). Cell-surface antigens of melanoma recognized by human monoclonal antibodies. Proc Nat Acad Sci 84:2416.
15. Kan-Mitchell J, Mitchell, MS (1988). Human monoclonal antibodies for the diagnosis of tumors. In Kupchik, HZ (ed): "Cancer Diagnosis In Vitro Using Monoclonal Antibodies, Vol. 39 of Immunology Series," New York: Marcel Dekker, p 289.
16. Larrick JW, Buck DW (1984). Practical aspects of human monoclonal antibody production. BioTechniques 2:6.
17. Cote RJ, Morrissey DM, Houghton AN, Beattie Jr EJ, Ottegen HF, Old LJ (1983). Generation of human monoclonal antibodies reactive with cellular antigens. Proc Natl Acad Sci USA 80:2026.
18. Schlom J, Wunderlich D, Teramoto YA (1980). Generation of human monoclonal antibodies reactive with human mammary carcinoma cells. Proc Natl Acad Sci USA 77:6841.
19. Kan-Mitchell J, Imam A, Kempf RA, Taylor CR and Mitchell MS (1986). Human monoclonal antibodies directed against melanoma tumor-associated antigens. Cancer Res 46: 2490.

20. Kan-Mitchell J, Andrews KL, Gallardo D, Mitchell MS (1987). Altered antigenicity of human monoclonal antibodies derived from human-mouse heterohybridomas. Hybridoma 6:161.
21. Imam A, Mitchell MS, Modlin RL, Taylor CR, Kempf RA and Kan-Mitchell J (1986). Human monoclonal antibodies that distinguish cutaneous malignant melanomas from benign nevi in fixed tissue sections. J Invest Dermatol 86:145.
22. Formenti SC, Mitchell MS, Rosen F, Kempf RA, Imam A, Taylor CR, Kan-Mitchell J (1985). Use of human xenografts to detect the binding of human monoclonal antibodies (MoAbs) to colon carcinoma. Proc Amer Assoc Cancer Res 26:297.
23. Formenti SC, Kan-Mitchell J, Jernstrom P, Taylor CR and Mitchell MS (1986). Imunohistochemical reactivity of a human monoclonal antibody (Hu-MAb) from a patient with colon cancer. Proc Amer Assoc Cancer Res 27:337.

Human Tumor Antigens and Specific Tumor Therapy, pages 115-126
© 1989 Alan R. Liss, Inc.

MELANOMA, GANGLIOSIDES AND HUMAN MONOCLONAL ANTIBODY[1]

Reiko F. Irie, Peter J. Chandler,
and Donald L. Morton

Division of Surgical Oncology, John Wayne Cancer Clinic,
Jonsson Comprehensive Cancer Center, UCLA School of
Medicine, Los Angeles, California 90024.

Gangliosides of Human Melanoma

Currently, the only effective therapy for malignant melanoma is surgical resection. While there have been many advances in chemo and radiation treatment of other forms of cancer, such therapy is not as effective against melanoma metastases. For this reason, immunologic approaches are currently being investigated. The potential effectiveness of immunotherapy in melanoma is encouraging since this tumor contains large quantities of antigenic glycolipid molecules called gangliosides. Gangliosides are glycosphingolipids bearing sialic acids, are found in the plasma membrane of Deuterostomia and are synthesized most abundantly by neural tissues. Gangliosides are most commonly embedded in the lipid bilayer of the outer membrane by a ceramide group (a sphingosine with a long chain fatty acid), with a carbohydrate portion protruding into the extracellular environment. The carbohydrate portion is composed of 2 to 8 sugars. Of these sugars, the sialic acids (a family of hexose sugars) are an important component in determining antigenic diversity. While there are 18 different sialic acids isolated in animals and man, only one, N-acetyl neuraminic acid, is found in normal human tissue. The diversity and immunologic specificity of gangliosides are determined by the number, position, linkage of the oligosaccharide chain and nature of this unique sugar family.

[1]Supported by NIH grants CA30647, CA42396 and CA12582.

Heterogeneity of gangliosides is observed among different
species, intraspecies, and among different tissues; likewise, cell
surface ganglioside expression changes at different points in
the cell cycle, at different differentiation points and during
cellular transformation. Melanoma is distinct from other types
of human malignancies and normal melanocytes as it contains
large quantities of many different gangliosides. These
qualitative and quantitative differences of ganglioside expression
between normal melanocytes and melanoma is the basis for
immunotherapy in melanoma. Carubia et. al. explored the
ganglioside expression of melanocytes and human melanoma (1),
and determined that while normal melanocytes contain primarily
GM3 (90%) and GD3 (5%), melanoma cells express these
gangliosides as well as GD2, GM2, GM1, GD1a, GD1b, and
GT1b. In 1987, we analyzed the ganglioside composition of 80
melanoma specimens, including 52 biopsies and 28 cultured cell
lines. This study demonstrated the heterogeneity of both the
prevelance and quantity of gangliosides between melanoma
specimens (2) (Figure 1). The four most commonly expressed
gangliosides of human melanoma are GD3, GM3, GD2 and GM2
with ganglioside GD3 composing about 50% of the total
membrane-associated gangliosides.

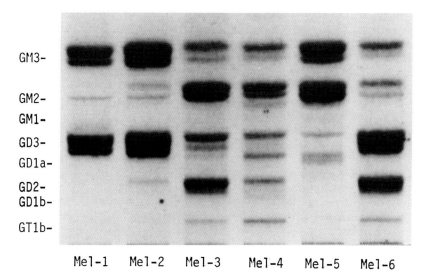

Figure 1. Thin-layer chromatogram of gangliosides isolated
from six melanoma specimens. Heterogeneity of ganglioside
expression is depicted.

Immunogenicity of Melanoma-Associated Gangliosides

In 1975 our laboratory demonstrated that sera of melanoma patients contained antibodies reactive to a tumor-associated membrane antigen, OFA-I (oncofetal antigen–immunogenic), that is cross-reactive between human cancer and fetal brain tissues (3,4,5). When the survival of Stage II melanoma patients was studied retrospectively, it was found that those patients with a high titer of anti-OFA-I antibody had a significantly prolonged survival as compared to those with low titers (p < 0.001) (6). The majority of the anti-OFA-I antibodies found in these patients were later demonstrated to be specific to a cell surface ganglioside GM2, and further studies of the serum reactivity determined that antibodies reacting to GD2 were also present (7). Demonstrating the immunogenic nature of these gangliosides enabled us and other investigators to explore the therapeutic potential of active and passive immunization to melanoma. During the last several years our group has been engaged in two major clinical immunotherapy studies on melanoma: the use of human monoclonal antibodies in passive immunotherapy (8) and the use of ganglioside-rich tumor cell vaccine (TCV) in active specific immunotherapy (9). Although the heterogeneity of melanoma has been a considerable obstacle in these clincial trials, this problem is potentially surmountable if several immunogenic gangliosides can be targeted as antigens for such immunotherapy. Our group has demonstrated that four different melanoma-associated gangliosides are immunogenic in man. These include GD2, GM2, O-acetyl GD3 and gangliosides containing N-glycolyl neuraminic acid.

The extracellular portion of ganglioside GD2 consists of 5 carbohydrates including 2 sialic acids. GD2 is not found on normal melanocytes, whereas 71% of biopsied melanoma cells contain this ganglioside (2). GD2 comprised an average of 2% of the total ganglioside composition in biopsied samples (n=52) and 9.8% in cultured melanoma cells (n=28). Eventhough GD2 is a relatively small part of the total ganglioside content, the immunogenic nature and its prevelance makes it a very appealing target for immunotherapy. In 1982 two groups of investigators, Irie et al (10,11) and Watanabe et al (12), demonstrated the presence of anti-GD2 antibody (or anti-OFA-I-2) antibody in melanoma patients and showed that anti-GD2 production could be induced in melanoma patients immunized with a GD2 positive tumor cell vaccine (13). The most convincing argument for the immunogenicity of ganglioside GD2 is that we were able to produce HuMAb to GD2 in vitro from B-lymphoctes from a patient with melanoma (10,11).

The carbohydrate portion of ganglioside GM2 is similar to that of GD2 except GM2 bears one less sialic acid. Ganglioside GM2 is found on all melanoma cells and comprises an average of 3.2% of biopsied tissue and 13.6% of cultured tumor cells (2). This ganglioside appears to be capable of stimulating not only humoral immune responses but cellular responses as well.

Our first indication that GM2 was immunogenic was the detection of anti-GM2 antibody in sera of melanoma patients (10,14). Further evidence of the immunogenicity of GM2 was demonstrated as anti-GM2 antibody was induced in 10 of 26 patients who received a GM2-positive TCV (13). Recently, Livingston et al. demonstrated that anti-GM2 antibody could be induced by immunization with purified ganglioside GM2 in conjunction with appropriate adjuvants (15). GM2 immunogenicity was demonstrated in vitro when we successfully produced human monoclonal antibody to GM2 by EBV transformation of the lymphocytes of a patient with serum antibodies to GM2 (10,14).

Our group has shown that GM2 might be responsible for stimulation of natural killer (NK) activity in man (16,17). The erythroblastoid cell line K562 had been known to be sensitive to NK lysis and when the cell surface ganglioside expression of K562 was examined, GM2 was found as a predominant ganglioside (10). We also found that human sera containing IgM auto-anti GM2 antibody reacted to K562 cells in serologic assays. Hypothesizing that human NK effector cells might recognize GM2 on target cell lines, we tested GM2 expression and NK sensitivity of 14 lymphoid tumor target cell lines with varying quantities of GM2. A positive correlation (r = .83) was found between GM2 content and NK sensitivity. The specificity of NK lysis was confirmed by inhibition studies using pure GM2. This hypothesis supports our previous finding that patients receiving GM2-rich TCV displayed heightened levels of NK activity (18).

Another ganglioside of melanoma which is particular interest is O-acetylated GD3. This ganglioside constitutes 3 to 18% of the total gangliosides in melanoma and is found in 83% of biopsied tumors (n=52) and 54% of UCLA-melanoma cultured cell lines (n=28) (2). O-acetyl sialic acids are found only in alkali-labile gangliosides of melanoma. Using murine monoclonal antibodies and a lectin specific for O-acetyl sialic acids, our group (19) and others (20,21) have identified the alkali-labile gangliosides to be O-acetyl GD3. O-acetylated GD3 is also immunogenic in man since antibodies to this ganglioside have been detected in the sera of melanoma patients (19). While GD3 is found widely in human normal tissues, O-acetyl GD3 is restricted to neoplastic cells in man. In light of the large prevelance in biopsied specimens and the restriction to transformed cells this ganglioside is a promising target for immunotherapy.

Recently, our laboratory as well as others have identified melanoma tumors which contain a sialic acid that is normally not found in humans (22,23). This sialic acid called N-glycolyl neuraminic acid (NeuGc) is distributed in all mammals except humans. Unlike the 3 aforementioned sialyloligosaccharides, immunogenic NeuGc containing oligosaccharides can be found on protein moeities. In melanoma gangliosides NeuGc is found on GM3, GM2, and GD3, and composes from 0-0.07% of total gangliosides (23). One of the human heterophile antibodies (anti-Hanganutziu-Deicher antigen antibody; H-D antibody) recognizes specifically glycoconjugates containing NeuGc. Using this antibody we found that both biopsied melanoma and culture melanoma cell lines contained NeuGc bearing glycoconjugates (22).

The immunogenicity of NeuGc was indirectly demonstrated by our group, by comparing the anti-NeuGc antibody titers of melanoma patients with that of undiseased individuals. In this study melanoma patients had a much higher prevelance of IgG antibody against NeuGc than non-melanoma patients (22). The uniqueness of NeuGc containing glycoconjugates in man and its immunogenic qualities make it another potential target for immunotherapy.

Gangliosides as Antigens for Passive Immunotherapy with Human Monclonal antibody

Utilizing both hybridoma and viral transformation techniques, murine and human monoclonal antibodies have been produced to all of the major gangliosides of human melanoma; GM2, GD2, GD3, O-acetylated GD3, and GM3. Houghton et al. (24) and Cheung et al. (25) have successfully used murine monoclonal antibodies to GD3 and GD2, respectively, in Phase I clinical trials. In 1986, our laboratory reported the clincial use of human monoclonal antibody (8). This Phase I trial with 8 Stage III recurrent melanoma patients suggested the therapeutic potential of human monoclonal antibody. The effectiveness of HuMAb and murine monoclonal anti-ganglioside antibodies has generated optimism about the efficacy of an additional human monoclonal antibody developed in this laboratory, anti-GM2, of which clinical trials are in progress.

There are several methods currently used to establish human anti-tumor antibody-producing cells lines in vitro. These include Epstein-Barr virus (EBV) transformation of human B-lymphocytes, the hybridoma technique, and its modified versions. Our laboratory has successfully used the EBV transformation technique to establish 3 stable lymphoblast cell lines that secrete IgM class antibody to gangliosides GD2 (L72), GM2 (L55) and monosialogangliosides containing terminal NeuAc-Gal-GlcNAc (L87). Yamaguchi et al have reported the production of human monoclonal antibodies to ganglioside antigens by fusion of human lymphoblastoid cells (EBV transformed) with mouse (NS-1) cells (26): Mab-HJM1 reacted strongly with GD3, and weakly with GD2 and GD1b; Mab-FCMI reacted strongly with GM3 and GD1a, and weakly with GD3 and GD2; and MAb-32-27 reacted with di and tri-sialogangliosides.

The first HuMAb clinically applied in our laboratory was L72, an anti-ganglioside GD2 antibody. L72 is an IgM class antibody containing kappa light chains and electrofocusing analysis has shown that this HuMAb precipitated around pH 8.0. Prior to clinical use, the antibody was rigorously analyzed in order to predict clinical efficacy. Initially the cytotoxicity of the antibody was tested in vitro. Using the complement dependent cytotoxcity assay with GD2 positive and negative cell lines, L72 only lysed GD2 positive cells in the presence of complement (27). L72 was ineffective in killing tumor cells in antibody-dependent cell mediated (ADCC) assays. In vivo testing was performed using a nude mouse model (28,29). Tumor-free intervals were compared among six groups of mice: those receiving GD2 positive tumor cells, L72 with or without complement, those injected with GD2-positive tumor cells, non-specific IgM with or without complement, and those injected with a GD2-negative tumor cell line, L72 with or without complement. The antibody and complement were injected locally or systemically. The mice injected with GD2-positive tumors, L72 and complement had significantly longer tumor-free intervals than the control groups. This experiment demonstrated both the cytotoxicity and the specificity of L72.

Subsequently, HuMAb L72 was intralesionally administered to 8 recurrent cutaneous melanoma patients, marking the first clinical testing of HuMAb (8). Of these 8 patients, 6 significantly responded (greater than 50% tumor reduction) within 4 weeks after the last administration. Figure 2 demonstrates the histopathology of pre and post treatment biopsies of a patient's tumor that completely regressed. The post treatment biopsy (Figure 2b) was taken 37 days after the last human monoclonal antibody injection. Pathological examination revealed no evidence of viable melanoma. The upper picture (Figure 2a) is a melanoma biopsy from the same patient before monoclonal antibody treatment. No side effects were observed in any patient. The tumors of the two patients that did not respond were biopsied and ganglioside expression was biochemically analyzed. Both of these patient's tumors did not contain any ganglioside GD2. Biochemical analysis of the remaining tumors of the other patients was also performed and all of the tumors tested contained ganglioside GD2. This initial clinical trial not only demonstrated the clinical efficacy and the specificity of HuMAb L72 but it also demonstrated the need for a more comprehensive panel of HuMAbs which are specific to many different cell surface structures on melanoma. As mentioned previously our laboratory has developed two other HuMAbs specific to gangliosides found on melanoma: HuMAb L55, anti-GM2 and L87 which reacts with monosialogangliosides having the terminal structure, NeuAc-Gal-GlcNAc, such as GM3 and sialylparagloboside (SPG). Although HuMAb L87 reacts strongly in vitro to melanoma cells which contain ganglioside GM3, it does not react to normal tissues which contain GM3 and/or SPG. Both of these antibodies are cytotoxic to melanoma cells containing the corresponding antigen in the complement dependent cytotoxicity assay (Figure 3 and 4). In our current clinical trials with L55, no adverse effects or toxicity to normal tissue have been observed.

In light of the precise specificity of human monoclonal antibodies the heterogeneic expression of gangliosides on melanoma poses a significant problem. To circumvent this problem our laboratory is continuing to research the immunogenicity of human melanoma and developing new HuMAbs which will increase the scope of passive immunotherapy. Our present research is aimed at the development of HuMAb to O-acetyl GD3 and gangliosides containing N-glycolyl neuraminic acid. With the successful production of these antibodies, we will potentially have a comprehensive panel of HuMAbs which will offset the heterogeneous nature of melanoma-associated gangliosides.

Figure 2

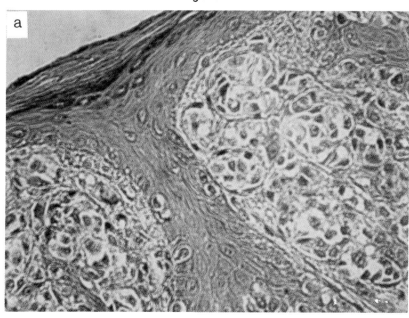

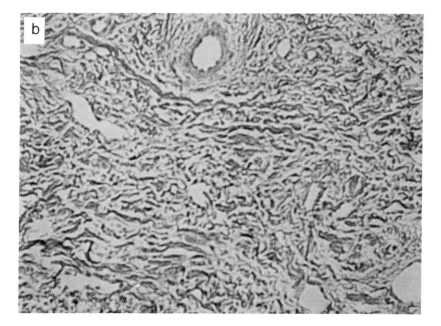

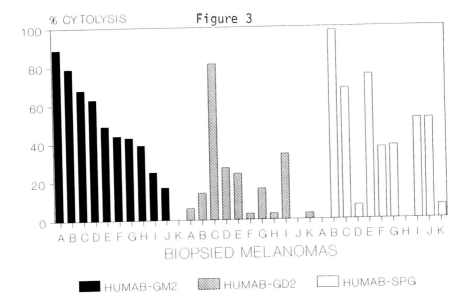

Figure 3

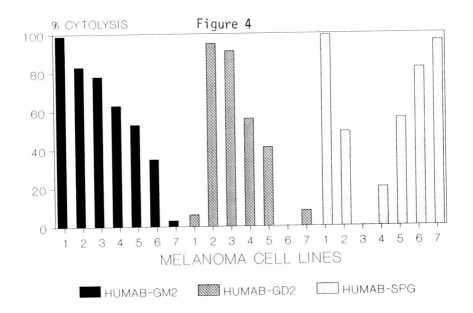

Figure 4

REFERENCES

1. Carubia JM, Yu RK Macala LJ, Kirkwood JM, and Varga JM (1984). Gangliosides of normal and neoplastic human melanocytes. Biochem Biophys Res Commun 120:500-504.
2. Tsuchida T, Saxton RE, Morton DL, and Irie RF (1987). Gangliosides of human melanoma. J Natl Cancer Inst 78:45-54.
3. Irie RF, and Morton DL (1975). A new membrane antigen on human cultured cells. Proc Am Assoc Cancer Res 16:171.
4. Irie RF, Irie K, Morton DL (1976). A membrane antigen common to human cancer and fetal brain tissues. Cancer Res 36:3510-3517.
5. Irie RF (1980). Oncofetal antigen (OFA): A human tumor-associated fetal antigen immunogenic in man. IN: Serologic Analysis of Human Cancer Antigen. (Ed.) S. Rosenberg, Pub. Academic Press (N.Y.), pp. 493-513, 1980.
6. Jones PC, Sze LL, Liu PI, Morton DL, Irie RF (1981). Prolonged survival for melanoma patients with elevated IgM antibody to oncofetal antigen. J Natl Cancer Inst 66:249-254.
7. Irie RF, Tai T, Morton DL (1985). Antibodies to tumor-associated gangliosides (GM2 and GD2): Potential for suppression of melanoma occurrence. IN "Basic Mechanisms and Clinical Treatment of Tumor Metastasis" M. Torisu and T. Yoshida, (Eds.) Pub., Academic Press: San Diego, pp 371-384.
8. Irie RF, Morton DL (1986). Regression of cutaneous metastatic melanoma by intralesional injection with human monoclonal antibody to ganglioside GD2. Proc Natl Acad Sci USA, 83:8694-8698.
9. Morton DL, Nizze JA, Gupta RK, Famatiga E, Hoon DSB, Irie RF (1987). Active specific immunotherapy of malignant melanoma. IN "Current Status of Cancer Control and Immunobiology" Eds and Pub. J.P. Kim, Kim, J-G. Park, pp.152-161, 1987.
10. Irie RF, Sze LL, Saxton RE, (1982). Human antibody to OFA-I, a tumor antigen, produced in vitro by EBV-transformed human B-lymphoblastoid cell lines. Proc Natl Acad Sci 79:5666-5670.
11. Cahan LD, Irie RF, Singh R, Cassidenti A, Paulson JC (1982). Identification of a human neuroectodermal tumor antigen (OFA-I-2) as ganglioside GD2 Proc Natl Acad Sci 79:7629-7633.
12. Watanabe T, Pukel CS, Takeyama H, Lloyd KO, Shiku H, Li LTC, Travassos LR, Oettigen HF, OLD LJ (1982). Human melanoma antigen AH is an autoantigenic ganglioside related to GD2 J Exp Med 156:1884-1889.

13. Tai T, Cahan LD, Tsuchida T, Saxton RE, Irie RF, Morton DL (1985). Immunogenicity of melanoma-associated gangliosides in cancer patients. Int J Cancer 35:607-612.
14. Tai T, Paulson JC, Cahan LD, Irie RF (1983). Ganglioside GM2 as a human tumor antigen (OFA-I-1) Proc Natl Acad Sci 80:5392-5396.
15. Livingston PO, Natoli EJ, Calves MJ, Stockert E, Oettgen HF, and Old LJ (1987). Vaccines containing purified GM2 ganglioside elicit GM2 antibodies in melanoma patients. Proc Natl Acad Sci USA 84:2911-2915.
16. Ando I, Hoon DSB, Pattengale PK, Golub SH, Irie RF (1987) Ganglioside GM2 as a target structure recognized by human natural killer cells. J Clin Lab Analysis 1:209-213.
17. Ando I, Hoon DSB, Suzuki Y, Saxton RE, Golub SH, Irie RF (1987). Ganglioside GM2 on the K562 cell line is recognized as a target structure by human natural killer cells. Int J Cancer 40:12-17.
18. Moy PM, Golub SH, Calkins E, Morton DL (1985). Effect of intralymphatic immunotherapy on natural killer activity in malignant melanoma patients. J Surg Oncol 29:112.
19. Ravidranath MH, Paulson JC, Irie RF (1988). Human melanoma antigen O-acetylated ganglioside GD3 is recognized by Cancer antennarius lectin. J Biol Chem 263:2079-2086.
20. Cherish DA, Varki AP, Varki NM, Stallcup WB, Levine J, and Reisfeld RA (1984). A monoclonal antibody recognizes an O-acetyl sialic acid in a human melanoma-associated ganglioside. J Biol Chem 259:7453-7459.
21. Thurin J, Herlyn M, Hindsgaul O, Stromberg N, Karlsson K-A, Elder D, Steplewski Z, Koprowski H (1985). Proton NMR and fast-atom bombardment mass spectrometry analysis of the melanoma-associated ganglioside 9-O-acetyl GD3. J Biol Chem. 260:14556-14563.
22. Nakarai H, Saida T, Shibata Y, Irie RF, Kano K (1987). Expression of heterophile, Paul-Bunnell and Hanganutziu-Deicher antigens on human melanoma cell lines. Int Archs Allergy Appl Immun 83:160-166.
23. Hirabayashi Y, Higashi H, Kato S, Taniguchi M, and Matsumoto M (1987). Occurrence of tumor-associated ganglioside antigens with Hanganutziu-Deicher antigenic activity on human melanomas. Jpn J Cancer Res 78:614-620.

24. Houghton AN, Mintzer D, Cordon-Cardo C, Welt S, Fliegel B, Vadhan S, Carswell E, Melamed MR, Oettgen HF, Old LJ (1985). Mouse monoclonal IgG3 antibody detecting GD3 ganglioside: A phase I trial in patients with malignant melanoma. Proc Natl Acad Sci USA 82:1242-1246.
25. Cheung NV, Lazarus H, Miraldi FD, Abramowsky CR, Kallick S, Saarinen UM, Spitzer T, Strandjord SE, Coccia PF, Berger NA (1987). Ganglioside GD2 specific monoclonal antibody 3F8: A phase I study in patients with neuroblastoma and malignant melanoma. J Clin Oncol 5:1430-1440.
26. Yamaguchi H, Furukawa K, Fortunato SR, Livingston PO, Lloyd KO, Oettgen HR, Old LJ (1987). Cell surface antigens of melanoma recognized by human monoclonal antibodies. Proc Natl Acad Sci USA 84:2416-2420.
27. Katano M, Saxton RE, Irie RF (1984). Human monoclonal antibody to tumor-associated ganglioside GD2. J Clin Lab Immunol 15:119-126.
28. Katano M, Jien M, Irie RF (1984). Human monoclonal antibody to GD2 inhibited human melanoma xenograft. Eur J Cancer Clinic Oncol 20:1053-1059, 1984.
29. Katano M, Irie RF (1984). Suppresed growth of human melanoma in nude mice by human monoclonal antibody to ganglioside GD2. Immunology Letters, 8:169-174.

Human Tumor Antigens and Specific Tumor Therapy, pages 127–136
© **1989 Alan R. Liss, Inc.**

IDENTIFICATION AND CHARACTERIZATION OF A HUMAN COLON TUMOR-ASSOCIATED ANTIGEN, CTAA 16-88, RECOGNIZED BY A HUMAN MONOCLONAL ANTIBODY

Nicholas Pomato, James H. Murray, Ebo Bos[1], Martin V. Haspel, Richard P. McCabe, and Michael G. Hanna, Jr.

Bionetics Research Institute/Organon Teknika 1330-A Piccard Drive, Rockville, Maryland 20850. and [1]Organon International B.V., 5340 BH, Oss, The Netherlands

ABSTRACT   A colon tumor-associated antigen, CTAA 16-88, was identified with the human monoclonal antibody MCA 16-88. Based on immunochemical reactivity, the antigen is related to intermediate filament proteins and shares epitopes with cytokeratins 8, 18, and 19. Based on solubility and molecular size differences, the antigen appears to represent altered forms of these cytokeratins. MCA 16-88 can differentiate between colon tumor and normal tissue by immunohistochemical analysis and selective localization in clinical colon metastasis. This indicates that there are quantitative or qualitative differences in the expression of CTAA 16-88. The differences may be related to transcriptional or posttranslational events associated with neoplastic transformation.

INTRODUCTION

Based on the assumption that there is a differential expression of antigens on tumor versus normal cells, methods for the control of cancer have been explored (1). Even if these antigens are present in human tumor cells, the question arises as to the capability of these antigens to elicit immune responses in patients causing the abrogation in development of tumor metastases. Although the immunogenicity of experimentally induced tumors in animal models is well documented, the relevance of these systems to spontaneous human tumors is still uncertain (2). We have developed methods for the identification and characterization of potentially immunogenic tumor-associated antigens by using human monoclonal antibodies (3). These antibodies were generated from the peripheral blood lymphocytes of colorectal cancer patients who have been immunized with autologous cells (4). Two of the human monoclonal antibodies, MCA 16-88 and MCA 28A32, when radiolabeled, have been found to localize in human colorectal cancer xenografts in nude mice in (5,6) and in metastatic colorectal cancer lesions in patients (7,8).

This report summarizes the data on the biochemical isolation and preliminary characterization of the antigen, CTAA 16-88, recognized by MCA 16-88.

RESULTS

Distribution of CTAA 16-88 as Determined by Immunohistochemical Analysis.

Distribution of CTAA 16-88 in human colon tumor tissue and normal tissue as well as its expression in human colon tumor cell lines was determined by indirect and direct immuno-histochemical techniques (3,5). Indirect analysis with MCA 16-88 showed reactivity with nine of 13 patients' formalin-fixed colon tumor tissue but no reactivity with paired autologous normal colon tissue. The antibody also reacted with enzymatically dissociated, unfixed preparations of colon carcinoma cells from 6 of 9 patients and 7 colon tumor cell lines.

Direct staining of frozen tumor tissues with biotinylated MCA 16-88, demonstrated significant reactivity with colon tumor. Reactivity with normal tissues was quantatively less than that seen with colon tumor and was confined to tissues of epithelial origin (5). The minimal normal tissue reactivity seen on tissue sections in vitro was not observed on the patients in the

clinical studies (8) where no cross-reactivity
with normal tissues was observed by radioimmuno-
scintigraphy.

Purification of CTAA 16-88.

    HT-29 human colon adenocarcinoma cells were
extracted in a buffer containing NP-40 and the
antigen was precipitated with 20% ammonium
sulfate. The redissolved antigen was subjected
to size-exclusion high performance liquid
chromatography (HPLC) using a TSK-4000SW column.
The presence of antigen was monitored by EIA
using MCA 16-88. The antigen chromatographed as
a 900 Kda molecular weight (MW) polypeptide. All
fractions containing CTAA 16-88 were pooled and
applied directly to a thiopropyl sepharose
column, washed with a high salt containing
buffer, and eluted with 10 mM dithiothreitol.
The purification is summarized in Table 1.

Purity and Molecular Size Characteristics of CTAA
16-88.

    The purity of the antigen was determined by
anion exchange HPLC, size exclusion HPLC, native
polyacrylamide gel electrophoresis (PAGE), and
agarose isoelectric focusing (IEF). Both of the
analytical HPLC procedures resulted in a single
protein peak comprising greater than 95% of the
eluted protein. The native (non-denaturing)
gradient PAGE and the IEF gave a single, diffuse
protein band after staining with Coomassie
brilliant blue with an isoelectric point of
approximately $5.5 \pm .5$ and a molecular weight of
about 140 Kda. The discrepancy in size observed
between PAGE and size exclusion chromatography
could be due to aggregation during the
chromatographic step. However, minimizing these
interactions using size exclusion chromatography
in the presence of 9 M urea or in the presence of
buffers containing high salt concentrations
resulted in no change in the molecular weight of
CTAA 16-88. Sucrose density gradient analysis of
the antigen gave a sedimentation coefficient of
approximately 4.5S, indicative of a low density
molecule.

TABLE 1

PURIFICATION OF CTAA 16-88

Purification Step	Activity[a] (units/ml)	Protein[b] (mg/ml)	Volume (ml)	Specific[c] Activity	Yield (%)
Crude Extract	141	2.73	52	52	100
20% Ammonium Sulfate	446	1.34	12	333	73
TSK-4000 SW	412	0.14	8.0	2943	45
Thiopropyl Sepharose	1170	0.29	2.4	4034	38

[a]Determined by EIA. Represents total optical density units at A$_{450}$ at the indicated protein concentration.
[b]Determined by the method of Lowry et al. (9).
[c]Units/mg protein.

The apparent high molecular weight of this antigen of 900 Kda as determined by size exclusion chromatography, the lower molecular weight of 140 Kda determined by native PAGE, and the low density obtained by sucrose density gradient centrifugation indicates that this protein exists as a linear molecule in aqueous solution.

Under denaturing conditions, using SDS-PAGE, the antigen appears as a series of closely-migrating polypeptide chains in the molecular weight range of 43 to 35 Kda. The proteins in this complex, separated by SDS-PAGE and electroeluted, were found to be individually immunoreactive to MCA 16-88. The biochemical characteristics of this molecule are summarized in Table 2.

TABLE 2
PHYSICOCHEMICAL CHARACTERISTICS OF CTAA 16-88

Procedure	M.W.	$S_{20,w} \times 10^{13}$	pI
Size Exclusion HPLC	900 Kda	-	-
Native PAGE	100-140 Kda	-	-
Sucrose Density	-	4.5	-
SDS-PAGE	35-43 Kda	-	-
IEF	-	-	$5.5 \pm .5$

The Relationship of CTAA 16-88 to Intermediate Filament Proteins.

MCA 16-88 was tested for immunoreactivity to a series of intermediate filament proteins using EIA. Confirmation was performed using Western blot analysis. The antibody reacted with both cytokeratin 8 and desmin. It was less reactive with cytokeratin 18 and unreactive with vimentin. It can be concluded that the epitope recognized by MCA 16-88 can be found on certain intermediate filament proteins although reactivity of MCA 16-88 with cytokeratins 8, 18, and desmin was much less than with the cognate antigen CTAA 16-88 (Table 3).

Using CTAA 16-88 as the antigen, a panel of antibodies directed to the intermediate filament proteins, cytokeratins 8, 10-11, 13, 18, and 19,

TABLE 3

RELATIONSHIP OF CTAA 16-88 TO INTERMEDIATE FILAMENT PROTEINS

Monoclonal Antibody	Antigen				
	CTAA 16-88	Cyto 8	Cyto 18	Desmin	Vimentin
MCA 16-88	50[a]	2.0	0.25	4.0	-[b]
Anti-Cyto 8	8	0.13	-	-	-
Anti-Cyto 10, 11	-	-	-	-	-
Anti-Cyto 13	-	-	-	-	-
Anti-Cyto 18	50	-	1.25	-	-
Anti-Cyto 19	50	-	-	-	-
Anti-Desmin	-	-	-	200	-
Anti-Vimentin	-	-	-	-	200
Anti-GFAP	-	-	-	-	-

[a]Results are expressed as total A_{450} units obtained at an antibody concentration of 1.0 ug/ml.

as well as vimentin, desmin and glial fibrillary
acidic protein (GFAP) were analyzed by EIA. The
murine monoclonal antibodies specific for cytokeratins 8, 18 and 19 were found to be immunoreactive with CTAA 16-88. Interestingly,
antibodies to cytokeratins 8 and 18 were more
immunoreactive with CTAA 16-88 than they were to
cytokeratin 8 or 18, respectively (Table 3).
These results indicate that CTAA 16-88 share
epitopes with cytokeratins 8, 18 and 19.

DISCUSSION

The results presented in this paper provide
evidence for the existence of a colon tumor-
associated antigen, designated CTAA 16-88, which
is recognized by the a human colon tumor reactive
monoclonal antibody, MCA 16-88. Based on
biochemical and immunological evidence, this
antigen is related to intermediate filament
proteins but seems to represent altered forms of
these proteins. The aqueous solubility of this
protein as well as its lower molecular weight
range (35-43 Kda) under denaturing conditions
indicate that this protein complex is not related
to native cytokeratins which are insoluble in
aqueous solution and have lower molecular
weights. N-terminal protein sequence analysis of
CTAA 16-88 indicates that although this protein
has homology with various intermediate filament
proteins, especially the cytokeratins, this
homology is low enough (< 65%) to demonstrate
that at least some of the polypeptides in the
CTAA 16-88 complex are not derived directly from
native cytokeratin but represent altered forms
related to these cytokeratins.
The immunological characterization of CTAA
16-88 with a panel of monoclonal antibodies
specific for various intermediate filament
proteins indicate that this antigen represents a
complex of closely related polypeptides sharing
some of the same epitopes with cytokeratins 8, 18
and 19. The biochemical properties of this
antigen relative to the native cytokeratins,
which include differences in solubility
properties, lack of correlation of molecular
weights, and lack of absolute amino acid sequence
homology, indicate that CTAA 16-88 represents a

complex of polypeptides which are altered forms
related to these proteins.

It has previously been demonstrated that
certain intermediate filament proteins are
susceptible to proteolytic degradation which
result in smaller yet discrete proteins (10,11).
In addition, it has been shown that there are
increases in proteolytic activity which
accompanies neoplastic transformation (12).
Altered forms of cytokeratins 18 and 19 have been
described from other tumor cells (13) and may be
related to changes in the biological profile of
the tumor.

The purification and characterization of
CTAA 16-88 is a significant step in identifying
relevant human tumor antigens with potential
application in the immunological management of
various types of carcinoma. Successful treatment
of colon cancer using active-specific
immunotherapy has been described (4). By
definition, monoclonal antibodies obtained from
the lymphocytes of these actively immunized
patients recognize epitopes immunogenic in man
and those antibodies with specificity for cancer
cells may recognize true human tumor antigens.
Using one of these antibodies, MCA 16-88, a
tumor-associated antigen, immunogenic in cancer
patients, has been identified. Because this
antigen has been found to be present in the sera
of colon cancer patients, as well as in primary
and secondary tumor tissue, it has potential use
for in vitro diagnostic and prognostic
applications and in vivo applications in cancer
detection and therapy. CTAA 16-88 is also being
tested, both in vivo and in vitro, for its
ability to elicit cellular immune responses to
determine whether this antigen will have
therapeutic value either alone or as a supplement
to the autologous tumor cells used in active
specific immunotherapy.

REFERENCES

1. Hewitt, HB (1982). Animal tumor models and
their relevance to human tumor immunology. J
Biol Resp Modif 1:107.

2. Herberman, RB (1983).   Counterpoint: Animal
tumor models and their relevance to human
tumor immunology.   J Biol Resp Modif 2:39.
3. Haspel, MV, McCabe, RP, Pomato, N, Janesch,
NJ, Knowlton, JV, Peters, LC, Hoover, HC, Jr,
and Hanna, MG, Jr (1985). Generation of
tumor cell-reactive human monoclonal
antibodies using peripheral blood lymphocytes
from actively immunized colorectal carcinoma
patients. Cancer Res 45:3951.
4. Hoover, HC, Jr, Surdyke, MG, Dangel, RB,
Peters LC, and Hanna M.G Jr (1985).
Prospectively randomized trial of adjuvant
active specific immunotherapy for human
colorectal cancer. Cancer 55:1236.
5. McCabe, RP, Peters, LC, Haspel, MV, Pomato,
N, Carrasquillo, JA, and Hanna, MG, Jr
(1988). Development and characterization of
human monoclonal antibodies and their
application in the radioimmunodetection of
colon carcinoma. In Srivastava. S (ed):
"Radiolabeled Monoclonal Antibodies for
Imaging and Therapy, New York": Plenum
Press.
6. McCabe, R.P, Peters, LC, Haspel, MV, Pomato,
N, Carrasquillo, JA, and Hanna, MG Jr (In
Press).   Preclinical pharmacokinetic and
tumor localization studies with human
monoclonal antibodies to colorectal cancer.
Cancer Res.
7. Del Vecchio, S, Carrasquillo, JA, Steis, R,
Bookman, M, Smith, J, Reynolds, J,
Perentesis, P, McCabe, R, Hanna, MG, Jr
Haspel, M, Longo, D, and Larson, SM (1987).
Imaging of colon cancer with I-131 human
monoclonal antibody. J Nucl Med 28:333.
8. Carrasquillo, JA, Steis, RG, Mccabe, R,
Reynolds, JC, Bookman, M, Del Vecchio, S,
Smith, JW, Perentesis, P, Daily, V, Paris, E,
Rotman, M, Hanna, MG, Jr, Haspel, MV, Longo,
D, and Larson, SM (1988). Imaging of colon
cancer with I-131 16-88 human monoclonal
antibody. J Nucl Med 29:833.
9. Lowry, OH, Rosenbrough, NJ, Farr, AL, and
Randall, RJ (1951). Protein measurement with
folin phenol reagent. J Biol Chem 193:265.

10. Pruss, RM, Mirsky, R, and Raff, M (1981).
    All classes of intermediate filaments share a
    common antigenic determinant defined by a
    monoclonal antibody. Cell 7:419.
11. Schiller, DL and Franke, WW (1983). Limited
    proteolysis of cytokeratin A by an endogenous
    protease: Removal of positively changed
    terminal sequences. Cell Biol Int Reports
    7:3.
12. Lioth, LA (1976). Mechanisms of cancer
    invasion and metastasis. In VT DeVita, Jr, F
    Hellman, and SR Rosenberg (eds): "Important
    Advances in Oncology, pp 29-41": New York:
    JP Lippincott.
13. Chan, R, Rossitto, PV, Edwards, BF, and
    Cardiff, RD (1986). Presence of
    proteolytically processed keratins in the
    culture medium of MCF-7 cells. Cancer Res
    46:6353.

Human Tumor Antigens and Specific Tumor Therapy, pages 137–146
© 1989 Alan R. Liss, Inc.

BIOCHEMICAL ANALYSIS OF A NOVEL MELANOMA CELL SURFACE ANTIGEN DEFINED BY A HUMAN MONOCLONAL ANTIBODY [1]

Dirk Schadendorf[2], Hiroshi Yamaguchi, Lloyd J. Old, and Pramod K. Srivastava [3,4]

Memorial Sloan-Kettering Cancer Center
New York , New York 10021

ABSTRACT Human monoclonal antibodies have identified glycolipid and glycoprotein antigens on the surface of human melanoma cells. One such antigen, identifed by a monoclonal antibody hmAb DSM1 derived from lymphocytes of a melanoma patient immunized with autologous and allogeneic melanoma cells, is expressed on a range of cultured tumor cell lines, including those of neuroecto-dermal and urothelial orgin. This antigen has been purified by lectin affinity, ion exchange and Mono P FPLC chromatography. Detergent solubilization studies indicate existence of water soluble, detergent soluble and detergent insoluble forms of antigen. Western blots of antigen extracts show size heterogeneity in membrane (60 – 65Kd) and cytosolic forms (52 – 62Kd) of antigen. The structural basis of this heterogeneity is presently unclear. Sequences of tryptic peptides generated from gp60 do not bear significant homology with any known protein. Current evidence also raises the possibility that this antigen is an alloantigen. This communication reports the first instance of purification of a cell surface glycoprotein defined by a human monoclonal antibody.

[1] This work was supported by the National Cancer Institute grant CA-08748, and the Oliver S. & Jennie R. Donaldson Charitable Trust, Inc.
[2] D.S. is the recipient of Deutsche Forschungsgemeinschaft fellowship (Scha 1-1-).
[3] P.K.S. is a recipient of the First Independent Research Support and Transition Award of the NIH (CA-44786).
[4] To whom correspondence should be addressed.

INTRODUCTION

The central premise of cancer immunology is the belief
that malignant transformation is associated with
immunologically detectable changes in cell phenotype (1).
Individually distinct transplantation antigens of chemically
induced mouse sarcomas provided early evidence for this
idea. The antigens responsible for the specific
immunogenicity of these tumors are being isolated and
characterized (2). Over the past several years, this
laboratory has been analyzing the humoral immune response to
human cancer by autologous and allogeneic typing. This
involves testing of patients` sera and more recently,
monoclonal antibodies generated from lymphocytes of cancer
patients,on cultured tumor cells and normal tissues. Several
immunogenic cell surface antigens have been identified with
this technique (3 - 9) and have been classified as class 1
(restricted to autologous tumors), class 2 (present on autologous and some allogeneic tumor cells) and class 3 (widely
distributed) antigens (1). The present report describes the
biochemical characterization of a class 3 cell surface
antigen, expressed widely on human melanomas (10).

METHODS

Cell lines and human monoclonal antibodies were
described earlier (10). Serological techniques for the
detection of cell surface antigens have been reported
previously (4 - 7). Sodium dodecyl sulfate polyacrylamide
gel electrophoresis (SDS-PAGE) was performed according to
Laemmli (11) and gels were silver stained by the method of
Oakley et al. (11a). Protein blotting was carried out by the
method of Tobwin et al.(12). Chromatographic procedures were
performed according to manufacturer`s instructions.

RESULTS

The monoclonal antibody DSM1 was derived from a cancer
patient`s EBV-transformed peripheral blood lymphocytes fused
with mouse myeloma NS-1. The antigen defined by DSM1 is
expressed on several tumor types including those of neuroectodermal (11/14 melanomas, 6/8 astrocytomas) and urological
origin as determined by Protein A - rosetting assays(Table 1).

TABLE 1
DISTRIBUTION OF THE ANTIGEN DEFINED BY HUMAN MONOCLONAL
ANTIBODY DSM1 ON TUMORS AND NORMAL CELLS

Cells	Titer
MELANOMAS	
SK-MEL-28, -29, MeWo	40,000
SK-MEL-13, -130, -173	10,000
SK-MEL-31, -61, -177, -189	2,560
SK-MEL-93	640
SK-MEL-23, -37, -94	0
ASTROCYTOMAS	
SK-MG-3, -11	10,000
U-251-MG	6,400
SK-MG-4	2,560
SK-MG-1, -14	640
SK-MG-21, -23	0
NEUROBLASTOMAS	
SK-NMC	40,000
SK-NSH, IMR-32	0
LEUKEMIAS	
HL-60	2,560
K-562, NALL-1, NALM-1	0
CCRF-HSB-2, CCRF-CEM	0
T-45, DAUDI, SK-LY-16	0
RENAL CANCERS	
SK-RC-7, -9	40,000
SK-RC-54	10,000
SK-RC-6	2,560
SK-RC-45, -48	0
BLADDER CANCERS	
235-J	40,000
T-24	10,000
5637, Scaber	0
LUNG CANCERS	
SK-LC-8	40,000
SK-LC-6, -7, -12	0
BREAST CANCERS (n=4)	0
COLON CANCERS (n=4)	0
other epithelial CANCERS (n=4)	0
NORMAL TISSUES	
EBV-transformed B-cells (n=3)	0
(including patient's own B-cells)	
Erythrocytes (A,B,AB,O)	0
PBL (n=4)	0
melanocytes (n=3)	0 or 2,560
fibroblasts (n=3)	0 or 5,000
normal kidney epithelium (n=3)	0 or 40,000

Biochemical identification of the antigen defined by
DSM1 was achieved using western blotting. Sub-cellular
fractions of SK-MEL-13 were blotted and probed with antibody
DSM1. The pattern of polypeptide binding to the monoclonal
antibody was complex. Distinctive polypeptides of
approximatly 60,000 d were detected in cytosolic and crude
membrane preparations (Figure 1). For this reason, we refer
to this antigen as gp60.

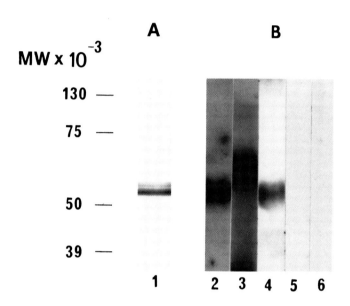

FIGURE 1.   Biochemical identification of the antigen
defined by human monoclonal antibody DSM1. Panel A: SDS-PAGE
of purified antigen from cytosol after Mono P FPLC chromatofocussing (Fig. 2C), followed by silver staining (lane 1).
Panel B: Western blot analysis of SK-MEl-13 cytosol (lane
2), detergent soluble membrane preparation (lane 3) and
detergent-insoluble matrix (lane 4) under non-reducing
conditions and cytosol under reducing condition (lane 6)
probed with DSM1; Western blot of SK-MEL-13 cytosol under
non-reducing condition probed with unrelated human
monoclonal antibody Ri37 (lane 5).

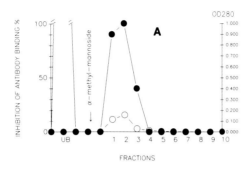

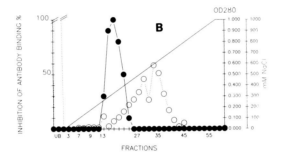

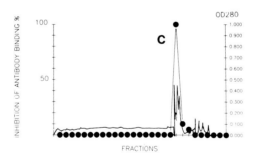

FIGURE 2.   Purification of gp60 from cytosol from SK-MEL-13 cells by sequential (A) Con A - Sepharose chromatography, (B) Q - Sepharose chromatography and (C) Mono P FPLC chromatofocussing. Solid circles represent gp60 activity and hollow circles (in A and B) and continuous line (in C) represent protein profile.

Purification of the gp60 antigen was initiated from cell line SK-MEL-13. Inhibition of rosetting of DSM1 on live SK-MEL-13 cells or inhibition of antibody binding on fixed SK-MEL-13 cells in a radioimmunoassay were used to assay the antigen. Figure 2 shows the results of purification of gp60 from SK-MEL-13 cytosol by sequential application of lectin affinity, ion exchange and Mono P FPLC chromatography. The purified antigen has a molecular weight of approximatly 60,000 d judged by SDS-PAGE (Figure 1, lane 1). This is consistent with the molecular size of the antigen as detected by western blotting .

DISCUSSION

The gp60 antigen can be isolated from membranes as well as cytosol of melanoma cells. Properties of the membrane and the soluble antigen suggest considerable heteromorphism: the cytosolic antigen is water soluble , while the membrane antigen requires the presence of detergent for solubility. Yet another form of gp60 remains with the detergent insoluble matrix. A similar multi-compartment distribution of other proteins has been desribed previously (13 - 15).

There is considerable heterogeneity in the molecular weight of this antigen within a sub-cellular compartment. The cytosolic and the detergent insoluble forms occur in the 52 - 62 Kd range and the detergent soluble form in the 60 - 64 Kd range. A significant portion of this heterogeneity may be due to differences in carbohydrate moieties on the protein, but its precise structural basis is presently unclear.

The gp60 antigen is distinct from other purified human melanoma antigens reported previously on the basis of molecular weight and other properties (Table 2). Also, sequences of tryptic peptides generated from gp60 do not bear significant homology with any known protein (D.S., L.J.O. & P.K.S. unpublished observation). These observations suggest that we have identified and biochemically characterized a novel melanoma cell surface antigen.

The gp60 antigen, as defined by DSM1, is present on the allogeneic melanoma cells used for vaccination as well as other allogeneic melanoma cells, but not on autologous melanoma cells. This observation raises the possibility that it is an alloantigen. Resolution of this question will require generation of molecular and polyclonal (as opposite to monoclonal) serological probes for gp60.

TABLE 2

COMPARISON OF GP60 WITH OTHER PURIFIED MELANOMA ASSOCIATED ANTIGENS

Name	Nature	Molecular weight	pI	Localization	Distribution	Immunogenicity in humans	Reference
gp60	glycoprotein	60 kd	4.4	cell surface	11/14 melanomas; 12/16 neurological and urological cancer; 2/28 leukemia and epithelial cancer	Yes	present report
FD	glycoprotein	90 kd	5.5	cell surface	unique	yes	8
gp90	glycoprotein	90 kd	5.5	cell surface	abundant on most melanomas and sarcomas; poorly ex-pressed on most normal tissues	yes	16
M-TAA	lipoprotein	180/190 kd	6.4	cell surface	most melanomas and small percentage of other tumors	yes	17
MAA	glycoprotein	75 kd	n.d.[a]	cell surface	most melanomas; poor or nc expression on other tumors	yes	18
Melanotrans-ferrin	glycoprotein	97 kd	5.0	cell surface	widely expressed on tumors; rarely on normal tissues	n.d.[a]	19 – 22
gp94	glycoprotein	94 kd	n.d.[a]	n.d.[a]	6/6 melanomas; 0/7 other tumors	n.d.[a]	23 , 24
gp240	glycoprotein	240 kd	n.d.[a]	n.d.[a]	6/6 melanomas; 4/7 other tumors	n.d.[a]	
gp15	glycoprotein	15 kd	3.5	cell surface	19/27 melanomas; 1/9 other tumors	yes	25

[a] n.d. - not determined

REFERENCES

1. Old LJ (1981) Cancer Immunology : The search for specificity . Cancer Res 41: 361 - 375.
2. Srivastava PK, Old LJ (1988) Individually distinct transplantation antigens of chemically induced mouse tumors. Immunology Today 9: 78 - 83.
3. Carey TE, Lloyd KO, Takahashi T, Travorros LR, Old LJ (1976) AU—Cell surface antigen of human malignant melanoma. Proc Natl Acad Sci USA 76: 2898 - 2902.
4. Shiku H,Takahashi T, Oettgen HF, Old LJ (1976) Serological typing with immune adherence assays and definition of two new surface antigens. J Exp Med 144: 873 - 881.
5. Shiku H, Takahashi T, Resnick LA, Oettgen HF, Old LJ (1977) Cell surface antigens of human malignant melanoma. J Exp Med 145: 784 - 789.
6. Carey TE, Takahashi T, Resnick LA, Oettgen HF, Old LJ (1976) Cell surface antigens in malignant melanoma . Proc Natl Acad Sci USA 73: 3278 - 3282.
7. Pfreundschuh M, Shiku H, Takahashi T, Ueda R, Ransohoff J, Oettgen HF, Old LJ (1978) Serological analysis of cell surface antigens of malignant human brain tumors. Proc Natl Acad Sci USA 75: 5122 - 5126.
8. Real FX, Mattes MJ, Houghton AN, Oettgen HF, Old LJ (1984) Class 1 (unique) tumor antigen of human melanoma J Exp Med 160: 1219 - 1233.
9. Irie RF, Irike K, Morton DL (1976) A membrane antigen common to human cancer and fetal brain. Cancer Res 36: 3510 - 3517.
10. Yamaguchi H, Furukawa K, Fortunato SR, Livingston PO, Lloyd KO, Oettgen HF, Old LJ (1987) Cell surface antigens of melanoma recognized by human monoclonal antibodies. Proc Natl Acad Sci USA 84: 2416 - 2420.
11. Laemmli UK (1970) Cleavage of structural proteins during the assembly of the head of bacteriophage T4 Nature 227: 417 - 422.
11a.Oakley BR, Kirsch DR, Morris NR (1980) A simplified ultrasensitive silver stain for detecting proteins. Anal Biochem 105: 361 - 363.
12. Tobwin H, Staehelin T, Gordon J (1979) Electophoretic transfer of proteins from polyacylamide gels to nitrocellulose sheets.Proc Natl Acad Sci USA 76: 4350-4354.
13. Flanagan J,Koch GLE (1970) Cross-linked surface immunoglobulin attaches to actin. Nature 273: 278 - 281.

14. Mescher MF, Jose MJL, Balk SP (1981) Actin-containing matrix associated with the plasma membrane of murine tumor and lymphoid cells. Nature 289: 139 - 144.

15. Shashikant CS, Srivastava PK, Das MR (1983) A DNA polymerase activity with the skeletal framework of the plasma membranes of a rat hepatoma. Biochem Biophys Res Comm 114: 571 - 577.

16. Real FX, Furukawa KS, Mattes JM, Gusik SA, Cordon-Cardo C Oettgen HF, Old LJ, Lloyd KO (1988) Class 1 (unique) tumor antigens of human melanoma : Identification of unique and common epitopes on a Mr 90,000 glycoprotein Proc Natl Acad Sci USA in press

17. Gupta RK, Morton DL (1984) Studies of a melanoma tumor associated antigen detected in the culture medium of a human melanoma cell line by allogeneic antibody JNCI 72: 67 - 92.

18. Heaney-Kieras J, Bystryn JC (1982) Identification and purification of a Mr75,000 cell surface human melanoma-associated antigen . Cancer Res. 42: 2310 - 2316.

19. Woodbury RG, Brown JP, Yeh MY, Hellstrom I, Hellstrom KE (1980) Identification of a cell surface protein, p97,in human melanomas and certain other neoplasmas Proc Natl Acad Sci USA 77: 2183 - 2187.

20. Brown JP, Wright PW, Hart CE, Woodbury RG, Hellstrom KE, Hellstrom I (1980) Protein antigens of normal and malignant human cells identified by immunoprecipitation with monoclonal antibodies. J Biol Chem 255: 4980-4983.

21. Dippold WG , Lloyd KO, Li T, Ikeda H, Oettgen HF, Old LJ (1980) Cell surface antigens of human malignant melanoma: Definition of six antigenic systems with mouse monolonal antibodies. Proc Natl Acad Sci USA 77: 6114 - 6118.

22. Rose TM, Plowman GD, Teplow DB, Dreyer WJ, Hellstrom KE, Brown JP(1986) Primary structure of the human melanoma-associated antigen p97 (melanotransferrin) deduced from the mRNA sequence.Proc Natl Acad Sci USA 83:1261 - 1265.

23. Gallaway DR, McCabe RP, Pellegrino MA, Ferone S, Reisfeld RA (1981) Tumor-associated antigen in spent culture medium of human melanoma cells: Immunochemical characterization with xenosera. J Immunol 126: 62 - 66.

24. Reisfeld RA, Gallaway DR, McCabe RP, Morgan AC (1982) Molecular and immunological characterization of human melanoma antigens. In: Reisfeld RA, Ferrone S (eds) "Melanoma antigens and antibodies" New York: Plenum Press, pp 317- 337.

25. Hersey P, Murray E, Werkmeister J, McCarthy WH (1979) Detection of a low molecular weight antigen on melanoma cells by a human antiserum in leukocyte-depedent antibody assay. Br J Cancer 40: 615 - 627.

Human Tumor Antigens and Specific Tumor Therapy, pages 147–156
© 1989 Alan R. Liss, Inc.

PRODUCTION OF HUMAN MONOCLONAL ANTIBODIES BY IN VITRO IMMUNIZATION

Paula Boerner and Ivor Royston

University of California San Diego, Cancer Center, T-011
La Jolla CA. 92093

ABSTRACT At present, no method is available for the
routine production of human monoclonal antibodies
directed against tumor associated antigens. In an
effort to produce human monoclonal antibodies directed against specific antigens on a routine basis, our
laboratory is attempting to develop methods for in
vitro immunization of human lymphocytes. Once developed, these methods may be applied to immunization of
human lymphocytes using purified human tumor associated antigens as well as intact human tumor cells
as immunogens. In our recent work, described below,
horse spleen ferritin was used as a model antigen to
investigate the immune response of human splenocytes
to a high molecular weight, complex protein. Using
an anti-ferritin ELISA as a semi-quantitative measure
of specific anti-ferritin responses by human lymphocytes in culture, we identified conditions which
supported specific IgG as well as IgM anti-ferritin
responses in vitro. Fusion of lymphocytes immunized
under optimized culture conditions allowed production
of human hybridoma cell lines which produced either IgM
or IgG ferritin-reactive antibodies. It is hoped that
application of these conditions, which supported human
anti-ferritin responses, to in vitro immunization with
tumor-associated antigens will lead to development of
tumor antigen reactive human monoclonal antibodies.

INTRODUCTION

Tumor reactive monoclonal antibodies have been generated by immunizing rodents with cells or extracts prepared

from human tumors. Some of the monoclonal antibodies generated by this method have proven useful for research into
the biology of tumor associated antigens (1) and for clinical application, either for tumor imaging or for directed
killing of tumor cells in vivo (2). However, attempts to
produce antibodies reactive with human tumors by xenogeneic
immunization may result in lack of detection of some tumor-
associated antigens because of masking by the many cell
surface molecules recognized as foreign by the non-human
host. The potential immunodominance of normal membrane
antigens such as blood group glycoproteins and histocompatibility antigens may prevent reactivity by the xenogeneic
host to the often subtle structural changes which distinguish a tumor antigen from a normal membrane protein. A
second limitation to the usefulness of monoclonal antibodies
transcribed from non-human genes is that therapy has often
been compromised by a human immune response to the therapeutic agent itself (3).

The need for development of monoclonal antibodies of
human origin for use in therapy and the impossibility of
deliberate immunization of human subjects with most antigens
of interest has led to efforts to immunize human lymphocytes
in vitro. Mishell and Dutton (4) first demonstrated the
feasibility of in vitro immunization in 1967 using murine
lymphocytes. Hoffman et al. (5) successfully applied this
approach to human lymphocytes in 1973 and several groups
have now demonstrated that human monoclonal antibodies reactive with an immunizing antigen can be generated from exposure to antigen in vitro (6-8). However, many of the human
monoclonal antibodies produced from in vitro immunizations
have resulted from a primary exposure to antigen in vivo
followed by a secondary exposure in vitro. Or, if the in
vitro response has been a true primary immunization rather
than a secondary boost in vitro, the majority of antibodies
produced have been of the IgM rather than the IgG isotype.
The goal of our current work is to identify culture conditions which will support a primary immune response to T
cell-dependent antigens followed by development of antigen
specific IgG as well as IgM secreting plasma cells, which
can then be fused to produce the desired hybridoma cell
lines. Conditions which support specific IgG and IgM responses to the immunizing antigen used in these initial
studies, horse spleen ferritin, are described below.

METHODS

Preparation of Human Lymphocytes.

Tissue acquisition and reproducibility of results are two problems often encountered when working with human lymphocytes. Human spleen is the only lymphatic organ which provides sufficient numbers of cells for performing a series of experiments using lymphocytes prepared at one time from one individual. When a spleen became available from an accident victim whose condition necessitated splenectomy, our laboratory received 50-100 grams of tissue through the UCSD Tissue Bank. Small chunks of tissue were diced and forced through a wire mesh screen to form a single cell suspension. RBCs were osmotically lysed and the remaining cells were frozen in liquid nitrogen in aliquots of 50-200 x 10(6) cells/vial. 1-3 vials were thawed in a 37 degree water bath prior to each experiment.

Quantitation of Specific anti-Ferritin Responses.

The number of B lymphocytes which secrete antibody reactive with the immunizing antigen can be quantitated using the ELISA-plaque assay of Sedgwick and Holt (9). Alternatively, a semi-quantitative measure of the specific response can be obtained by assay of ferritin-reactive antibody in the immunization culture supernatants by standard ELISA techniques. The lymphocytes were exposed to 0.1 ug/ml ferritin in a standard medium consisting of RPMI + 10% FCS (fetal calf serum) for 1-5 days. The cells were then washed to remove the ferritin and resuspended in antigen-free medium for 1-5 days to allow secretion of detectable levels of antibody. Culture supernatants were assayed for specific anti-ferritin IgM and IgG class antibodies by ELISA using Immulon 96 well plates coated with 50 ug/ml ferritin. IgG antibodies showed no detectable plastic binding but values for nonspecific binding were subtracted for quantitation of IgM secretion. Because supernatants from non-immunized, control cultures showed significant binding to ferritin coated wells, all reported OD values represent the difference between reactivity of immunized cultures minus the reactivity of control cultures. Therefore, all values shown represent ferritin-dependent antibody production. Each condition was assayed in duplicate or triplicate and the standard deviations depicted in the figures represent the sum of the standard deviations for immunized + control cultures.

RESULTS

Anti-Ferritin Antibody Production by in Vitro Immunization Cultures.

Lymphokines are required for activation and differentiation of resting B cells (10). In vitro immunization cultures usually require supplementation with purified lymphokines or with supernatants produced from allogeneic cultures of lymphocytes obtained from 2-4 individuals (11). These supernatants are likely to contain all the known as well as possible yet unknown factors necessary for plasma cell development. Since allogeneic stimulation is known to induce lymphokine secretion, we attempted to immunize allogeneic cultures, consisting of lymphocytes obtained from 2 individual spleens, without addition of exogenous lymphokine preparations. Ferritin-specific responses were compared for splenocytes from spleen A, spleen D, and cells from spleens A + D mixed in a 1:1 ratio (Fig. 1). Responses were compared at 2 cell densities, 1.5 and 3.0 x 10 (6) cells/ml, in the presence or absence of additional factors as shown. A small ferritin specific IgM signal was induced in spleen A. This response was enhanced in the presence of the adjuvant, muramyl dipeptide (MDP). No IgG signal was observed with this spleen under any conditions tested. Spleen D exhibited a barely detectable ferritin-specific IgG signal when immunization occurred in the presence of either 2-mercaptoethanol (BME) or MDP. No ferritin-specific IgM signal was

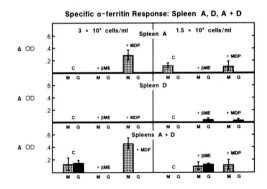

FIGURE 1. Comparison of anti-ferritin IgM (M) and IgG (G) responses by syngeneic and allogeneic cultures of human splenocytes.

observed with this spleen. Co-cultures of cells from spleens
A + D at 3 x 10(6) cells/ml gave both IgG and IgM responses.
The IgM response was usually best observed at the higher
cell density except in the presence of BME, which, in this
experiment, shifted the response from the higher to the
lower cell density. The IgM response was again enhanced by
MDP but not by BME or by pokeweed mitogen (PWM). In contrast, the ferritin-specific IgG signal was most often observed at the lower cell density, especially in the presence
of added factors.

The data shown in Figure 2 represent a second experiment using cells of spleens A + D co-cultured at a 1:1
ratio. IgG and IgM responses were compared at cell densities of 1.5 and 3.0 x 10(6) cells/ml in the presence or
absence of PWM, BME, MDP, and a mixed lymphocyte culture
supernatant (MLR) prepared from a 72 hour co-culture of
cells from 4 spleens. It was again observed that the IgM
responses were most evident at the higher cell density,
whereas the IgG responses occurred most often at the lower
density. At 3 x 10(6) cells/ml, the IgM and IgG responses
were relatively high and of similar magnitude. Addition of
MDP again enhanced the IgM response but none of the other
additions provided significant improvement over the non-
supplemented cultures. Addition of more than one factor at
the higher cell density usually eliminated the IgG response.
Addition of any combination of more than 2 factors suppressed all responses (data not shown). At a density of
1.5 x 10(6) cells/ml, the IgM and IgG responses were not

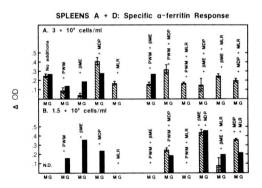

FIGURE 2. Comparison of anti-ferritin IgG (G) and IgM
(M) responses by allogeneic cultures at (A) 3 x 10(6)
cells/ml and (B) 1.5 x 10(6) cells/ml.

significant (see Fig. 1). Supplementation with additional
factors, especially MDP and BME, substantially aided the IgG
response, whereas few combinations of factors significantly
enhanced the IgM response at the lower cell density. These
data again indicated that, when allogeneic cultures were
supplemented with additional factors, the IgM response was
best observed at higher cell densities, whereas the IgG
response was better supported in lower density cultures.

The magnitude of the specific anti-ferritin response
was compared with the amount of polyclonal stimulation observed for each of the conditions shown in Figure 1. No
correlation was observed between secretion of polyclonal
immunoglobulin (Ig) and level of secretion of specific anti-
ferritin antibody (Table 1). For example, PWM stimulated
IgG and IgM secretion by spleen A more than 5-fold, but no
specific response was observed. A specific anti-ferritin
IgG response was seen with unsupplemented cultures of
spleens A + D. Addition of PWM or MDP to these cultures
stimulated polyclonal IgG secretion 2 to 3-fold, but the
specific response was suppressed.

Five million lymphocytes from spleens A + D were immunized in the absence of added factors with 0.1 ug/ml ferritin. These were fused to the heteromyeloma cell line,
K6H6/B5 (12), according to standard fusion techniques (13).
Fusion frequencies were 40-75 clones/million lymphocytes
fused. Between 2-20 % of the clones produced initially reacted by ELISA with ferritin. The number of ferritin-reactive
clones obtained depended upon time of antigen exposure.
Equivalent numbers of IgG and IgM clones were produced with
the protocol described, but the ratio of specific IgM/IgG
secreting hybridomas was influenced by culture conditions.
Neither IgG nor IgM anti-ferritin antibodies bound significantly to plastic, but preliminary characterization of the
clones obtained from one series of fusions revealed that
approximately 60% of the clones initially identified as
binding to ferritin produced antibody which bound with low
affinity to ferritin unrelated proteins. Non-specific protein binding was not as efficient as ferritin binding in the
ELISA assay, but clones were not considered specific unless
the level of non-ferritin protein binding was less than 20-
30% of the level of ferritin binding. An example of the
protein binding characteristics of a clone characterized as
ferritin-specific is shown in Figure 3. Binding to plates
coated with beta-galactosidase or with cytochrome c reductase was relatively low relative to ferritin binding with
this clone. Cross-reactivity with another iron-binding

TABLE 1
COMPARISON OF SPECIFIC AND TOTAL Ig PRODUCTION
IN HOMOGENEIC AND ALLOGENEIC SPLEEN CULTURES

	Total IgM	IgG (ug/ml)	Anti-ferritin IgM	IgG (ΔOD)
A. Spleen A:				
no additions	1.7±0.1	0.7±0.3	-	-
+ PWM	15.6±2.5	15.2±1.2	-	-
+ BME	1.7±0.1	0.5±0.2	-	-
+ MDP	5.0±1.1	0.8±0.3	.29±0.08	
B. Spleen D:				
no additions	0.2	0.4±0.1	-	-
+ PWM	0.3	2.3±1.0	-	-
+ BME	ND	0.4	-	.05±.02
+ MDP	1.1±0.1	2.9±0.9	-	.04±.02
C. Spleens A+D:				
no additions	8.2±0.4	4.1±1.1	.13±.10	.15±.04
+ PWM	7.5±0.2	12.6±0.6	.13±.08	-
+ BME	7.3±0.8	2.5±0.4	-	-
+ MDP	14.4±0.8	7.1±1.0	.46±.09	-

protein, human transferrin, was also tested. Some ferritin-specific antibodies showed equivalent or greater binding to transferrin than to ferritin (Figure 3), whereas other ferritin-binding antibodies did not significantly crossreact with transferrin (data not shown).

DISCUSSION

Using a semi-quantitative ELISA we have compared numerous conditions for in vitro immunization of human lymphocytes with a high molecular weight, complex, T cell-dependent antigen. We have found human spleen to be an excellent source of lymphocytes for immunization in vitro. Reproducibility was observed from experiment-to-experiment when cells of the same spleens were used. Reproducibility was not observed from one spleen to another (see Figure 1), suggesting that the in vitro immune response can be heavily influenced by the cellular composition of the lymphatic organs from

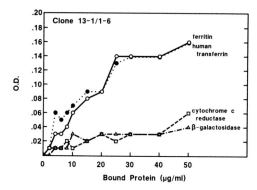

FIGURE 3. Protein binding characterization of anti-
ferritin antibody produced by clone 1/1-6.

which the cells were obtained. It is apparent from the data
presented here and from cell marker analysis of spleen populations (data not presented) that individual spleens differ
significantly in their composition of cell types, which can
influence the immune response. No matter which conditions
were applied to spleen A, a ferritin-specific IgG response
was not observed. With spleen D an IgM response was never
observed and the IgG response was barely detectable. However, when mixtures of cells from spleens A and D were immunized, both responses were observed in the same culture and
were significantly stronger than in cultures of either
spleen alone. Immunization of allogeneic cultures in vitro
may therefore reduce experimental variation as well as boost
specific responses.

Exogenous supplementation with lymphokines has been
reported as necessary for many successful in vitro immunization protocols (11). We conclude from the enhanced specific response observed with mixed cultures that sufficient
lymphokine production can be induced by allogeneic stimulation within the immunization culture without need for additional factors. Indeed, when lymphokines were added in the
form of an MLR or when PWM was added to stimulate production
of lymphokines by T cells, the responses were either not
changed or were reduced. The amount of lymphokine secretion
may be tightly regulated in allogeneic cultures and use of
such cultures for in vitro immunization may avoid possible
suppression due to overexposure.

In vitro immunization cultures of murine lymphocytes
have routinely been supplemented with BME (4) and sometimes

with MDP (14), but these agents have not been widely used with human lymphocytes. Pollock and d'Apice (15) have recently reported successful production of specific IgM but not IgG human monoclonal antibodies from lymphocytes cultured with MDP. Their result corresponds to our observation that MDP primarily enhanced the anti-ferritin IgM response but had little effect on the IgG response. The mechanisms by which MDP and BME influence immune responses are not clear. MDP is the active agent in Freund's adjuvant, but the basis for the apparent specificity observed with this agent for IgM production is unknown.

The many hybridoma clones which secreted broadly reactive antibody may reflect the high ferritin-binding backgrounds observed in our control, non-immunized cultures. These hybrids and this background may arise from resting B cells, which express low affinity surface Ig which has not yet undergone affinity maturation. If so, these cells have not yet been specifically activated by antigen and do not represent the products of true in vitro immunization. Our initial ELISA screens indicated that ferritin-reactive clones were produced at a rate of approximately 2 clones/10(6) lymphocytes fused. However, only 2-4 of every 10 ferritin-reactive clones initially identified were highly ferritin-specific.

Analysis of in vitro immunization cultures and the hybridoma clones produced from fusions of immunized lymphocytes indicate that immunization of allogeneic splenocyte cultures can lead to production of both IgG and IgM human monoclonal antibodies of predetermined specificity at an approximate level of 0.2 clones/10(6) lymphocytes fused.

REFERENCES

1. Lennox ES, Sikora K (1982). Definition of human tumor antigens. In McMichael AJ, Fabre JW (eds): "Monoclonal Antibodies in Clinical Medicine," London: Academic Press.

2. Sikora K, Smedley H, Thorpe P (1984). Tumour imaging and drug targeting. Br. Med. Bull. 40:240.

3. Miller RA, Oseroff AR, Stratte PT, Levy R (1083). Monoclonal antibody therapeutic trials in seven patients with T-cell lymphoma. Blood 62:988.

4. Mishell RI, Dutton RW (1966). Immunization of normal mouse spleen cell suspension in vitro. Science 153:1004.

5. Hoffmann MK, Schmidt D, Oettgen HF (1973). Production of antibody to sheep red blood cells by human tonsil cells in vitro. Nature 243:408.

6. Strike LE, Devens BA, Lundak RL (1978). Production of human-human hybridomas secreting antibody to sheep erythrocytes after in vitro immunization. J. Immunol. 132: 1789.

7. Ho M-K, Rand N, Murray J, Kato K, Rabin H (1985). In vitro immunization of human lymphocytes. I. Production of human monoclonal antibodies against bombesin and tetanus toxoid. J. Immunol. 135:3831.

8. Wasserman RL, Bodens RD, and Thaxton ES (1986). In vitro stimulation prior to fusion generates antigen binding human-human hybridomas. J. Immunol. Methods 93:275.

9. Sedgwick JD, Holt PG (1986). The ELISA-plaque assay for the detection and enumeration of antibody-secreting cells. J. Immunol. Methods 87:37.

10. Jelinek DF, Lipsky PE (1987). Regulation of human B lymphocyte activation, proliferation, and differentiation. Adv. Immunol. 40:1.

11. Reading CL (1982). Theory and methods for immunization in culture and monoclonal antibody production. J. Immunol Methods 53:261.

12. Carroll WL, Thielemans K, Dilley J, Levy R (1986). Mouse X human heterohybridomas as fusion partners with human B cell tumors. J. Immunol. Methods 89:61.

13. Burnett KG, Hayden JN, Hernandaz R, Waldron KM, Oh E (1987). Radiolabeled human antibodies that localize breast cancer in vivo: Selecting antibodies for clinical applications. In Strelkauskas AJ (ed): "Human Hybridomas: Diagnostic and Therapeutic Applications," New York: Marcel Decker, p 253.

14. Leclerc C, Juy D, Chedid L (1979). Inhibitory and stimulatory effects of a synthetic glycopeptide (MDP) on the in vitro PFC response: Factors affecting the response. Cell. Immunol. 42:336.

15. Pollock BJ, d'Apice AJF (1988). Production of human monoclonal antibodies against specific antigens by in vitro immunization. In Borrebaeck CAK (ed): "In Vitro Immunization in Hybridoma Technology," Amsterdam: Elsevier, p 277.

Human Tumor Antigens and Specific Tumor Therapy, pages 157–166
© 1989 Alan R. Liss, Inc.

SPECIFIC RECOGNITION OF HUMAN TUMOR ASSOCIATED

ANTIGENS BY NON-MHC-RESTRICTED CTL[1]

O.J. Finn, D.L. Barnd, L.A. Kerr[2],
M.C. Miceli, and R.S. Metzgar

Department of Microbiology and Immunology
Duke University, Durham, NC 27710

ABSTRACT Cytotoxic T cell lines with specific anti-tumor reactivity but exhibiting no MHC restriction, have been established from lymph node cells of patients with pancreatic adenocarcinoma. They can be propagated continuously on IL-2 and allogeneic pancreatic tumor lines. Unlike natural killer (NK) cells, these tumor specific CTL are CD3 antigen positive and their cytotoxicity is blocked by OKT3 antibody. Their tumoricidal activity is restricted to tumors of the same tissue site. This appears to be due to the expression of a pancreatic adenocarcinoma associated antigen DU-PAN 2 which is able to stimulate the proliferation of these T cells and serve as their target in the absence of MHC restriction.

INTRODUCTION

Recent development of new methods and reagents for maintenance of human lymphoid cells in vitro has raised again the possibility of identifying in tumor bearing hosts cells with

1. Supported by a grant from Cytogen Corp. (OJF), NIH grant 5T32GM07184 (DLB), Stead Fellowship (LAK), and NIH grant PO1-CA-32672 (RSM)
2. Present address: Dept. of Urology, Mayo Clinic, Rochester, MN 55902

antitumor reactivity and expanding their numbers
for study or therapeutic use. Peripheral blood,
although the most accessible source, has proven to
have very low incidence of antitumor reactive
cells. Concentration of effector cells at the
tumor site has been observed to lead to a
corresponding depletion in the periphery.
Expansion of peripheral blood lymphocytes in vitro
in the presence of interleukin-2 (IL-2), has
given rise to cells with broad tumoricidal
activity, lymphokine activated killers (LAK) (1).
In addition, in vitro propagation of a small
number of cytotoxic T cell clones highly specific
for autologous tumors has been reported in melanomas,
sarcomas, and breast carcinomas (2-4). These
malignancies are usually surgically treated and
excised tumors provide an adequate source of both
autologous target cells and tumor infiltrating
lymphocytes (TIL). Some tumor types, however, are
rarely resected and this fact must be acknowledged
when considering the use of TIL as a practical
antitumor immunotherapeutic approach. In such
cases other reservoirs of tumor reactive
lymphocytes must be identified. We were
interested in detecting an immune response to one
such tumor, pancreatic adenocarcinoma, by
analyzing the draining lymph nodes from patients
with this malignancy for the presence of tumor
reactive lymphocytes.

A number of pancreatic adenocarcinoma
associated antigens have been identified by us
and found to be expressed on exocrine pancreatic
tumor sections as well as on in vitro established
pancreatic tumor cell lines. If some of these or
similar tumor associated antigens were stimulating
a population of T cells residing in the draining
lymph nodes, we reasoned that such a population
could be expanded in vitro using our previously
described culture methods (5), IL-2, and
antigenically cross-reactive allogeneic pancreatic
adenocarcinoma cell lines as a continuous
antigenic stimulus. Because of a number of
reports documenting the isolation of rare
cytotoxic T cell clones which killed autologous as
well as allogeneic tumors (2,4), we

designed experiments to search for the presence of pancreatic tumor reactive but non-MHC-restricted T cells in patients with pancreatic adenocarcinoma.

MATERIALS AND METHODS

Cell lines and culture conditions: Lymph nodes draining the pancreatic carcinoma were obtained at the time of exploratory laparotomy. Lymphocytes were sedimented on a ficoll-hypaque discontinuous gradient and plated at 4-6 x 10^5 cells/ml in 24 well plates in RPMI-1640 medium with 10% human serum, 2 mM fresh glutamine, 100 U/ml penicillin, 100 ug/ml streptomycin, and 5 units/ml recombinant IL-2 (gift from Dupont, Glenolden, PA) at 37 C, 5% CO_2 humidified atmosphere. Lymhocytes were cultured with IL-2 alone or IL-2 and an irradiated monolayer of one of three allogeneic pancreatic adenocarcinoma cell lines, HPAF, T3M4, or CAPAN-2 (gift from Dr. Jorgen Fogh, New York, NY). One x 10^6 irradiated tumor cells/ml were added every 14 days. Additional tumor cell lines used in these studies were the pancreatic tumor cell lines CAPAN-1 (gift from Dr. Fogh); BXPC-3, HS766T, ASPC-1, and HGC-25 (gifts from Dr. Martina Schessler, New York, NY); QGP-1, SW979, PT45-P1, and PANC-89 (gifts from Dr. Holger Kalthoff, Hamburg, FGR); COLO-357 (gift from Dr. George Moore, Denver, CO); RWP-1 (gift from Dr. Jade Chin, New York, NY); and PANC-1. Nonpancreatic tumor cell lines used were Du-145 and PC-1 (gifts from Dr. Joy Ware, Durham, NC); SK-MEL, DuMel-12, DuMel-92, DuOs-1 and SW13 (gifts from Dr. Timothy Darrow, Durham, NC); MF and MT (gifts from Dr. Susan Slovin, Philadelphia, PA).
Cytotoxicity, immunofluorescence and proliferation assays: Four hour ^{51}Cr release assays and indirect immunofluorescence assays were performed as described (5). Proliferation assays were performed as described (5) using irradiated (6000 rad) pancreatic tumor cell lines or affinity purified Dupan 2 mucin (6) as stimulating antigen.

<u>Inhibition of cytotoxicity by MoAb</u>: Effector cells
were preincubated with indicated amounts of
affinity purified antibodies for 45 min at 37 C.
Labeled targets were then added and the
cytotoxicity assay was performed as described
above. Percent inhibition was calculated as
follows: %inhibition =
        percent cytotoxicity with antibody
1 - -------------------------------- X   100
     percent cytotoxicity without antibody

<u>Immunoprecipitation and SDS-PAGE analysis</u>: ^{125}I-
labelling, chemical crosslinking, and
solubilization was performed as described (7)
Immunoprecipitation was performed using either
control antibody, anti-T cell receptor (TCR)
antibody, BF1, or anti-CD3 antibody, Leu 4.
Immunoprecipitates were analyzed by SDS-PAGE.

                   RESULTS

<u>Effector Function, Phenotype and Specificity of
in vitro Expanded Lymphocytes</u>.

        Lymph node cell cultures from fourteen
patients were initiated as described and all
exhibited proliferation when stimulated with IL-2
plus allogeneic tumor cells as compared to IL-2
alone. Cells plated in IL-2 alone slowly
decreased in number and died over a period of
seven to fourteen days. Cells maintained on any
one of the three allogeneic tumor lines and IL-2
proliferated indefinitely, requiring feeding every
2-3 days and frequent subculture. In addition,
the cells appeared to be destroying the
stimulating tumor monolayers. A four-hour
chromium release assay was used to measure the
ability of <u>in vitro</u> expanded lymphocytes from one
patient, J.H., after 5 wks. of culture, to kill
the stimulating tumor targets. As expected, the
lymphocytes were strongly cytotoxic for the T3M4
tumor cells on which they were expanded. More
importantly, they exhibited similar reactivity
against another pancreatic adenocarcinoma line,

CAPAN-2 (Fig. 1A). A much lower level of lysis
was observed of the standard natural killer target
cell lines, K562 (myelogenous leukemia) and MOLT4
(T cell leukemia). The pancreatic cell line,
HPAF, which had previously been noted to be
resistant to antibody/ complement mediated
cytolysis, was also resistant to cell mediated
lysis. However, J.H. cells expanded and
maintained on HPAF killed both CAPAN-2 and T3M4
cells (Fig. 1B).

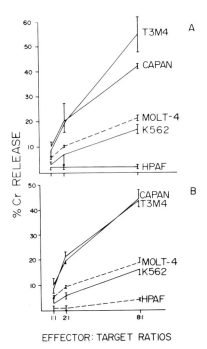

FIGURE 1

Lymph node cell culture from another patient,
W.D., was characterized with respect to the T cell
related cell surface markers expressed as culture
time progressed (Table 1).

PHENOTYPIC ANALYSIS OF CULTURED LYMPH NODE CELLS FROM
PANCREATIC CARCINOMA PATIENT W.D.

Days in Culture	Stimulated with	% Positive Cells :								
		Leu 1	T3	T4	T8	T11	Leu 11b	Leu 7	Tac	HLA-DR
0	IL-2	16	15	7	6	12	0	3	0	67
4	IL-2	37	31	16	7	26	6	18	9	57
7	IL-2	50	52	31	18	37	3	10	5	46
42	IL-2+CAPAN	90	97	16	80	NT	0	1	30	92
42	IL-2+T3M4	84	97	23	71	NT	1	3	45	96

Table 1

% ^{51}Cr RELEASE

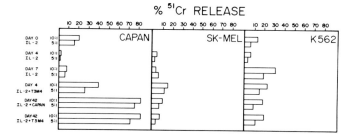

FIGURE 2

Figure 2 reflects the cytotoxic potential of
the same cells at the same time periods in culture
as were shown in Table 1. Cells cultured in the
presence of T3M4 tumor cells yielded lymphocytes
as early as day 4 which killed pancreatic tumor
cells at levels approaching those seen after one
month in culture. At the same time less than 10%
lysis of K562 cells and the melanoma line SK-MEL
was seen.   Although we have not examined all
patient lymph node cultures to the same extent
that we have studied W.D., in every case after one
month in culture the lymph node cells expanded on
the pancreatic tumor monolayers became
phenotypically and functionally homogeneous
cytotoxic T cell lines with unlimited, IL-2
dependent, growth potential and a stable,

pancreatic tumor directed, non-MHC-restricted cytotoxicity. We were unable to expand cells with a similar reactivity, using the same in vitro conditions, from either lymph nodes of nontumor bearing donors (transplant patients) or from peripheral blood.

T Cell Receptor and CD8 Accessory Molecule are Involved in Antigen Recognition.

The fact that these cytotoxic cells demonstrate phenotypic and functional characteristics of an antigen specific CTL but apparently lack the MHC restriction exhibited by other CTL raises questions about the role of CD4 and CD8 molecules, as well as the CD3 complex, in target recognition and lysis by these cells. We employed specific antibody blocking studies to address these questions, the results of which are shown in Fig. 3. Incubation of effector cells

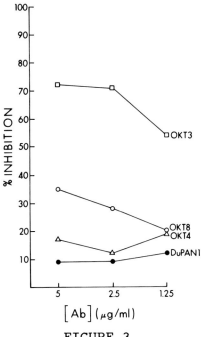

FIGURE 3

with OKT3 antibody, prior to their use in a
cytotoxic assay, resulted in up to 72% inhibition
of their lytic activity (Fig. 3). Preincubation
with OKT8 antibody also inhibited lysis by these
CTL, but to a lesser extent (up to 35%) than did
OKT3. The inhibitory effect of both antibodies
titered out as a function of decreasing antibody
concentration. In contrast, OKT4 antibody, as
well as a control antibody (Dupan1), had little
effect on cytotoxic activity of these cells.
     The nature of the receptor was examined by
immunoprecipitation and SDS-PAGE analysis using
antibodies directed to the CD3 complex and the TCR
α and β chains. No γ chain was precipitated
either with anti-CD3 or anti-γ antibodies (data
not shown). In contrast, anti-CD3 and anti- β
antibodies both precipitated α/β chain heterodimer
as shown in Figure 4.

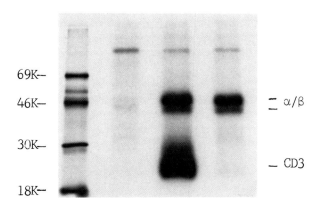

FIGURE 4

Pancreatic Mucin as the CTL Target Antigen.

     The specificity of these T cells for
pancreatic adenocarcinoma was evaluated by
cytotoxic and proliferation assays on a panel of
tumor cell lines, listed in Materials and Methods,
derived from pancreatic adenocarcinomas and from
solid tumors of other tissue types. The ability of
a tumor cell line to stimulate T cell proliferation

or serve as a target for cytotoxicity was compared with the expression of various pancreatic adenocarcinoma associated antigens. Results of these studies (not shown) indicated that DU-PAN 2 antigen may play a role in the recognition of the tumor cells.

DU-PAN 2 antigen was purified on antibody affinity columns by Dr. Micheal S. Lan, Duke University and used to stimulate proliferation of the cell line W.D.-CAPAN. As is shown in Table 2, purified DU-PAN 2 antigen stimulates proliferation of W.D.-CAPAN as well as does the cell from which it was purified, HPAF.

Table 2. Proliferation Assay

Responders	Stimulators	^{3}H incorp. (cpm)
W.D.-CAPAN	---	719
"	CAPAN-2	3750
"	T3M4	3351
"	HPAF	2249
"	K562	654
"	DU-PAN 2 (125 ug/ml)	2489

DISCUSSION

Investigation of cellular anti-tumor effector mechanisms is critically important for understanding the role of these cells in tumor recognition, rejection, and possibly nonspecific recruitment of other effector cells into the tumor site. Tumoricidal activity of lymphocytes has generally been associated with three distinct cell populations: antigen nonspecific, non-MHC-restricted natural killer cells; antigen specific, MHC-restricted cytotoxic T cells; and the recently described lymphokine activated killers (1). In this report we have described a population of T cells, isolated from pancreatic tumor bearing patients, which exhibit tumor antigen specificity and a high degree of cytotoxicity but apparently lack MHC restriction.

This non-MHC restricted function is not due
to the presence of a γ/δ receptor for antigen.
Expression of the α/β heterodimer on the surface
of these T cells raises the possibility that the
tumor antigen they recognize may be capable of
stimulating their proliferation in solution,
independent of MHC molecules. Binding of nominal
antigen by α/β bearing T cells has been reported
previously for human T cell clones specific for
fluorescein-5-isothiocyanate (8). High antigen
valence was required for binding and activation.
Pancreatic mucins, detected in part by a
monoclonal antibody DU-PAN 2, are very large,
highly glycosylated molecules (6) that could be
expected to form highly multivalent antigen forms
in solution. Our preliminary results suggest that
the pancreatic mucins may be the stimulating and
target antigens specifically recognized by the
CTL. Our future studies are designed to better
understand the molecular nature of this CTL-tumor
antigen interaction.

REFERENCES

1. Mazumder A (1985) Lymphokine Res 4: 215
2. De Vries JE, Spits H (1984) J Immunol 132:
   510
3. Sato T, Sato N, Takahashi S, Koshiba H,
   Kikuchi K (1986) Cancer Res 46: 4384
4. Slovin S, Lachman RD, Ferrone S, Kiely PE,
   Mastrangelo MJ (1986) J Immunol 137: 3042
5. Miceli C, Metzgar RS, Chedid M, Ward F,
   Finn OJ (1985) Hum Immunol 14: 295
6. Lan MS, Khorrami A, Kaufman B, Metzgar RS (1987)
   J Biol Chem 262: 12863
7. Ioannides CG, Itoh K, Fox FE, Pahwa R, Good RA,
   Platsoucas CD (1987) Proc Natl Acad Sci USA 84:
   4244
8 . Siliciano RF, Hemesath TJ, Pratt JC, Dintzis
   RZ, Dintzis HM, Acuto O, Shin HS, Reinherz EL
   (1986) Cell 47: 161

Human Tumor Antigens and Specific Tumor Therapy, pages 167–179
© 1989 Alan R. Liss, Inc.

HUMAN TUMOR ANTIGENS DEFINED BY CYTOTOXIC AND PROLIFERATIVE
T CELLS

Michael T. Lotze, Shohken Tomita and Steven A. Rosenberg

Surgery Branch, National Cancer Institute
Bethesda, MD 20892

ABSTRACT We have developed autologous T cell lines
and clones with unique reactivity to human tumor
antigens. The tumor which we have studied most
intensively is human melanoma for which specific
proliferative and cytotoxic clones and lines of both
CD4 and CD8 phenotype have been generated. In current
experiments 3/6 parental cytolytic lines cultured
directly from tumor in the presence of Interleukin-2
(IL-2) were specific for the autologous fresh tumor
and not reactive with allogeneic tumor or autologous
nontumor targets (fibroblasts, B cell lines).
Autologous tumor specific cloids could be generated by
limiting dilution techniques with clonal frequency
varying from 1/156 to 1/30,529 depending on the time
that cloning was performed relative to the initial
culture. Cultured tumor was susceptible to lysis by
cloned T cell lines and increased from 0.1 to 8.7 with
one clone/tumor combination when targets were stimulated with 1000 U/ml of gamma interferon for 3 days. No
lysis of the other cultured target was observed in the
criss-cross experiment. Lysis of tumor 560 by cloid 12
(CD8+) was completely blocked by an anticlass I MHC
antibody, W6/32. No apparent bystander toxicity was
observed of allogeneic tumor targets cocultured with
autologous tumor cells lysed in these assays.
Interleukin-4 (BSF-1) is a T cell derived glycoprotein
(M.W. 20 kd, pI 6.2) which has multiple biologic
functions including serving as a T cell growth factor.
Preliminary experiments in our laboratory indicate
that IL-4 is also capable of stimulating the growth of
both antitumor clones and lines alone and in conjunc-

tion with IL-2 (stimulation indices of 32.6 and 314,
respectively). These combinations may be helpful in
growing specific cytolytic cells. At low doses of
IL-2, IL-4 inhibits the expansion of NKH1[+] cells. In
5/5 experiments IL-4 decreased the IL-2 induced
generation of cells with lymphokine activated killing
(LK) from normal peripheral blood. Patients pretreated
with IL-2 however on immunotherapy protocols could be
demonstrated to produce cells with LAK activity with
IL-4 alone in 6/6 individuals. We are evaluating the
adoptive transfer of expanded tumor infiltrating
lymphocyte (TIL) clones and lines in murine and human
studies. Objective responses in patients treated with
combinations of IL-2, cyclophosphamide and TILs have
been observed in several patients.

INTRODUCTION

   Based on extensive studies in the mouse (1) we have
developed strategies for the treatment of human tumors
using IL-2 alone or in conjunction with transferred IL-2
activated peripheral blood mononuclear cells (PBMC) which
we have operationally defined as lymphokine activated
killer cells (LAK). Treatment with IL-2 alone (2-7) or in
conjunction with LAK (8) has been associated with significant antitumor responses in patients with melanoma, renal
cell cancer, colorectal carcinoma and lymphoma. Studies
in rodents have demonstrated that combinations of IL-2,
cyclophosphamide and adoptively transferred tumor-sensitized
lymphocytes taken directly from the tumor (9) induce tumor
regression. In our studies (10,11) these cells were as
much as 100-fold more effective in inducing an antitumor
response as LAK cells. We have demonstrated (12-14) that
expanded tumor infiltrating lymphocytes (TILs), in some
cases with specificity for the autologous tumor, can be
generated from human tumors. Their application following
adoptive transfer in the therapy of human tumors has begun.
In the studies reported here we have evaluated cloned
populations derived from human TILs obtained from melanomas.
Based on previous work (15-20) we used these reagents to
evaluate tumor antigens and mechanism of tumor recognition.
Further, we have employed IL-4 (21-27) to expand T cells
from human tumors. These approaches coupled with more
recent advances in our understanding of T cell recognition
(28) of cellular antigens (Figure 1) and requirements for

tumor cell susceptibilty to lysis (29) could allow more
sophisticated application of nascent immunotherapies.

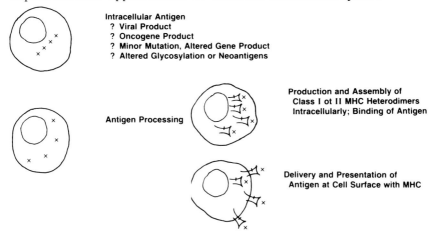

FIGURE 1. Presentation of Cellular Antigens for T
Cell Recognition of Tumor Postulated mechanisms could lead
to strategies accessible to manipulation for therapy.

MATERIALS AND METHODS

Media and Lymphokines. Cell lines were maintained in
culture using RPMI 1640 supplemented with 10% fetal bovine
serum, 100 g/ml penicillin, 100 g/ml streptomycin and 1%
glutamine as previously described (30). Recombinant
lymphokines were generously provided by Cetus (IL-2;
Emeryville, CA), Biogen (interferon gamma; Cambridge, MA)
and Immunex (IL-4; Seattle, WA). All cytokines were kept
in concentrated form at −80°C and then diluted immediately
prior to used.

Cellular reagents and assays. PBMC and tumor cells
were obtained as previously described (3,4,30). Fresh
tumors were harvested directly from operation, enzymatically
digested and cryopreserved as single cell suspensions. All
phenotyping and cytolytic assays were conducted as
previously described (3,4,30). Cloning was carried out as
previously described (19).

RESULTS

Generation of Tumor Specific TILs and Cloning.

Cloning of TILs was carried out immediately (Day 0) or after 3-5 weeks of initial culture with IL-2. Apparently tumor specific clones could be obtained in 3/6 instances as shown below in Table 1.

TABLE 1

ANTI-HUMAN MELANOMA CLONES CAN BE GENERATED DIRECTLY FROM TUMOR INFILTRATING LYMPHOCYTES

Tumor No.	Source of Melanoma Metastasis	% Initial Preparation		Growth of TIL	Specific tumor killing	Day Cloned	Clonal Frequency	Growth of specific clones
		MNC	Tumor					
468	Lymph node	30	70	(+)	(+)	Day 28	1/440	(+)
501	Lymph node	25	75	(+)	(+)	Day 23	1/156	(+)
560	Lymph node	28	72	(+)	(+)	Day 0	1/1,217	(+)
558	Skin	29	71	(+)	(-)	Day 36	1/510	(-)
544	Skin	40	60	(+)	(-)	Day 0	1/3,508	(-)
508	Skin	30	70	(+)	(-)	Day 0	1/30,529	(-)

All patients examined for incidence of clonal frequency are listed above. Condition for growth included 10% human AB sera, 1,000 u/ml of IL-2, irradiated autologous PBLs at 10^5/well and irradiated autologous tumor cells at 5×10^3/well. TILs were plated either uncultured (day 0) or at day 23-36 of culture. All viable cells were counted at the beginning of culture. Clonal frequency was determined using Poisson statistics on day 14-21 of growth.

When tested against autologous normal cell lines (EBV B cell, fibroblasts, PBL) or against allogeneic tumor little or no lysis was observed with the cloned line (Figure 2) whereas excellent lysis of the autologous tumor was demonstrated. Cloids from this TIL could not be successfully recloned but were obtained under conditions in which the probability of representating a clone was $\geq$90% and therefore are likely to represent clonal or oligoclonal populations.

SPECIFIC LYSIS OF AUTOLOGOUS MELANOMA
BY CLONED TIL

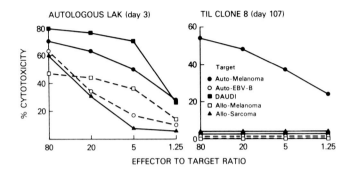

FIGURE 2. Tumor specific lysis by a T cell clone. Whereas only lysis of the autologous fresh tumor cell was noted (right) by TILs, LAK could lyse other cultured autologous targets and allogeneic targets.

When clone 8 was tested against the cultured B cell tumor Daudi or an allogeneic melanoma (560) no lysis was observed (Table 2). Excellent lysis of the fresh autologous tumor or the cultured tumor stimulated by interferon gamma could be seen.

TABLE 2.

INTERFERON GAMMA TREATMENT INCREASES LYSIS OF AUTOLOGOUS
TUMOR BY A CLONED T CELL LINE

Target Cells	Condition	EFFECTOR CELLS		
		LAK (Day 3)	560-TIL	468-TIL:Clone 8
		Lytic Units 30/10^6 Effector Cells		
DAUDI	CULTURED B Cell Line	54.7	<0.1	<0.1
TU 468	FRESH Melanoma	54.1	<0.1	105.0
TU 560	FRESH Melanoma	<0.1	4.8	<0.1
TU 468	CULTURED (-IFN)	51.8	<0.1	<0.1
	CULTURED (+IFN)	68.6	<0.1	8.7
TU 560	CULTURED (-IFN)	45.8	40.3	<0.1
	CULTURED (+IFN)	7.3	54.1	<0.1

Fresh or cultured autologous tumor lines were tested for lysis by allogeneic LAK or TIL lines or clones in a 4 hour ^{51}Cr release assay. Cultured cell lines were incubated without (-IFN) or with (+IFN) recombinant gamma interferon for three days (100 Units/ml).

Similarly when tested in proliferation assays for 5 days the TIL cell line could proliferate with Irradiated autologous tumor cells in the absence of IL-2 (stimulation index; SI,6) with IL-2 alone (SI,61), and to the combination (SI,107). With a cloned TIL obtained from Tumor 560 (cloid 12) MHC class I restricted lysis could be demonstrated (Table 3).

TABLE 3.
LYSIS OF AN AUTOLOGOUS TUMOR BY TIL IS BLOCKED BY
ANTIBODIES TO CLASS I MOLECULES

Group		% Specific Lysis (+/- SEM) AUTOLOGOUS Tumor			
	EiT Ratio	40	8	1.6	0.32
1.	No antibody	33.0(3.4)	29.4(0.5)	16.6(3.1)	1.8(3.6)
2.	W6/32: Anti MHC-1	-2.0(0.4)	-1.6(2.6)	1.6(2.9)	0.2(2.6)
3.	Anti HLA-DR: Anti MHC-II	41.5(1.5)	29.5(1.3)	8.0(4.7)	12.3(2.8)
4.	P3X63: Control murine ascites	29.6(4.3)	26.7(1.9)	9.7(1.8)	5.4(4.5)

Antibody from ascites (10 l) was added to a 4 hour ^{51}Cr release
assay. Final dilutions of antibody were 1:20 for W6/32 and 1:150 for
anti HLA-DR and P3X63.

Thus both lines and clones of specific tumor reactive cells
demonstrated many of the classical features of T cell
mediated recognition.

IL-4 Inhibits LAK Generation by IL-2 Stimulation and
Induces LAK Activity from IL-2 Pretreated Patients.

Using IL-4 alone or in conjunction with IL-2 no induction or augmentation of LAK generation could be identified
from human peripheral blood lymphocytes or splenocytes. IL-4
usually suppressed IL-2 induced LAK generation (for example
35.09 to 9.85 L.U. against Daudi and 18.85 to 0.32 against
fresh tumor in a representative experiment). IL-4 could
however stimulate proliferation of cloned TILs (468-Clone
8: IL-2 1U, SI 8.6; IL-4 1000U, SI 15.1; Both, SI 54.3)
and TIL lines. When PBMC were pretreated with IL-2 in vitro
or obtained from patients treated with IL-2 in vivo, IL-4
induced LAK generation could be demonstrated (Table 4).
LAK activity was usually much lower than IL-2 induced
activity and combinations of IL-2 and IL-4 often generated
less activity than IL-2 alone.

TABLE 4.

IL-4 GENERATES LAK FROM IL-2 PRETREATED PATIENTS

	(U/ML) IL-2	IL-4	TU 587	DAUDI Lytic Units$_{30}$/10^6 Cells	% YIELD
PATIENT 3 PBMC	–	–	<0.01	0.01	56.0
	1	–	0.10	8.06	73.8
	1000	–	239.80	311.45	88.8
	–	1000	0.01	0.73	92.5
	1	1000	1.83	11.89	62.5
PATIENT 3 NULL	–	–	0.03	0.91	38.8
	1	–	169.33	535.78	73.8
	1000	–	1281.04	7201.42	137.5
	–	1000	75.99	74.62	81.3
	1	1000	56.27	174.04	99.0
PATIENT 4 PBMC	–	–	<0.01	0.47	42.5
	1	–	12.11	36.23	67.5
	1000	–	170.69	419.73	87.5
	–	1000	2.39	21.83	53.8
	1	1000	14.80	79.03	41.3
PATIENT 3 NULL	–	–	<0.01	0.97	28.8
	1	–	51.66	106.06	83.8
	1000	–	778.53	>10000.00	101.3
	–	1000	2.70	15.04	47.5
	1	1000	4.34	30.00	82.5

PBMC obtained by leukophoresis from patients treated with IL-2
1-2 days following discontinuation of IL-2 were placed in culture for
3-5 days alone or with various concentrations of IL-2 and IL-4. Null
cells were prepared from PMBC vigorously depleted of B, T and monocytes
by rosetting with sheep red blood cells, adherence depletion, and
antibody and complement lysis with antibodies to CD3 and DR. TU 587
is a fresh allogeneic melanoma tumor target.

IL-4 Decreases the Relative Growth of NKHI[+] Cells from TILs and Enhances the Growth of Specific T Cells.

In our earliest experiments evaluating the ability of IL-4 to augment TIL growth from melanomas we were able to demonstrate that short term (20 day) cultures of TIL grew at an accelerated rate and that NKHI[+] cells were decreased (Figure 3). We have confirmed the enhanced growth of TIL from melanomas in several other cases (26).

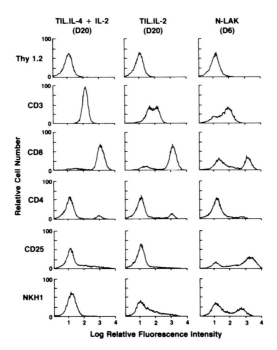

FIGURE 3. Phenotype of Cells Grown from Human Melanoma with IL-2 +/- IL-4. Decreased NKHI[+] cells are noted from the TIL grown in IL-4 compound to that without or 6 day LAK cultures from PBMC.

DISCUSSION

T cells from human melanomas may be grown in IL-2 or in combination with IL-4. These cell lines and clones demonstrate apparent classical T cell mediated recognition and MHC restriction. Further clinical efforts employing treatment of patients with these lymphokines or the adoptive transfer of cultured ($1-7.5 \times 10^{11}$ cells/treatment) TILs are in progress and should help answer questions regarding the in vivo effectiveness of such treatments and the role of these cells.

ACKNOWLEDGEMENTS

Careful preparation of this manuscript by Ethel M. House and ADP CONSULTANTS is appreciated, as well as excellent technical assistance by Mary C. Custer.

REFERENCES

1. Rosenberg SA (1986). Adoptive Immunotherapy of Cancer Using Lymphokine Activated Killer Cells and Recombinant Interleukin-2. Important Advances in Oncology 2:55.
2. Lotze MT, Rosenberg SA (1988). Interleukin 2 as a pharmacologic reagent. In Smith EK (ed): "Interleukin 2," Orlando: Academic Press, p 237.
3. Lotze MT, Frana LW, Sharrow SO, Robb RJ, Rosenberg SA (1985). In vivo administration of purified human interleukin 2. I. Half-life and immunologic effects of the Jurkat cell line-derived interleukin 2. J Immunol 134:157.
4. Lotze MT, Matory YL, Ettinghausen SE, Rayner AA, Sharrow SO, Seipp CA, Custer MC, Rosenberg SA (1985). In vivo administration of purified human interleukin 2. I. Half-life, immunologic effects, and expansion of peripheral lymphoid cells in vivo with recombinant IL-2. J Immunol 135:2865.

5. Lotze MT, Chang AE, Seipp CA, Simpson C, Vetto JT, Rosenberg SA (1986). High-dose recombinant interleukin 2 in the treatment of patients with disseminated cancer. Responses, treament-related morbidity, and histologic findings. JAMA 256:3117.

6. Lotze MT, Custer MC, Rosenberg SA (1986). Intraperitoneal administration of interleukin-2 in patients with cancer. Arch Surg 121:1373.

7. Lotze MT, Rosenberg SA (1986). Results of clinical trials with the administration of interleukin 2 and adoptive immunotherapy with activated cells in patients with cancer. Immunobiol 172:420.

8. Rosenberg SA, Lotze MT, Muul LM, Chang AE, Avis FP, Leitman S, Linehan WM, Robertson CN, Lee RE, Rubin JT, Seipp CA, Simpson CG, White DE (1987). A progress report on the treatment of 157 patients with advanced cancer using lymphokine-activated killer cells and interleukin-2 or high-dose interleukin-2 alone. N Eng J Med 316:889.

9. Evans R (1983). Combination therapy by using cyclophosphamide and tumor-sensitized lymphocytes: a possible mechanism of action. J Immunol 130:2511.

10. Rosenberg SA, Spiess P, Lafreniere R (1986). A new approach to the adoptive immunotherapy of cancer with tumor-infiltrating lymphocytes. Science 233:1318.

11. Spiess PJ, Yang JC, Rosenberg SA (1987). In vivo antitumor activity of tumor-infiltrating lymphocytes expanded in recombinant interleukin-2. JNCI 79:1067.

12. Muul LM, Spiess PJ, Director EP, Rosenberg SA (1987). Identification of specific cytolytic immune responses against autologous tumor in humans bearing malignant melanoma. J Immunol 138:989.

13. Tomita S, Lotze MT, Rosenberg SA (1987). Clonal analysis of tumor infiltrating lymphocytes (TIL) against human malignant melanoma. Fed Proc 46:1195.

14. Belldegrun A, Muul LM, Rosenberg SA (1988). Interleukin 2 expanded tumor-infiltrating lymphocytes in human renal cell cancer: isolation, characterization, and antitumor activity. Cancer Res 48:206.

15. Baker PE, Gillis S, Smith KA (1979). Monoclonal cytolytic T-cell lines. J Exp Med 149:273.

16. Lotze MT, Strausser JL, Rosenberg SA (1980). In vitro growth of cytotoxic human lymphocytes. II. Use of T cell growth factor (TCGF) to clone human T cells. J Immunol 124:2972.

17. Mukherji B, MacAlister TJ (1983). Clonal analysis of cytotoxic T cell response against human melanoma. J Exp Med 158:240.
18. de Vries JE, Spits H (1984). Cloned human cytotoxic T lymphocyte (CTL) lines reactive with autologous melanoma cells. I. In vitro generation, isolation, and analysis to phenotype and specificity. J Immunol 132:510.
19. Lotze MT, Rayner AA, Grimm EA (1985). Problems with the isolation of lymphoid clones with reactivity to human tumors. Behring Inst Mitt 77:105.
20. Anichini A, Fossati G, Parmiani G (1986). Heterogeneity of clones from a human metastatic melanoma detected by autologous cytotoxic T lymphocyte clones. J Exp Med 163:215.
21. Paul WE (1987). Interleukin 4/B cell stimulatory factor 1: one lymphokine, many functions. FASEB J 1: 456.
22. O'Garra A, Warren DJ, Holman M, Popham AM, Sanderson CJ, Klaus GGB (1986). Interleukin 4 (B-cell growth factor II/eosinophil differentiation factor) is a mitogen and differentiation factor for preactivated murine B lymphocytes. Proc Natl Acad Sci USA 83:5228.
23. Spits H, Yssel H, Takebe Y, Arai N, Yokota T, Lee F, Arai K-I, Banchereau J, de Vries JE (1987). J Immunol 139:1142.
24. Widmer MB, Acres RB, Sassenfeld HM, Grabstein KH (1987). Isolation of cytolytic cell populations from human peripheral blood by B cell stimulatory factor 1 (interleukin 4). J Exp Med 166:1447.
25. Kawakami Y, Custer M, Rosenberg SA, Lotze MT (1988) Human interleukin 4 (IL4) inhibits interleukin 2 (IL2) induction of human lymphokine activated killer (LAK) activity from peripheral blood and spleen cells. FASEB Jl 2:A660
26. Kawakami Y, Rosenberg SA, Lotze MT. Interleukin 4 promotes the growth of tumor infiltrating lymphocytes specific for human autologous melanoma. Submitted for publication.
27. Kawakami Y, Kasid A, Custer M, Rosenberg SA, Lotze MT. Interleukin 4 suppresses IL-2 induction of human lymphokine activated killer activity from naive cells. Submitted for publication.

28. Bjorkman PJ, Saper MA, Samraoui B, Bennett WS, Strominger JL, Wiley DC (1987). Structure of the human class I histocompatibility antigen, HLA-A2. Nature 329:506.

29. Wiebke EA, Lotze MT, Rosenberg SA (1987). Tumor cell susceptibility to lysis: marked increase in lysis by tumor-infiltrating lymphocytes following target stimulation with interferon-and tumor necrosis factor--implications for immunotherapy. Surg. Forum 38:436.

30. Roberts K., Lotze MT, Rosenberg SA (1987). Separation and functional studies of the human lymphokine-activated killer cell. Cancer Res 47:4366.

Human Tumor Antigens and Specific Tumor Therapy, pages 181–190
© 1989 Alan R. Liss, Inc.

MONOCLONAL ANTIBODIES IN CANCER THERAPY: SELECTION OF THE
MOST APPROPRIATE REAGENT FOR DIFFERENT APPROACHES[1]

Delia Mezzanzanica, Silvana Canevari, Patrizia Casalini,
Gabriella Della Torre[2], and Maria I. Colnaghi

Division of Experimental Oncology E and [2]A,
Istituto Nazionale Tumori, Via Venezian 1, 20133 Milano,
Italy

ABSTRACT - Six murine monoclonal antibodies (MAbs)
MBr1, MOv17, MOv18, MOv19, MLuC1 and MLuC2, raised
against human tumors of epithelial origin, were
selected, due to their restricted pattern of
reactivity, for therapeutic applications. To define
the most appropriate application for each one, the
fate of the antigen-antibody complex after binding to
the cell surface was analyzed.
Immunoelectronmicroscopy (IEM) and pH 2.8 desorption
indicated that MBr1, MOv17 and MLuC1 induced 30-60%
internalization of the bound antigen, whereas the
other three MAbs were quite incapable of inducing
internalization. Accordingly, when linked to
restrictocin, a ribosome-inactivating protein, MBr1,
MOv17 and MLuC1 yielded active immunoconjugates. On
the other hand, the stability of the MOv18-recognized
antigen enabled us to efficiently retarget cytotoxic
T lymphocytes using the bispecific
anti-tumor/anti-CD3 MAb.

[1] This work was partially supported by grants from the
Italian CNR Special project "Oncology" and from AIRC.

INTRODUCTION

Over the past few years numerous efforts have been made regarding the generation of MAbs which are suitable for clinical applications in oncology. Many of the available anti-tumor MAbs can only now be considered valid diagnostic tools, whereas the successfull application of MAbs in cancer therapy is still limited by several different problematic aspects (1). Besides the tumor specificity, many other factors such as the binding kinetic and affinity of the MAbs and the fate of antigen-antibody complex after MAb binding at the cell surface, could deeply affect the MAb's therapeutic efficiency. The analysis of the latter parameter was therefore considered a crucial step in the characterization of MAb suitability for therapy.

Six murine MAbs were selected for therapeutic approaches, due to their restricted pattern of reactivity on mammary and/or ovarian carcinoma. From current therapeutic applications, the production of immunoconjugates and the retargeting of cytotoxic T lymphocytes by bispecific MAbs were chosen. The efficiency of the former approach could depend both on the quantity and the pathway of MAb-induced internalization, whereas that of the latter, mainly depended on the stability of the MAb-recognized antigen on the cell surface.

RESULTS

The main characteristics of the selected MAbs are summarized in Table 1. The reactivity and the target antigen on the immunizing tumors have previously been described for MBr1, MOv18, MOv19 and MLuC1 and the relevant references are reported in Conde et al. (2). MOv17 was found to recognize a different epitope on the same molecule defined by MOv18 and MOv19, whereas MLuC2 was directed against a 75 KDa glycoprotein. To determine for each MAb the most appropriate therapeutic application,

the fate of antigen-antibody complexes after MAb binding
to the cell surface was evaluated. This parameter was
analyzed quantitatively as percentage of cell uptake (3)
and qualitatively as pathways of internalization (4).

TABLE 1

CHARACTERISTICS OF MABS USED IN THE INTERNALIZATION
STUDIES

MAb/isotype	Target reference cells [a]	Reactivity on mammary ca.	ovary ca.
MBr1/IgM	MCF-7	80%	50%
MOv17/IgG1	OVCA 432/MCF-7/HT-29	60%	65%
MOv18/IgG1	OVCA 432	2%	80%
MOv19/IgG2a	OVCA 432	2%	80%
MLuC1/IgG2a	MCF-7, SW626	70%	60%
MLuC2/IgG2a	HT-29	72%	30%

a Origin of human target cell lines: MCF-7 = mammary ca.;
  OVCA 432 and SW626 = ovary ca.; HT-29 = colon ca.

In Figures 1 and 2 are reported in full the data
obtained with one of the MAbs (MOv17).
As shown in Figure 1, the total bound ^{125}I-MOv17
could be desorbed from fixed cells, whereas a significant
portion (about 50%) of the labelled MAb could not be
desorbed from live cells (thus indicating a good
internalization of the recognized antigen).
IEM examination indicated that the MOv17-recognized
antigen was internalized by both coated (Fig. 2a) and
uncoated vesicles (Fig. 2b).

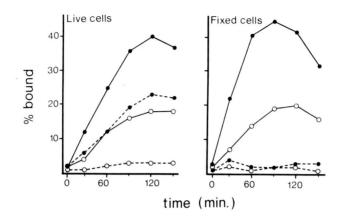

time (min.)

Figure 1.   OVCA 432 cell uptake of ^{125}I-MOv17 by pH
2.8 desorption method. (●): binding at 37°C; (O):
binding at 0°C; (——):total binding; (--): residual uptake
after pH 2.8 desorption.

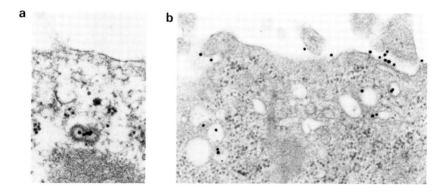

Figure 2.   Internalization of MOv17 in OVCA 432 cells
via coated vesicles (a, x 65000) and uncoated vesicles (b,
x 80000) by IEM.

The internalization data obtained with all six of the
selected MAbs are summarized in Table 2.   Both methods

indicate that the induced internalization of the recognized antigens was good for MBr1, MOv17 and MLuC1, poor for MOv18 and irrelevant for MOv19 and MLuC2.

TABLE 2

MAB-INDUCED INTERNALIZATION OF THE RECOGNIZED ANTIGENIC SITES

MAb	Target cells	% of cell uptake[a]	Internalization by[b] coated vesicles	uncoated vesicles
MBr1	MCF-7	28		+
MOv17	OVCA 432	54	+	+
	MCF-7	42	+	
	HT-29	60		+/-
MOv18	OVCA 432	25		+/-
MOv19	OVCA 432	17	ND[c]	
MLuC1	SW626	37	+	+
	MCF-7	53	ND	
MLuC2	HT-29	14	ND	

a Evaluated by pH 2.8 desorption method (3). The figures represent the % of cell uptake on live cells corrected by the % of cell uptake on fixed cells.

b Evaluated by IEM using biotinylated-MAb and avidin-colloidal gold (4).

c = not done.

Immunoconjugates have been generated with a new ribosome-inactivating protein, Restrictocin (2). In Table 3 are summarized their cytotoxic activity on the relevant

target cells, whereas their biochemical and biological
characterization has been described elsewhere (2). As
reported in the table, there was a direct correlation
between immunoconjugate efficiency and the ability of the
MAb to induce internalization. In fact, the
immunoconjugate obtained with MLuC2, which was unable to
induce internalization, showed no cytotoxic activity.

TABLE 3

CYTOTOXIC ACTIVITY OF IMMUNOCONJUGATES OBTAINED WITH
RESTRICTOCIN[a]

Type of conjugate	Target reference cells	IC_{50} (M)[b]	Specificity factor[c]
With MAbs which induced internalization:			
MBr1-Res	MCF-7	10^{-8}	1000
MLuC1-Res	MCF-7	$5x10^{-8}$	200
	SW626	$2x10^{-8}$	750
MOv17-Res	OVCA 432	$3.5x10^{-9}$	1140
With MAb which did not induce internalization:			
MLuC2-Res	HT-29	n.e.[d]	_[e]

a On adherent target cells treated for 20 hours
b IC_{50} = conjugate concentration required for 50% protein
   synthesis inhibition.
c Ratio of the toxin IC_{50} versus the immunoconjugate
   IC_{50}.
d n.e. = protein synthesis inhibition < 20% even at the
   maximum dose tested ($1.6x10^{-6}$ M).
e = calculation not possible.

Among the MAbs which did not induce internalization, MOv18, which exhibited the most specific pattern of reactivity, was chosen for the preparation of a bispecific MAb. This MAb, called αOC/TR, directed against both the tumor-associated antigen and the limphocyte CD3 molecule, was reported to be able to induce T cells to act against the tumor target (5-6). In Table 4 the specificity and the cytolytic activity triggered by αOC/TR, are summarized.

TABLE 4

ANALYSIS OF αOC/TR BISPECIFIC HYBRID ANTIBODY

Percent of binding activity related to parental MAbs	100%
Binding specificity[a]	yes
Hybrid MAb CC_{50} on OVCA 432[b] in presence of:	
CTL from T clone (E:T = 10:1)	7pM
CTL from PBMCs (E:T = 10:1)	26pM
CTL from PBMCs (E:T = 100:1)	1pM
Cytotoxic specificity[a] in presence of:	
CTL from T clone (E:T = 10:1)	intermediate
CTL from PBMCs (E:T = 100:1)	absolute

a Evaluated on OVCA 432 and various cell lines irrelevant according to immunofluorescence.

b CC_{50} = hybrid antibody concentration required for 50% cytotoxicity.

DISCUSSION

The qualitative and quantitative analysis of the MAb-induced internalization of tumor-associated antigens was performed to possibly define the most suitable therapeutic approach for each single MAb and tumor situation. As regards immunoconjugates with restrictocin, the quantitative analysis was proven useful to predict their cytotoxic activity, in agreement with previous reports on other toxins (7). However, no correlation was observed between the percentage of cell uptake and the specificity factors of the immunoconjugates, which could be considered a measure of the cytotoxic efficiency. Since the immunoconjugate efficiency, as already suggested (8), could mainly depend on the pathway of internalization, it was examined by IEM, but again no correlation was found during the early steps of the internalization process. Further analyses of the following steps, including the possible MAb-toxin degradation and/or the toxin translocation from endocytic vesicles through the cytosol, require different experimental approaches (8-10), which are now in progress. The information obtained from these experiments, together with a precise analysis of the MAb binding kinetics and affinity, should be very useful for predicting the efficiency of the relevant immunoconjugate.

On the other hand, the poor or irrelevant internalization induced by some MAbs, in the case of a good binding affinity, would result in a high stability of the antigen antibody complex on the cell membrane. In the case of MOv18, this characteristic was exploited to efficiently retarget cytotoxic T lymphocytes by bifunctional MAbs, but other therapeutic approaches could also be considered. In fact, the knowledge of the absence of internalization and therefore of degradation of labelled MAbs could possibly suggest the therapeutic use of nuclide as iodide.

ACKNOWLEDGEMENTS

The authors are grateful to Dr. F.P. Conde for kindly providing the restrictocin toxin and thank, Mrs. G. Pasquini and Mr. F. Sola for their excellent technical help, Ms. M. Hatton and Ms. P. Rocchi for manuscript preparation and Mr. M. Azzini for photographic reproduction.

REFERENCES

1. M.I. Colnaghi, S. Canevari, F. Conde, R. Fontanelli, F. Leoni, S. Ménard, R. Orlandi, P. Pizzetti, G. Porro and M. Ripamonti (1987). Monoclonal antibodies: perspectives for tumor therapy in Gallo R.C., Della Porta G., Albertini A. (eds.) "Monoclonals and DNA Probes in Diagnostic and Preventive Medicine", New York: Raven Press.

2. F. Conde, R. Orlandi, S. Canevari, D. Mezzanzanica, M. Ripamonti, S. Munoz, P. Jorge and M.I. Colnaghi (1988). The aspergillus toxin restrictocin is a suitable cytotoxic agent for generation of immunoconjugates with monoclonal antibodies directed against human carcinoma cells. In press in Eur. J. Biochem.

3. S. Matzku, E.B. Bröcker, J. Brüggen, W.G. Dippold and W. Tilgen (1986). Modes of binding and internalization of monoclonal antibodies to human melanoma cell lines. Cancer Res: 46, 3848.

4. G. Della Torre, S. Canevari, R. Orlandi and M.I. Colnaghi (1987). Internalization of a monoclonal antibody against human breast cancer by immunoelectron microscopy. Br. J. Cancer: 55, 357.

5. S. Canevari, S. Ménard, D. Mezzanzanica, S. Miotti, S.M. Pupa, A. Lanzavecchia and M.I. Colnaghi (1988). Anti-ovarian carcinoma anti-T3 heteroconjugates or hybrid antibodies induce tumor cell lysis by cytotoxic T cells. Int. J. Cancer: Supplement 2, 18.

6. D. Mezzanzanica, S. Canevari, S. Ménard, S.M. Pupa, E. Tagliabue, A. Lanzavecchia and M.I. Colnaghi (1988). Human ovarian carcinoma lysis by cytotoxic T cells targeted by bispecific monoclonal antibodies: analysis of the antibody components. In press in Int. J. Cancer: 41.

7. E.S. Vitetta, R. J. Fulton, R.D. May, M. Till, J.W. Uhr (1987). Redesigning nature's poisons to create anti-tumor reagents. Science: 238, 1098.

8. A. Godal, O. Fodstad, A. Pihl (1987). Studies on the mechanism of action of Abrin-9.2.27 immunotoxin in human melanoma cell lines. Cancer Res.: 47, 6243.

9. K. Sandvig, S. Olsnes, O.W. Petersen, B. Van Deurs (1987). Acidification of the cytosol inhibits endocytosis from coated pits. J. Cell Biol.: 105, 679.

10. S. Matzku, W. Tilgen, H. Kalthoff, W.H. Schmiegel, E.B. Bröcker (1988). Dynamics of antibody transport and internalization. Int. J. Cancer: Supp. 2, 11.

Human Tumor Antigens and Specific Tumor Therapy, pages 191–197

CONTROLLED LABELING OF MONOCLONAL ANTIBODIES FOR IMAGING METASTATIC CANCER: A PRELUDE TO THERAPY.

Paul Abrams, Robert Schroff, Alan Fritzberg,
A. Charles Morgan, D. Scott Wilbur, A. Srinivasan,
John Reno, Gowsala Sivam, Sudhakar Kasina,
J-L Vanderheyden, Paul Beaumier, Darrell Salk,
Mehmet Fer

NeoRx Corporation
410 W. Harrison
Seattle, Washington 98119

Antibody specific targeting allows delivery to cancer cells of potent cellular poisons that interfere with basic biologic processes. Development of controlled systems to radiolabel antibodies provides agents that can both image metastatic tumors and demonstrate appropriate delivery of therapeutic conjugates to the tumors.

Antibodies have been proposed as specific targeting vehicles since Paul Ehrlich coined the phrase "magic bullets" in 1901 (1). The concerted application of this concept, however, awaited Kohler and Milsteins's discovery of monoclonal antibodies in 1975 (2).

Since unconjugated antibodies have only rarely shown benefit (3), their principal use should be, as Ehrlich postulated, as targeting vehicles for cytotoxic agents and inducers such as drugs, toxins, radio-nuclides, and biologic response modifiers. Conjugating these agents to antibody, however, may alter the biodistribution of the antibody. Additional problems that have been encountered include insufficient stability and loss of potency of the cytotoxic agent after conjugation to the antibody. We have focused our efforts on addressing these issues.

A central feature of our approach has been the development of controlled chemistry for stably labeling antibodies with gamma–emitting radionuclides, specifi-cally ^{99m}Tc and ^{131}I. We have applied these systems to develop both clinically useful imaging agents to help stage cancer and parallel chemistries for treating the disease with antibody delivered radiotherapy. We have also shown that several highly potent drug conjugates localize nearly as effectively and specifically in tumors as unconjugated antibody, the latter serving as a "gold standard" for biodistribution.

Technetium-99m is the preferred radionuclide for imaging because its 140 keV photon provides excellent resolution with modern gamma cameras for both planar imaging and single photon emission computed tomography (SPECT); it is also safe, inexpensive and readily available so that it is used in more than 80% of conventional nuclear medicine scans. Because of its complex chemistry that prevented stable labeling of proteins and six-hour physical half-life that was considered too short for tumor localization and background clearance, most groups selected other radionuclides such as ^{111}In and ^{131}I despite their inherent difficulties of stability or image degradation.

A stable, gentle controlled chemistry for labeling proteins with ^{99m}Tc has been previously described (4). Briefly, a diamide dithiolate ligand was discovered not to require the participation of a carboxylate group for stable chelation of reduced ^{99m}Tc, and thus was available as a "handle" for linking the ligand or chelate to the antibody via an active ester. The chelate ($C_5N_2S_2$-Tc) in was shown to bind technetium stably when challenged at pH 2-13 and 0-100°C.

Analysis of labeled antibody revealed monomeric fragment [Fab or F(ab')$_2$] that showed no loss of ^{99m}Tc over 24 hours incubation in serum whether challenged by an excess of DTPA, urea or free ligand. Comparison of labeled preparation by HPLC gel sieving of serum drawn from a patient at 2 and 20 hour post injection showed monomeric peaks with identical retention times as the pre-injection sample, demonstrating that no transfer of ^{99m}Tc to other proteins occurred. Comparison of the immunoreactivities of metabolically or extrinsically labeled control antibodies with ^{99m}Tc-$C_5N_2S_2$ labeled preparations revealed absolutely no loss of immunoreactivity.

Having solved the chemical obstacles in employing ^{99m}Tc for labeling antibodies, it was now critical to determine if its six-hour half-life was, in fact, compatible with satisfactory tumor imaging. The line 10 (L-10) guinea pig hepatocellular carcinoma (5) was established in the flank of strain-2 guinea pigs. Technetium-99m (50 uCi) on 100 ug of the D_3 murine antibody F(ab')$_2$ were injected and imaging was conducted at 0, 4, 10, and 20 hours later using a gamma camera with a pinhole collimator. As early as 4 hours, specific tumor localization was clearly demonstrated; by 10 hours blood pool and normal organs all cleared with the exception of some excretion into the intestine and the tumor could be plainly seen. At 20 hours the tumor was excised and placed alongside the animal; virtually all the radioactivity resided in the tumor.

With these results, human clinical studies were performed with F(ab')$_2$ and Fab fragments of several antibodies directed to melanoma (NR-ML-05), lung (NR-LU-10), colon and breast cancer-associated antigens (NR-Co-02). Imaging was performed at 0, 3, 6-8, and 15-24 hours after injection.

Several observations were noteworthy. Tumor imaging with the Fab fragment occurred as early as three hours although, to be sure, the quality of the images was superior at later time points due to clearance of background. Secondly, there was no hepatic, splenic or bone marrow localization observed with any of these antibodies as has been observed with In-111 labeled antibodies. Tumors were detected in virtually every organ including brain, bone, liver, spleen, adrenal, lymph node, ovary, skin, lung and bowel. Of the important visceral organs, detection in the lung appeared worst (approximately 60%) and liver best (greater than 95%). The reasons for the poor detection rates of metastases in lung remain obscure. Administration of the murine antibody was safe with only three minor allergic reactions in more than 200 patients.

Two problems were observed. The first, and most critical (for imaging colon and ovarian cancer) was that the N_2S_2-Tc labeled antibodies were excreted into the intestine via the hepatobiliary route. Although cathartics could be used to clear the bowel, thus proving the counts to be intraluminal, they were not invariably successful. Thus, imaging of retroperitoneal lymph nodes especially could be obscured or misinterpreted.

Secondly, the Fab fragments accumulated in the
kidney; this was the only organ where the total dose
increased beyond the initial post-infusion levels.
They then declined over the 4-20 hours. While not
itself a major problem for imaging, it does represent a
potential second organ (after bone marrow) of toxicity
for therapeutic applications.

As a single, safe test that can detect tumors in
multiple sites simultaneously, this imaging technique
is sensitive, simple and cost effective. Its application will vary with tumor type and stage, but would
include screening for distant disease prior to
contemplated surgery, staging prior to chemotherapy,
or analysis of a particular anatomic sites. It is
important to note that while the radiolabeled antibody
technique and the other diagnostic imaging modalities
generally detect the same number of metastatic sites
of disease, they are not congruent. The radiolabeled
antibody often detects sites of lymph node and other
soft tissue metastasis not routinely surveyed by other
techniques but missed about 40% of pulmonary lesions.

We have evaluated two radiotherapeutic, B-emitting
radionuclides conjugated to antibodies by two different
ligand systems. Rhenium lies directly under technetium
in the periodic table and has two beta-emitting
isotopes suitable for therapeutic applications. Its
chemistry is nearly identical to technetium's and it
may be chelated by the same diamide dithiolate ligand
as used for the technetium imaging. Biodistribution
of rhenium and technetium labeled antibodies in a nude
mouse/human xenograft model Figure is identical.

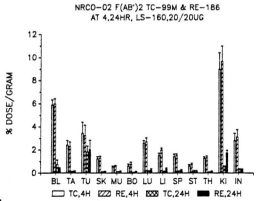

NRCO-02 F(AB')2 TC-99M & RE-186
AT 4,24HR, LS-160,20/20UG

Figure 1.

Isotopes of iodine (-123, -125, -131) have also been used for imaging, for radioimmunoassays and for therapy for many years. Iodine is easily incorporated into tyrosyl residues on proteins, but a major obstacle to the in vivo application of such iodinated proteins is dehalogenation. We have developed a method for incorporating halogens into non-activated rings that resist dehalogenation in vivo (6).

Briefly, halogens are introduced into meta- or para- positions on phenyl rings via organometallic substitution. The labeled material is incorporated onto antibody by aminoacylation with an active ester. Using unblocked thyroid as a "bioassay" for dehalogenated elemental iodide, para-iodophenyl (PIP) labeled antibody reveals virtually no radioactivity in thyroid over seven days compared to chloramine-T labeled material that showed substantial radioactivity in thyroid over the same period. PIP-labeled antibodies show identical uptake in tumor and normal tissues in animals as do their Tc-labeled counterparts, except the intestine where $Tc-N_2S_2$ accumulates and PIP-labeled conjugate does not.

The PIP system was applied to label drug conjugates to determine whether such conjugates, which were potent and selective in vitro, accumulated in normal organs such as the liver. Trichothecenes are a family of mycotoxins that inhibit protein synthesis that are isolated from fungi imperfecta and have in common a sesquiterpeniod ring structure. They are the most toxic agents known that contain only hydrogen, oxygen and carbon, and have no selectivity for tumor compared to normal cells. While 25 ug of one such trichothecene, Verrucarin A, kills mice (LD_{100}), 25 ug conjugated to the whole NR-LU-10 antibody shows no toxicity.

Between 5-8 molecules of Verrucarin A were conjugated to NR-LU-10 antibody using an amide linkage. The PIP label (I-131) was then added and the labeled conjugate (50 ug) injected into nude mice bearing the LS174 colon tumor. At the same time, unconjugated NR-LU-10 (50 ug) labeled with PIP (I-125) was coinjected. Animals were followed up to seven days with sacrifice at 15 minutes, 4 hours, 24 hours, 72 hours, and 168 hours. The results showed virtually identical biodistribution of the conjugate and

unconjugated antibody at 24 hours and greater. The
conjugate showed more early accumulation in liver and
lung at 15 minutes and 4 hours, but this was
insufficient to have a negative effect on serum
half-life or bioavailability of conjugate for the
tumor. The percent injected dose per gram in tumor
(0.3 – 0.5 gm) was 20% and remained elevated at
similar levels for the entire period. Therapeutic
experiments are now under way.

In summary, controlled, stable radiolabeling
systems for proteins have been developed and characterized. Both ^{99m}Tc and halogens can now be linked to
antibodies in a controlled, stable fashion. The ^{99m}Tc
labeled antibodies provide excellent diagnostic imaging
tools to evaluate metastatic disease in multiple organs
simultaneously. Rhenium has two beta-emitting isotopes
and its chemistry is closely akin to technetium. This
was demonstrated by comparing technetium and rhenium
labeled antibodies in nude mice/xenograft models.
Finally, stable iodine labeling, which may itself
prove useful for antibody-guided radiotherapy, permits
tracking of drug conjugates. Trichothecene drug
conjugates were shown to be potent and to exhibit
similar biodistribution as unconjugated antibody.

Specific targeting will soon change the strategy of
treating cancer. Imaging will become an essential tool
for selecting patients most likely to benefit from
treatment and calculating the anti-tumor dose and
predicting likely toxicity.

Targeting also offers the potential of delivering
agents that interfere with basic biologic processes
rather than some part of the cell cycle. Thus, some of
the observed problems of resistance that arise from the
current generation of chemotherapy agents directed to
dividing cells can be overcome by switching to this new
class of agents.

References

1. Ehrlich P. (1957) The Collected Papers of Paul Ehrlich, II, pp. 550-557.

2. Kohler, G. and Milstein C. (1975): Continuous cultures of fused cells secreting antibody of pre-defined specificity. Nature 256:495-97.

3. Miller R.A., Maloney D.G., Warnke R., Levy R. (1982): Treatment of a B-cell lymphoma with monoclonal anti-idiotype antibody. N. Engl. J. Med. 306:517-22.

4. Fritzberg, A.R., Abrams, P.G., Beaumier P.L., et al., Specific and stable labeling of antibodies with technetium-99m with a diamide dithiolate chelating agent. (1988) Proc. Natl. Acad. Sci. (USA) 85:4025-29.

5. Bernhard M.I., Foon K.A., Oeltmann, T.N. et al. Guinea pig line 10 hepatocarcinoma model: characterization of monoclonal antibody and in vivo effect of unconjugated antibody and antibody conjugated to diptheria toxin A chain. (1983) Cancer Res. 43:4720-28.

6. Wilbur, D.S., Jones, D.S., Fritzberg, A.R., and Morgan A.C. Radioiodination of monoclonal antibodies Labeling with para-iodophenyl (PIP) derivatives for in vivo stability of the radioiodine label. J. Nucl. Med. 27:959 (1986) Abstr.

Human Tumor Antigens and Specific Tumor Therapy, pages 199–208

TARGETING MONOCLONAL ANTIBODIES TO MICROMETASTATIC CELLS IN COLON AND BREAST CANCER PATIENTS[1]

I. Funke, G. Schlimok, B. Bock, B. Schweiberer
and G. Riethmüller

Institute for Immunology, University of Munich
D-8000 Munich 2

ABSTRACT Targeting monoclonal antibodies to micro-metastatic cells

A monoclonal antibody (MoAb CK2) recognizing cytokeratine component No. 18, appeared to be the most suitable reagent for the detection of epithelial tumor cells in bone marrow. Its specificity was confirmed in a double-marker assay (combination of APAAP-technique and radio-autography). CK2 positive cells were demonstrated not to reveal any cross-reactivity with an antibody directed against the "leucocyte common antigen" expressed on cells of hematopoetic origin. A significant correlation between the presence of epithelial tumor cells in bone marrow and certain conventional risk factors was found. A more detailed phenotypic characterization could demonstrate the expression of proliferation associated antigens on these cells. Furthermore, in an immunotherapeutic approach with monoclonal antibody 17-1A, labeling of the disseminated tumor cells on bone marrow after infusion of the antibody was shown.

Key words: Antibodies, monoclonal· Cytokeratine ·
            Micrometastases · Tumor markers

[1] This work was supported by Deutsche Krebshilfe, Wilhelm-Sander-Stiftung and Maria-Albrecht-Stiftung

INTRODUCTION

Early micrometastases, which occurs in certain carcinomas even before clinical diagnosis, poses a special challenge for oncology. While the majority of all primary tumors can be treated locally, present diagnostic and therapeutic methods fail in the case of early disseminated tumor cells. The therapeutic challenge posed by early micrometastases in the most common tumors, i.e. mammary, stomach and rectal carcinomas, has not been adequately met with conventional chemotherapy.

DIAGNOSIS OF EPITHELIAL TUMOR CELLS
IN BONE MARROW

Monoclonal antibodies can be used for the early diagnosis of single disseminated tumor cells. In a broad study, an attempt was made to detect the early hematogenic spread of tumor cells in mammary, stomch and colon carcinomas using monoclonal antibodies. Bone marrow has proved to be the most accessible place for such a search. In the investigations presented here, immune cytochemical and immune radioautographical methods were implemented to identify tumor cells in the bone marrow of patients with actually diagnosed tumors. Antibodies characterized by a high tissue specificity and recognizing a cytoskeleton component present in all tumor cells of epithelial origin were decisive for the success of these investigations. The selection of the antibody CK2, which reacts with a cytokeratine polypeptide (Polypeptide No. 18), proved to be especially suitable since this cytokeratine polypeptide occurs only in epithelial cells in the single layer of the epithel and represents an especially strong intercellular protein (1).
It could be concluded that cytokeratine positive cells are not present in patients with non-malignant diseases. For this purpose, the bone marrow of patients

with non-malignant diseases was examined in a series of 75 different aspirations with the same anti cytokeratine antibody. Cytokeratine positive cells of this type could not be immunocytologically detected in any of the aspirations using the APAAP-technique (2). Since cytokeratine positive cells were often detected with a frequency of only 10^{-5} in patients with mammary carcinoma or colorectal tumors, the next step was to methodically rule out a false positive reaction on such isolated cells. For this purpose a double-marker technique was developed combining an immunoenzymatical staining technique (APAAP) with immune radioautography using ^{125}Iodine labeled antibodies. By using an antibody against the "Leukocyte

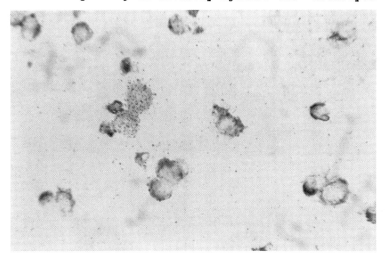

FIGURE 1. Double staining of bone marrow preparation after isolating the mononuclear cells with Ficoll-Hypaque-Density-Centrifugation. ^{125}Iod anti cytokeratine radioautography combined with anti T200 alkaline phosphatase staining.   Note, that the cytokeratine positive cells are T200 negative.

Common Antigen" (also called CD45 or T200), the question
was raised whether cytokeratine positive cells in bone
marrow simultaneously carry antigens of the hemopoetic
cell line. In a series of more than 30 patients it could
be shown that the CD45 antigen was detected in nearly 100%
of the mononuclear cells in bone marrow, but the
cytokeratine positive cells were consistently negative for
the CD45 antigen (see photograph). The origin of
cytokeratine positive cells from organ systems other than
the bone marrow was established.

    In a group of 155 patients with mammary carcinoma,
57 patients with colorectal carcinoma and 56 with stomach
carcinoma, cytokeratine positive cells could be identified
with varying frequency in bone marrow (Table 1).
    Since the biological and clinical implications of
tumor cells in bone marrow cannot be derived from their
presence alone, we attempted to evaluate the clinical
implications of disseminated cells in mammary carcinoma by
comparison with conventional risk factors.

TABLE 1
CYTOKERATINE POSITIVE CELLS IN THE BONE MARROW
OF TUMOR PATIENTS

Tumor	n	Positive Reactions	%
Mammary Ca	155	28	18,1
Colorectal Ca	57	12	21,0
Stomach Ca	56	18	32,1

TABLE 2
CORRELATION OF THE DETECTION OF CYTOKERATINE
POSITIVE CELLS IN BONE MARROW WITH CLINICAL
STAGES IN MAMMARY CARCINOMA

Conventional Risk factors	Cytokeratine cells in bone marrow
Stage M_0[a]	12/122 (9,8)
Stage M_1[b]	16/37 (43,2)
Stage M_0	
Tumor size $\leq$ 2 cm	2/47 (4,3)
Tumor size $>$ 2 cm	10/73 (13,7)
Stage M_0	
Lymph node negative	6/73 (8,2)
Lymph node positive	6/47 (12,8)
	n.s.

[a] No clinical detection of distant metastasis.
[b] Detection of distant metastasis.

As is shown in Table 2, the frequency of epithelial tumor cells can be correlated with risk factors such as spread to the regional lymph nodes, the size of the tumor and the detection of distant metastasis. The correlation with tumor size and distant metastasis were statistically significant.

COMPARISON OF CONVENTIONAL PROGNOSIS PARAMETERS

Since disseminated tumor cells in bone marrow are not homogenetically distributed, the correlation can be notably increased if bone marrow is aspirated in several locations. In a group of 20 patients with positive tumor cells, the influence of the number of aspirations on

cytokeratine positive cells was tested. Sixty-five percent
of the positive results were obtained from a one-sided
aspiraton at the iliac crest, whereas 95% were obtained
from a double-sided aspiration. The use of the
cytokeratine marker and double-sided aspiration at the
iliac crest guarantee reliable results. Increasing the
number of aspirations, as is sometimes recommended (3), is
not necessary for the cytokeratine method. For example, in
the case of stomach carcinoma, the clinical implications
of tumor cells can be emphasized by correlating the
prognostically varying histological forms of the tumor. As
is shown in Table 3, in the diffuse type of stomach
carcinoma according to the Laurén classification (4) the
detection of cytokeratine positive cells was significantly
more frequent than in the intestinal type of carcinoma.

TABLE 3

CORRELATION OF TUMOR CELL DETECTION IN BONE MARROW
AND HISTOLOGICAL TYPE OF STOMACH CARCINOMA

Histological Type according to Laurén [3]	Positive Reactions MAK CK2[a] (%)	
Intestinal Type	7/33	(21,2)
Diffuse Type	9/19	(47,4)
	$p < 0,05$	

[a] MAK CK2: monoclonal antibodies against the
cytokeratine component No. 18, which is expressed only in epithelial cells and their resulting tumors.

EXPRESSION OF PROLIFERATION-ASSOCIATED ANTIGENS

The double-marker technique, developed to establish the origin of cytokeratine positive cells from outside the bone marrow system is also useful for the characterisation of additional properties on these epithelial tumor cells. The main interest was to ascertain whether or not antigens are present in these cells which lead to an active proliferation. For this purpose, double staining was performed in a group of aspirations to detect the Transferrin Receptor, the Epidermal-Growth-Factor-Receptor (EGF-R) and the nuclear proliferation asssociated antigen Ki 67. As is shown in Table 4, antigens which are associated with active proliferation are present in a

TABLE 4
EXPRESSION OF PROLIFERATION ANTIGEN MARKERS ON
CYTOKERATINE POSITIVE MAMMARY TUMOR CELLS IN
BONE MARROW

Marker[a]	Positive Tumor cells	%
EGF-Receptor	10/37	27,0
Transferrin-Receptor	17/59	28,0
Ki 67	11/28	39,4

[a] Detection with commercial antibodies (Sebak, Dako, Dianova). For further explanation see text.

surprisingly high percentage of disseminated tumor cells. Figure 2 demonstrates the expression of the Transferrin

Receptor on a cytokeratine positive cell. First attempts
to expand this epithelial cell population out of the bone
marrow aspirates through in vitro cell culture have been
successful. Further more their true metastatic potential
could be demonstrated with the induction of tumor growth
in the nude mouse liver six weeks after transplantation
into the peritoneal cavity. In this case the cells were
derived from a patient with colorectal carcinoma having no
clinical evidence for distant metastasis.

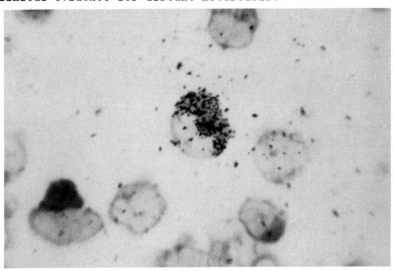

FIGURE 2. Expression of the transferrin-receptor
(stained in the APAAP-technique) on a cell of epithelial
origin as demonstrated through simultaneous staining with
the ^{125}J-labeled anti cytokeratin No. 18 antibody CK2.
Note that the surrounding bone marrow cells do not react
with mAb CK2.

OBSERVATION OF ADJUVANT THERAPY MEASURES

With the clear indication that these tumor cells play an important role in the process of metastasis, the next step was to determine whether monoclonal antibodies used in therapeutic approaches react with such cells in bone marrow. In a comparative study antibodies against the 17-1A antigen (5) were used. As is shown in Table 5, cytokeratine positive cells were stained with the anti 17-1A antibodies M77 and M79 (6). In conjunction with a

TABLE 5
CORRELATION BETWEEN ANTI CYTOKERATINE POSITIVE AND ANTI 17-1A POSITIVE TUMOR CELLS IN BONE MARROW

Tumor	n	Anti-cytokeratine positive	Anti-17-1A (M77 and M79)
Mammary carcinoma	50	11	5/11
Colorectal carcinoma	35	6	4/6

therapeutic study of the antibody 17-1A, it was possible to determine whether or not infused antibodies can reach disseminated tumor cells in bone marrow. in 3 out of 7 patients having cytokeratine positive cells and 17-1A positive cells before injection, it was shown that the infused 17-1A antibody (100-500mg/infusion) stained cells in the bone marrow (see Schlimok et al. [7]). This demonstrates that disseminated tumor cells in bone marrow are useful in passive antibody therapy. Of special interest is that the method described here for the early diagnosis of micrometastasis is suitable as well for the monitoring of an immunotherapeutic strategy.

AKNOWLEDGEMENTS

This work was supported by the Deutsche Krebshilfe, the Wilhelm-Sander-Stiftung and the Maria-Albrecht-Stiftung.

REFERENCES

1. Debus E, Moll R, Franke WW, Weber K, Osborn M (1984). Am J Pathol 114:121.
2. Cordell JL, Falini B, Erber WN, Ghosh AK, Abdulaziz Z, MacDonald S, Pulford KAF, Stein H, Mason DYJ (1984). Cytochem 32:219.
3. Redding HW, Coombes RC, Monaghan P, Clink HMD, Imrie SF, Dearnaley DP, Ormerod MG, Sloane JP, Gazet JC, Powles TJ, Neville AM (1983). Lancet II:1271.
4. Laurén P (1965). Acta path Microbiol Scand 64:31
5. Herlyn M, Steplewski Z, Herlyn D, Koprowski H (1979). Proc Natl Acad Sci USA 76:1438.
6. Göttlinger HG, Funke I, Johnson JP, Gokel JM, Riethmüller G (1986). Int. J Cancer 38:47.
7. Schlimok G, Funke I, Holzmann B, Göttlinger G, Schmidt G, Häuser H, Swierkot S, Warnecke HH, Schneider B, Koprowski H, Riethmüller G (1987). Proc Natl Acad Sci USA 84:8672.

Human Tumor Antigens and Specific Tumor Therapy, pages 209–219
© 1989 Alan R. Liss, Inc.

TARGETING FOR LYSIS BY CTL

Uwe D. Staerz

Basel Institute for Immunology[1]
Basel, Switzerland

ABSTRACT   An approach is discussed that uses antibody
constructs of dual specificity to target cells for
destruction by cytotoxic T lymphocytes (CTL). Heteroconjugated antibodies and hybrid antibodies, that focus
the T cell antigen receptor of CTL to antigens on any
chosen cells enable the destruction of these targets
as shown in vitro with virus infected cells and in vivo
with a tumor model system.

INTRODUCTION

Hybrid antibodies, composed of anti-T cell receptor and
anti-X antibodies, can confer the anti-X specificity of the
antibody to a cytotoxic T lymphocyte (CTL) response. This
technology is based on observations that antibodies reactive with any component of the T cell receptor (TCR)
complex can not only block all known functions of both
major T cell subsets (1-7) but under certain experimental
conditions can substitute for antigen-plus-MHC recognition
by the T lymphocyte. Clonotypic antibodies can drive proliferation of their corresponding T cell clone as well as
the release of interleukins (2,5,8). Antibodies reactive
with a broader T cell population, e.g. F23.1 and anti-CD3
reagents, activate resting peripheral T lymphocytes (9-13).
But, as in the case of cytotoxic T lymphocytes these
monoclonal antibodies can act as target structures for cell
mediated lysis. Whether they are carried on the surface of

[1]The Basel Institute for Immunology was founded and is
supported by F. Hoffmann-La Roche & Co. Limited.

a B hybridoma, inserted into the Fc receptor of a tumor
line or covalently fixed to the surface of a lymphoma they
always render this target susceptible to lysis by CTL
(14-17). After monoclonal antibodies against the TCR had
been defined as excellent targets for CTL recognition, the
hybrid antibody system was devised to enable these cellular
components of the immune system to act at diseased sites
without the complications imposed by MHC restriction
(17-20). Data will be presented that demonstrate the specificity and sensitivity of this approach, together with
its possible in vivo application to irradicate a lymphoma.

IN VITRO EXPERIMENTS

Heteroconjugates of Monoclonal Antibodies as Targeting
Agents.

    In one of the examined system targets could be discri-
minated on the basis of different expression of Fc receptors on their surface as attachment sites for the TCR
antibody, e.g. F23.1 (21). Thus, CTL can be specifically
focussed onto Fc receptor bearing cells, such as P815. The
exchange of the "IgGFc-to-Fc receptor" binding for a second
antibody created a construct that can focus a strong T cell
response to a wide variety of predetermined target cells.
The first heteroconjugated antibody examined for their
efficacy consisted of 19E12 (anti-Thy1.1) as targeting
antibody and either F9 (anti-idiotypic against CTL clone
G4) or F23.1 (anti-TCR Vβ8) as recruitment structure for
the CTL.
    As demonstrated in Table 1, the activity of the anti-
body heteroconjugate directly correlates to the specificity
of its components. Only if the TCR and the target antigen
is recognized by the antibody bridge, the CTL is triggered.
Thus, F9-19E12 can only recruit G4 [F9$^+$ F23.1$^-$] onto S.AKR
but not onto EL4, and F23-19E12 shows only activity for OE4
[F9$^-$ F23.1$^+$]. Real hybrid antibodies constructed by fusion
of B hybridomas secreting the parental antibodies have
corresponding characteristics. However, the specific activity of this material is much higher, so that hybrid antibody concentration as low as 0.5 ng/ml efficiently focus
CTL in vitro.
    Besides targeting tumors, one of the potential applica-
tions for hybrid antibody focussing of CTL is anti-viral
therapy. In a number of viral in vivo systems virus-

TABLE 1
ANTIGEN SPECIFIC TARGETING BY HETEROCONJUGATES

| Target[a] | Mediator | % specific release | |
		G4 Effector[a]	OE4 Effector[a]
EL4 [Thy1.2]	–	3	0
S.AKR [Thy1.1]	–	0	4
EL4	F9-19E12	8	2
EL4	F23-19E12	2	6
S.AKR	F9-19E12	62	2
S.AKR	F23-19E12	0	61

[a]The cloned CTL lines, G4 and OE4 (both H-2^b anti H-2^d) were used at effector target ratios of 6:1.
[b]The purified antibody, 19E12 specific for the Thy1.1 alloantigen was purified and coupled to F9, antiidiotype for G4 and F23.1 which reacts with the Vβ8 family, using the heterobifunctional cross-linked SPDP.

specific CTL seems to reduce the viral load of the animal, thus having beneficiary effects on the disease process. To examine the feasibility of the hybrid antibody approach in viral infection, we examined two systems. In the first, the VS virus, we produced heteroconjugates using the same antibodies against the TCR, F9 and F23.1, and as partner a monoclonal antibody, 8E11, specific for the VSV G protein that is known to be expressed on the surface of infected cells. Similar as in the previous example, the hetero-conjugates directed the lytic activity (Table 2). F9 encompassing heteroconjugates induced only G4, whereas F23.1 determined the activity of the CTL line 18D5 [F9⁻, F23.1⁺]. Although this experiment proved the feasibility of this technology in an in vitro viral system, it seemed necessary to examine at least a second system in more detail. In the influenza model, the specificity of targeting was tested using virus-strain specific monoclonal antibodies against hemagglutinin. Indeed, these constructs were able to distinguish between target cells infected with viruses of the two strains (18). However, it seemed more reasonable to attempt to aim at a virus structure with less strain variation than hemagglutinin, if one contemplates

Staerz

TABLE 2
HETEROCONJUGATES TARGET VIRUS INFECTED CELLS

Effector[a]	Target					
	EL4			EL4/VSV		
	−	F9-8E11[b]	F23-8E11[b]	−	F9-8E11	F23-8E11
G4	2[c]	12	8	4	58	0
18D5	1	−1	4	5	1	36

[a]The cloned CTL lines, G4 and 18D5 (both $H-2^b$ anti $H-2^d$) were used at effector target ratios of 13:1.
[b]The monoclonal antibody 8E11, which reacts with the G protein was bound to the TCR antibodies via SPDP.
[c]Values are given as % specific release.

adopting this model for therapeutic considerations. Nucleoprotein represents a very likely candidate. Although it is only expressed in very low abundance on infected cell surfaces it was, nevertheless, attempted to target CTL to this viral protein based on earlier results, suggesting that only a very small number of directly coupled antibodies were sufficient to recruit CTL. Prior to the killing assay, influenza virus [A/Puerto Rico/8/34]-infected cells were examined for surface expression of hemagglutinin and nucleoprotein via indirect immunofluorescence. As expected, large quantities of hemagglutinin could be detected on the cell surface by the monoclonal antibody 2A7, while staining for nucleoprotein resulted only in a very small shift compared to the background staining. Aliquots of the infected cells and uninfected cells were tested for antibody mediated lysis by two different hetero-constructs, F23-2A7 and F23-4B4. As could be expected from previous experiments, uninfected cells are not susceptible to lysis by OE4, either in the presence of the bivalent antibody or their unlinked constituents (Table 3). However, both heteroconjugates were equally efficient in targeting infected cells in spite of the much lower surface expression of nucleoprotein compared to hemagglutinin. In summary, the in vitro experiments demonstrate that bi-specific antibody constructs are powerfuul tools for targeting via a constitutive or a virally encoded marker,

TABLE 3

TARGETING SENSITIVITY OF VIRUS INFECTED CELLS

	Target	
Mediator	EL4	EL4/PR8[a]
F23 + 2A7 (αHA)[b]	18[c]	19
F23 + 4B4 (αNP)	17	15
F23 - 2A7	20	70
F23 - 4B4	16	62

[a]LE4 cells were infected with A/Puerto Rico/8/34 [HINI] prior to assay.
[b]The lymphomas were incubated either with a mixture of the monoclonal antibodies, F23.1 and IC5-2A7 (2A7, anti-hemagglutinin), F23.1 and IC6-4B4 (4B4, anti-nucleoprotein) or heteroconjugates of these antibodies at a final concentration of 500 ng/ml.
[c]The values are given as % specific release.

even if this surface structure can only be detected in very small numbers by conventional means.

IN VIVO EXPERIMENTS

Several groups have so far provided conclusive evidence that heteroconjugates of monoclonal antibodies were extremely efficient in vitro (17-20), it still had to be established whether this finding held true for in vivo models. Only then this technology would promise therapeutic applications. As heteroconjugates represent a rather unphysiological situation it was decided to produce bivalent antibodies with two distinct binding sites, i.e. hybrid antibodies. Since the behaviour of AKR/J-derived thymomas in AKR/Cu mice has been extensively studied as a tumor model, we exploited the allelic difference in Thyl as tumor markers. AKR/J carries Thyl.1 which is recognized by the monoclonal antibody 19E12 and the host, AKR/Cu bears the Thyl.2 allele. As shown in Table 1, heteroconjugates between F23.1 and 19E12 were very efficient in targeting

Thy1.1 bearing cells for lysis by F23.1$^+$ CTL. By fusing
the two hybridoma cell lines F23.1 and 19E12, both of which
secrete an IgG2a antibody, a hybrid hybridoma, H1.10.1.16,
was established which secretes a fraction of its total Ig
in the form of bispecific antibodies, composed of F23.1 and
19E12 chains that could be purified on a hydroxyapatite
high pressure liquid chromatography column (22). In control
experiments it was shown that the hybrid antibody shows the
exact behaviour as predicted from heteroconjugates of the
same components. Thus, the stable hybrid hybridoma line
provides a constant source of native, hybrid antibody.
Factors that determine the yield of the desired bispecific
antibodies have been discussed previously (22).

To determine the feasibility of hybrid antibody targeting in the AKR/Cu-AKR/J murine model systems, preliminary work was done in controlling the growth of two AKR/J-
derived [Thy1.1] thymomas in the genetically similar strain
AKR/Cu [Thy1.2] using the hybrid antibody H1.10.1.16 as
targeting agents. A lethal number of the AKR/J-derived
thymoma S.AKR was to be injected into the host, together
with the hybrid antibody H1.10.1.6. To provide active CTL,
the animals should either be primed with allogeneic cells,
or provided with in vitro activated alloreactive CTL in an
adoptive transfer. In both cases, approximately 25% of the
responding T cells would be positive for F23.1 and would be
able to bind the hybrid antibody. However, in titrating
S.AKR cells in AKR/Cu host, normal animals could resist
tumor growth. Prior irradiation was required to establish
a lethal tumor, since AKR/Cu mice are not truly congenic
with AKR/J. In the first tests of hybrid antibody targeting, AKR/Cu had to be sublethally irradiated before
injecting a dose of tumor which kills 90% of the animals.
As indicated in Figure 1, mice were irradiated on day 0,
followed by an i.v. injection of 10^5 S.AKR cells. On day 2
they received i.v. injections with either PBS, a mixture of
the two parental antibodies, or the purified hybrid antibody, H1.10.1.16. All antibodies were applied as F(ab')$_2$
preparations to prevent inference of Fc receptor bearing
cells that could capture the antibodies. Mixed lymphocyte
culture activated AKR/Cu cells were injected i.v. later on
the same day. The responses were boosted on day 9 with
allogeneic cells, and the antibody treatment was repeated
on day 12. Although the number of animals was very small,
the hybrid antibody treated animals showed a significant
better survival than either of the control groups (23).
In a second experimental set, the AKR/J-lymphoma SL2*

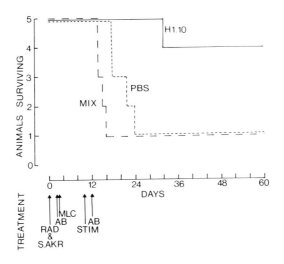

FIGURE 1 Young adult AKR/Cu (Thy1.2) female irradiated female mice irradiated on day 0 with 400r were i.v. injected with 10^5 S.AKR (Thy1.1) lymphoma cells. Animals were subsequently treated with purified H1.10.1.16 (-), with a mixture of 19E12 and F23 (-ı-), or PBS followed by $2x10^7$ cells of a 5 day mixed lymphocyte culture (AKR/Cu anti-C57Bl/6) with a 5 hour delay. Additional antibody was injected and the effector cell population was boosted as indicated. All antibodies were used as F(ab')$_2$ preparations at 18µg per animal and injection.

(provided by I.D. Bernstein) was chosen which had been selected for nonexpression of MHC molecules and, therefore, was not rejected by the AKR/Cu animals. SL2* was lethal within 24 days after i.v. injection of cell numbers as low as 10^3 cells without prior irradiation of the host. 10^5 SL2* cells were i.v. injected, followed by the hybrid antibody and mixed lymphocyte cells in 2 hour intervals (Figure 2). In addition the animals were treated as indicated in

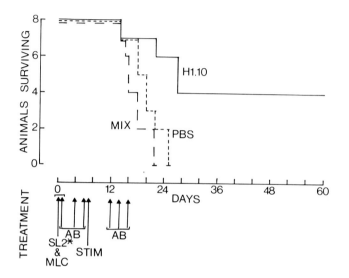

FIGURE 2   Similar as in the previous Figure, young adult AKR/Cu female mice used, but without prior irradiation since the AKR/J (Thy1.1) derived by lymphoma line SL2* does not bear MHC on its surface and is not subject to rejection by the host animal. The treatment protocol is indicated in the Figure.

the Figure. All mice that were only provided with PBS or unlinked antibodies died within 25 days after establishment of the tumor. However, 50% of the animals in the hybrid antibody group survived the regiment for more than 60 days. Again this experiment supports the idea that hybrid antibodies are active in vivo possibly protecting the animal from spread of the tumor.

DISCUSSION AND SUMMARY

It would be advantagous in the case of certain diseases to focus a T cell response at any chosen target, for example in treating cancer or infections that have evaded the normal host defence. However, at present it seems too difficult to conceive a situation when one could use antigen-specific lines or clones of effector cells due to complications of MHC restriction of T cell specificity and the problem of rejection of transplanted effector cell. It has previously been demonstrated that heteroconjugates of antibodies and hybrid antibodies can target cells for lysis by CTL without the interference of MHC molecules. As shown in Table 1, this effect is specific for the components of the bivalent construct rather than guided by the specificity of the CTL. In an extension of this system, virally encoded proteins provided as good an anchoring structure for bivalent constructs as constitutively synthesized cell surface structures. Even the nucleoprotein of influenza only expressed in very small abundance on the surface of infected cells proved to be an excellent site to focus CTL activity. Beyond the mere demonstration that basically any surface antigen can serve as a focus for hybrid antibody mediated lysis, an in vivo model system was explored that should give some information about the in vivo efficacy of hybrid antibodies. In these pilot studies it was demonstrated that hybrid antibodies can be effective in targeting tumors in vivo, most likely by the destruction mediated by CTL recruited to the disease foci. Although other activation markers found on T cells could possibly be used to induce resting T lymphocytes, it has to be established whether exogenously activated CTL always have to be transferred into the host (20). Furthermore, other in vivo systems, especially chronic infections, should be explored for the possible use of hybrid antibodies.

REFERENCES

1. Mauer SL, Fitzgerald KA, Hussey RE, Hodgdon JL, Schlossman SF and Reinherz EL (1983) Clonotypic structures involved in antigen-specific human T cell function. J Exp Med 157:705.
2. Haskins K, Kubo R, White J, Pigeon M, Kappler J and Marrack P (1983) The major histocompatibility complex-restricted antigen receptor on T cells. I.

Isolation with monoclonal antibody. J Exp Med 157: 1149.

3. Lancki DW, Lorber MI, Loken MR and Fitch FW (1983) A clone-specific monoclonal antibody that inhibits cytolysis of cytolytic T cell clone. J Exp Med 157:921.

4. Samuelson LE, Germain RN and Schwartz RH (1983) Monoclonal antibodies against the antigen receptor on a cloned T cell hybrid. Proc Natl Acad Sci USA 80:921.

5. Staerz UD, Pasternack MS, Klein JR, Benedetto JD and Bevan MJ (1984) Monoclonal antibodies specific for a murine cytoxic T-lymphocyte clone. Proc Natl Acad Sci USA 81:1799.

6. Landgren V, Ramstedt U, Axberg I, Ullberg M, Jondal M and Wigzell H (1982) Mechanisms of T lymphocyte activation by OKT3 antibodies. A general model for T cell induction. J Exp Med 15:1579.

7. Meuer SC, Hussey RE, Hodgdon JC, Hercend T, Schlossman SF and Reinherz EL (1982) Surace structures involved in target recognition by human cytotoxic T lymphocytes. Science 218:471.

8. Meuer SC, Hussey RE, Cantrell DA, Hodgdon JC, Schlossman SF, Smith KA and Reinherz EL (1984) Triggering of the T3-Ti antigen-receptor complex results in clonal T-cell proliferation through an interleukin 2 dependent autocrine pathway. Proc Natl Acad Sci USA 81:1509.

9. van Wauve FB, De May JR and Goosenes JG (1980) OKT3: A monoclonal anti-human T lymphocyte antibody with potent mitogenic properties. J Immunol 124:2708.

10. Chang TW, Kung PL, Gingras SP and Goldstein G (1981) Does OKT3 monoclonal antibody react with an antigen-recognition structure on human T cells?. Proc Natl Acad Sci USA 78:1805.

11. Burns GF, Boyd AW and Beverley PCL (1982) Two monoclonal anti-human T lymphocite antibodies have similar biologic effects and recognize the same cell surface antigen. Proc Natl Acad Sci USA 129:1451.

12. Lancki DW, Ma DI, Havran WF and Fitch FW (1984) Cell surface structures involved in T cell activities. Immunol Rev 81:65.

13. Staerz UD and Bevan MJ (1986) Activation of resting T lymphocytes by a monoclonal antibody directed against an allotypic determinant on the T cell receptor. Eur J Immunol 16:263.

14. Lancki DW and Fitch FW (1984) A cloned CTL demonstrates

different cell interaction requirements for lysis of two distinct target cells (Abstract). Fed Proc 43: 1659.

15. Hoffman RW, Bluestone JA, Oberdan L and Shaw S (1985) Lysis of anti-T3 bearing murine hybridoma cells by human allospecific cytotoxic T cell clones and inhibition of of that lysis by anti-T3 and anti-LFA1 antibodies. J Immunol 135:5.

16. Kranz DM, Tonegawa S and Eisen HN (1984) Attachment of an anti-receptor antibody to non-target cells renders them susceptible to lysis by a clone of cytotoxic T lymphocytes. Proc Natl Acad Sci USA 81:1922.

17. Staerz UD, Kanagawa O and Bevan MJ (1985) Hybrid antibodies can target sites for attack by T cells. Nature 314:628.

18. Staerz UD, Yewdell JW and Bevan MJ (1987) Hybrid antibody-mediated lysis of vitro-infected cells. Eur J Immunol 17:571.

19. Perez P, Hoffman RW, Shaw S, Bluestone JA and Segal DM (1985) Specific targeting of cytotoxic T cells by anti-T3 linked to anti-target cell antibody. Nature 316:354.

20. Jung G, Ledbetter JA and Müller-Eberhard HJ (1987) Induction of cytotoxicity in resting human T lymphocytes bound to tumor cells by antibody hetroconjugates. Proc Natl Acad Sci USA 84:4611.

21. Staerz UD and Bevan MJ (1985) Cytotoxic T lymphocyte-mediated lysis via the Fc receptor of target cells. Eur J Immunol 15:1172.

22. Staerz UD and Bevan MJ (1986) Hybrid hybridoma producing a bispecific monoclonal antibody which can focus effector T cell activity. Proc Natl Acad Sci USA 83:1453.

23. Staerz UD and Bevan MJ (1986) Use of anti-receptor antibodies to focus T cell activity. Immunol Today 128:241.

Human Tumor Antigens and Specific Tumor Therapy, pages 221–230
© 1989 Alan R. Liss, Inc.

INDUCTION OF LYSIS BY CROSSLINKED ANTIBODIES.

R.J. van de Griend,[1] J. van Dijk,[1] G.J. Fleuren,[1]
S.P. Goedegebuure[2] and R.L.H. Bolhuis,[2].

1) Department of Pathology, Wassenaarseweg 62
2300 RC Leiden. and 2) Dr. Daniel Den Hoed Cancer Center,
Groene Hilledijk 301, 3075 EA Rotterdam. The Netherlands.

ABSTRACT Antibodies can interfere with lytic processes in different ways. In "classic" antibody dependent cytolysis (ADCC), effector cells bind to Fc parts of antibodies on precoated target cells, which triggers the lytic machinery. Alternatively monoclonal antibodies (MAB) bound to an activation site on the effector cell can be bound by Fc receptor bearing target cells, resulting in cross linking and triggering the lytic process. Bispecific Heteroagregates off two MAB can bind both effector and target cells and trigger cytolysis and hence do not require FcR. The same occurs with bispecific MAB produced after fusion of CD3 and G250 (anti-kidney) hybridoma cells. Such bispecific antibodies were found to induce lysis at relative low concentrations and may therefore represent effective and selective reagents for immunotherapy in combination with activated CTL.

INTRODUCTION

MAB have been used to induce or enhance cytolytic activities by human cytotoxic lymphocytes (CTL). The best studied antibody-antigen interactions is that of anti-CD3 MAB to CD3 antigen. The CD3 antigen is physically associated with the T cell receptor (TCR) heterodimer (1). When the TCR binds to its complementary antigen on the target cell, the CD3 molecule delivers a signal that activates the T cell (2,3,4). Some anti-CD3 MAB deliver the same activating signal leading to cell proliferation, lymphokine production and cytotoxicity. Thus, these MAB mimic the activation that occurs upon TCR-antigen recognition (for review see 5). In addition, anti-CD3 MAB can induce cytolysis directly, provided that the target cell, expresses relevant IgG-Fc receptors, resulting in crosslinking of effector and target cell. Human CTL can be functionally and phenotypicaly divided in three categories.

1. "Classic" T cells, which show functional rearrangement of T cell receptor α and β chain genes, are $CD3^+ TCR\alpha\beta^+ FcR^-$.

2. A subset of T cells, expressing TCRγ and δ proteins and are $CD3^+ 4^- 8^- 16^+$ (6,7).

3. NK cells which are $TCR^- / CD3^- 16^+$ (8).

Several MAB recognizing activation sites present on one or more types of these cytotoxic effector cells have now been defined, for instance CD2,CD3,CD16 and CD28. However all these types of antibody induced cytotoxicity require. IgG-FcR on effector cells or on target cells (2)). Since most tumour cells do not express IgG-FcR receptors, we have developed bispecific antibodies, either chemically by crosslinking the Fc parts of two different MAB described by Karpovski (9) as well as bispecific MAb's generated by somatic hybridization of mouse hybridoma's described by Staerz (10). The bispecific antibodies bridge the effector cells to the target cells and simultaneously activate the T cells for instance their lytic machinery.

MATERIALS AND METHODS.

Cloning and expansion of cytotoxic lymphocytes.

T cell clones were derived from PBL by limiting dilution in round-bottomed microtiter plates with feeder cells as described in detail elsewhere (11) in the presence of lectin (leucoagglutinin, 1.0 ug/ml. To each well, 2×10^4 irradiated (20 GY) allogeneic PBL and 10^4 irradiated lymphoblastoid B-cell line (B-LCL) feeder cells were added (11). $CD3^-$ and $CD3^+$ clones were expanded by seeding 1000-3000 responder cells/well in the presence of leucoagglutinin and feeder cells. Clones were replated with new feeder cells weekly (2, 8, 11). The following clones and cell lines were tested: $TCR^- CD2^+ CD3^-$ NK cells cultured in bulk, obtained from $CD3^- CD16^+$ ($B73.1^+$) cells, purified by fluorescence activated cell sorting (purity 90% ($B73.1^+$

cells) without further cloning. TCRαβ$^+$CD3$^+$8$^+$16$^-$ clone CAK-11 and clone CTL9 were primed against B-LCL. Two TCRγδ$^+$/CD3$^+$ clones were tested: AK4, and AK925. These clones lack CD4 as well as CD8 antigens (6,7) express to some extend CD16 (IgG-FcR) and exert nonspecific cytolytic activity against a variety of tumour target cells and also exert antibody dependent cellular cytotoxicity (ADCC).

Target cells

The following tumour cell lines were used as target: K562, an erythro-myeloid cell line commonly used for the determination of NK cell activity; the T cell line MOLT; five B Cell lines, i.e., Daudi, Raji (Burkitt lymphoma), B cell leukemia (Capel, Nijmegen), LICR-LON (Leukemia plasma cell) and two EBV transformed B cell lines (B-LCL) APD and BSM. The latter two cells were also routinely used as feeder cells for the expansion of T clones (see above). One cell line derived from small cell lung carcinoma: (GLC2), A melanoma derived cell line IGR37; a renal cell carcinoma derived cell line A704, P815 mouse mastocytoma cells as well as normal fibroblast.

Antibody dependent cellular cytotoxicity.

Heteroaggregates were prepared between anti-CD2 (OKT11) or anti-CD3 (OKT3) MAb of IgG1 and IgG2a subclass, respectively, and rabbit anti-DNP IgG antibodies. The procedure has been described in detail elsewhere (9).
    Cytotoxicity assay was performed in round-bottom microtiter plates (Greiner). Briefly, varying numbers of viable effector cells were seeded to the wells before the addition of 100 µl ^{51}Cr-labelled target cells (10^3). Plates were incubated for 3 hr at 37°C, centrifuged, 100 µl of supernatant was collected, radioactivity was determined, and specific ^{51}Cr release was calculated. The effect of MAb, heteroaggregates and bispecific antibodies on lytic activity was determined as follows: Classical ADCC was performed by preatreatment of P815 or LICRON target cells with anti-P815 or anti human tumour antisera before assay. Anti-CD3 antibodies were tested by adding them to effector cells 30 minutes before target cells were added.

RESULTS.

"Classic" ADCC.

ADCC is defined as cytolytic activity exerted by IgG-FcR expressing Killer (K) cells against target cells coated by IgG antibody. For instance mouse mastocytoma P815 cells, or human leukemiaplasma cell derived cell line LICRON preatreated with appropiate rabbit IgG. In fig. 1 we have compared different types of cultured effector cells. $CD3^-$ TCR^- cells exert strong ADCC, activity, also et low (3:1) effector to target cell ratio's. Although some $CD3^+TCR\gamma\delta^+$ cells also exert ADCC, lytic activity is lower on a per cell basis. In addition ADCC activity is hardly detectable in other $CD3^+TCR\gamma\delta$ cells. It is likely that the density of IgG-FcR on the effector cells plays a role since $CD3^-$ cells show a more intensive staining with anti CD16 MAB; both B73.1 and VD2 are bound whereas most cloned $CD3^+$ $TCR\gamma\delta^+$ cells bind VD2 to some extend but virtually not B73.1. "Classic" ADCC activity is not exerted by $CD3^+TCR\alpha\beta^+FcR^-$ cells.

Induction of lysis by $CD3^+TCR\alpha\beta^+FcR^-$ cells using anti-CD3 MAB.

Binding of anti-CD3 MAB to CTL is known to result in blocking of lytic function, for instance MHC restricted lysis by clone CTL9 of its specific MHC class I Cw3 target cell BSM (fig. 2). However, when a target cell,which is not recognized by the effector cell, has IgG-FcR, it can bind the Fc portion of for instance the CD3 MAB which results in bridging of effector to target cells. The overal result is than enhancement (K562) or induction (Daudi) of cytolysis, rather than inhibition (fig.2). It is necessary that the MAB recognizes a cell surface structure that is involved in T cell activation ("activation site") e.g. CD2,CD3,CD16 or CD28 on the effector cell and that the target cell expresses IgG-FcR appropriate for binding the IgG subclass of the antibody.

ANTIBODY DEPENDENT CELLULAR CYTOTOXICITY

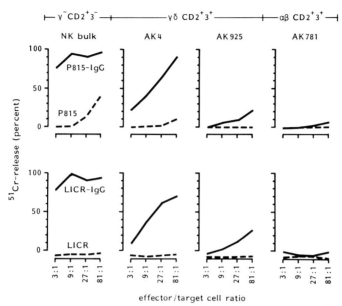

Fig 1   "Classic" ADCC by CD3⁻TCR⁻ NK cells and CD3⁻TCRγδ
clones using rabbit-IgG coated P815 (top) or LICRON
(bottom) cells.

INDUCTION OF LYSIS BY ANTI-CD3 X ANTI-DNP HETEROAGGREGATES.

Anti-CD3 x anti-DNP AB-heteroaggregates were tested for
their capacity to induce AB-lysis of TNP treated GLC2 (small
cell lung carcinoma derived) tumour cells. Clone CAK11,
which by itself does not lyse GLC2 cells, was incubated with
various amounts of anti-CD3 x anti-DNP heteroaggregates.
Concentrations as low as 0.01 µg/ml were found to be
effective to induce lysis of TNP treated target cells (fig
3). At higher concentrations (up to 5.0 µg ml), induction
was more efficient. Anti-CD3 MAB or TNP treatment of target
cells alone had no effect and non-TNP treated target cells
were also not affected by the AB-heteroaggregates. Next we
studied a number of tumour target cells for susceptability
of lysis by anti-CD3 x anti-DNP AB-heteroaggregates. As
shown in table 1 lysis was induced against various TNP
treated tumour cels of different histogenetic origin
including K562 but also against normal fibroblasts. Similar
results were obtained with CD3 cells with the TCRγδ
receptor. Anti-CD2 x anti-DNP AB-heteroaggregates were only
effective when IgG-FcR positive K562 target cells were used.
Therefore involvement of the FcR could not be excluded.

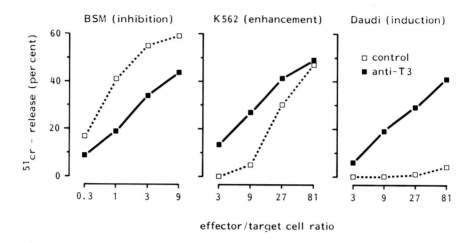

Fig 2 Anti-CD3 MAB inhibit allospecific lysis clone CTL9
against BSM but can induce non specific lysis against
IgG-FcR bearing target cells (e.g. K562 or Daudi
cells).

Table 1

INDUCTION OF LYSIS BY ANTI-CD3 X ANTI-DNP HETEROAGGREGATES.

Target cells

additions[1]	K562	MOLT	Raji	Leuk.	B cell mel IGR37	fibro- blast
clone CAK11						
none	23	0	0	5	0	0
CD2/DNP	42	6	0	0	2	0
CD3/DNP	66	53	58	35	25	32
clone AK4						
none	11	9	19	0	15	13
CD3/DNP	60	52	66	35	26	36

Results expressed as %[51] Cr-release. Effector to
target cell ratio 9:1. Tumour target cells were pretreated
with TNP for 15 min. [1] 0.1 µg/ml AB-hetero-aggregates.

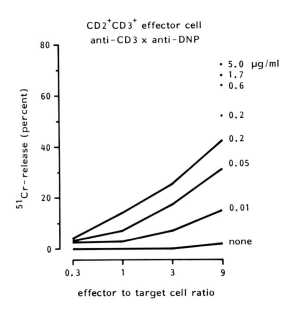

Fig3   Induction of cytolysis using anti-CD3 x anti-DNP
        heteroaggregates effector cells (clone CAK 11) were
        preincubated with the hetero-antibodies. Target cells
        (GLC 2) were ^{51}CR-labeled and treated with TNP (3mM,
        100µl/10^{5} cells) for 15 min at 37°C, washed and added
        to the assay.

CROSSLINKING OF EFFECTOR AND TARGET CELLS USING BISPECIFIC MAB
(OKT3 AND G250).

Bispecific MAB were developed by somatic hybridization of two
mouse hybridoma's producing OKT3 (IgG2) and G250 (IgG1)
respectively (against a renal cell carcinoma (RCC) associated
antigen (12). Hybrid MaB produced by these quadromas were
tested for their capacity to induce cytolytic activity by
CD3^{+} CTL (CAK11 and CTL9) against RCC cell line A704. As
shown in table 2, 26 out of 30 culture supernatants reacted
with both CD3 positive as well as G250 positive cells, were
capable to induce cytolysis up to 64% ^{51}Cr-release, of A704
RCC cells by clones CAK11 and CTL9. G250 MAB alone had no
effect whereas anti-CD3 MAB alone, as expected, was slightly
inhibitory.

Table 2.

Antibodies	induction of lysis	EFFECTOR CELLS CD3$^+$/TCRαβ		
		CAK11		CTL9
		expl	exp2	expl
CONTROLS				
None		11	2	9
G250		9	0	10
CD3		5	0	11
Bispecifics				
G250/CD3	+	34-52	9-28	29-64
		(n=6)	(n=26)	(n=26)
	−	7	1	3-9
		(n-1)	(n=4)	(n=4)

Results as % ^{51} Cr-release

DISCUSSION

Cytolysis can be triggered using (monoclonal) antibodies. Triggering of lysis can only occur after bridging target to effector cells by the antibody. This may result from one type of cell bound to the FAB portion of the MAB and the other cell via interaction with an FcR with subclass specificity for the IgG. In "classic" ADCC precoated target cells are recognized by IgG-FcR$^+$ effector cells. In case of FcR$^+$ target cells the FAB of the MAB must be directed against an "activation site" on the effector cells, for instance anti-CD3. The use of AB-heteroaggregates or bispecific antibodies enables to circumvent the requirement of IgG-FcR. CD3 proved to be an efficient "activation site". When crosslinked to anti-DNP antibodies efficient lysis of TNP treated target cells was observed by CD3$^+$ TCRαδ as well as by CD3$^+$ TCRγδ cells. Bispecific AB reagents used here, anti-CD$_3$ (IgG2a) x anti-G250 (IgG-1), proved to be very efficiently induce cytolysis by CD3$^+$TCRαβ as well as by CD3$^+$TCRγδ clones against kidney tumour derived cell line A704 (van Dijk et al submitted for publication). Dual specificity of the hybrid MAb's was confirmed by immuno histochemistry on tissue sections. Subclass identity between the fusion partners is not a prerequisite. In fact bispecific antibodies generated using heavy chain isotype switch variants of G250 e.g. IgG2a, IgG2 did not improve the results. Two IgG2a/IgG1 combinations were tested in more detail after purification by protein A and separation by ion-exchange chromatography (van Dijk et al, submitted for publication). Up to 40% of the antibody indeed showed dual specificity and the rest was mainly of parental origin.

Because bispecific antibodies are highly specific and active at low concentrations especially with activated effector cells, such antibodies may be of great value in combination with other types of immunotherapy.

REFERENCES

1. Meuer SC, Fitzgerald KA, Hussey RE, Hodgdon JC, Schlossman SF, Reinherz EL (1983). Clonotypic structures involved in antigen specific human T cell function: relationship to the T3 molecular complex. J Exp Med 157:705.

2. Bolhuis RLH, van de Griend RJ (1985). Phytohemagglutinin-induced proliferation and cytolytic activiy in T3$^+$ but not in T3$^-$ cloned T lymphocytes requires the involvement of the T3 antigen for signal transmission. Cell. Immunol 93:46.

3. Reinherz EL, Meuer SC, Schlossman SF (1983). The human T cell receptor: analysis with cytotxic T cell clones. Immunol Rev 74:83

4. Spits H, Yssel H, Leeuwenberg J, de Vries JE (1985). Antigen-specific cytotoxic T cell and antigen-specific proliferating T cell clones can be induced to cytolytic activity by monoclonal antibodies against T3. Eur J Immunol 15:88

5. Bolhuis RLH, Gravekamp C, van de Griend RJ (1986). Cell-cell interactions. In Clinics in immunology and allergy. Vol 6:29-90.

6. van de Griend RJ, de Bruin HG, Rumke HG, van Doorn, Roos D, Astaldi A (1982). Isolation and partial characterization of a novel subset of human T-lymphocytes defined by monoclonal antibodies. Immunology Vol 47:313-320.

7. van de Griend RJ, Tax WJM, van Krimpen BA, Vreugdenhil RJ, Ronteltap CPM, bolhuis RLH (1987). Lysis of tumor cells by CD3$^+$4$^-$8$^-$16$^+$ T cell receptor $\alpha\beta^-$ clones, regulated via CD3 and CD16 activation sites, recombinant interleukin 2, and interferon β. J Immunol 138:1627.
8. van de Griend RJ, van Krimpen BA, Ronteltap CPM, Bolhuis RLH (1984). Rapidly expanded activated human killer cell clones have strong antitumor cell activity and have the surface phenotype of either T gamma, T-non-gamma, or null cells. J Immunol Vol 132:3185-3191.
9. Karpovsky B, Titius JA, Stephany DA, Segal DM (1984). Production of target-specific effector cells using hetero-cross-linked containing anti-target cell and anti-Fc gamma receptor antibodies. J Exp Med 160:1686
10. Staerz UD, Kanagawa O, Bevan MJ (1985). Hybrid antibodies can target sites for attack by T cells. Nature 314:628.
11. van de Griend RJ, Bolhuis RLH (1984). Rapid expansion of all specific cytotoxic T cell clones using nonspecific feeder cell lines without further addition of exogenous IL-2. Transplantation Vol 38:401-406.
12. Oosterwijk E, Ruiter DJ, Hoedemaeker PhJ, Pauwels EKJ, Jonas U, Zwartendijk J, Warnaar SO (1986). Monoclonal antibody G 250 recognizes a determinant present in renal-cell carcinoma and absent from normal kidney. Int J Cancer 38:489-494.

Human Tumor Antigens and Specific Tumor Therapy, pages 231–241
© 1989 Alan R. Liss, Inc.

IMMUNOTOXINS CONTAINING POKEWEED ANTIVIRAL PROTEIN AGAINST B-LINEAGE RESTRICTED CD19 AND HMW-BCGF RECEPTORS FOR CELL-TYPE SPECIFIC ANTI-LEUKEMIC IMMUNOTHERAPY IN HUMAN B-LINEAGE ACUTE LYMPHOBLASTIC LEUKEMIAS[1]

Fatih M. Uckun[2], Dorothea Myers, Julian Ambrus, and James D. Irvin

Tumor Immunology Laboratory, Depts. of Therapeutic Radiology-
Radiation Oncology, Pediatrics, and
Bone Marrow Transplantation Program, UMHC, Minneapolis, MN ;
Laboratory of Immunoregulation, NIAID, Bethesda, MD;
Dept. of Chemistry, Southwest Texas State University, San Marcos, TX

ABSTRACT Immunotoxins against B-lineage restricted CD19 and HMW-BCGF receptors were prepared by covalently linking B43 and BA-5 monoclonal antibodies to the ribosome inhibitory protein PAP. Both immunotoxins are effective against leukemic B-lineage ALL progenitor cells and show potential for specific leukemia therapy in B-lineage ALL. While further studies are required to elucidate the immunotherapeutic potential of BA-5-PAP, extensive preclinical studies have demonstrated the clinical potential of B43-PAP in B-lineage ALL for 1) ex vivo elimination of residual leukemic progenitor cells from autologous bone marrow grafts as well as 2) more effective pretransplant conditioning and systemic treatment.

[1]This work was supported in part by R29 CA 42111, R01 CA 42633, P01 CA 21737 awarded by the National Cancer Institute, Special Grants from Minnesota Medical Foundation, Bone Marrow Transplantation Program Research Fund, Children's Cancer Research Fund, and Organized Research Funds from the State of Texas. F. M. Uckun is Recipient of a FIRST Award from the National Cancer Institute and Special Fellow of the Leukemia Society of America. This is publication #12 from the Tumor Immunology Laboratory, University of Minnesota.

[2]Address correspondence to : Fatih M. Uckun, M.D., Tumor Immunology Laboratory, Box 356 UMHC, Harvard Street at East River Road, Minneapolis, MN 55455.

INTRODUCTION

Acute lymphoblastic leukemia is the most frequent malignancy in childhood, accounting for 30% of childhood cancer. Chemotherapy is the primary treatment for ALL and introduction of multiagent chemotherapy has resulted in prolonged-disease free survival for many ALL patients. However, despite major improvements in the rate of initial achievement of remission by intensive induction chemotherapy, recurrence of leukemia is still encountered by a significant number of patients. For patients who relapse while receiving maintenance chemotherapy or shortly after elective cessation of chemotherapy, subsequent treatment has been unsatisfactory. Although second complete remissions are usually attained, the median duration of such remissions has been less than 6 months, and the 2-4 year disease free survival rates are below 10% in most series. Bone marrow transplantation (BMT), generally using marrow grafts from matched sibling donors, has been successfully applied for poor risk ALL. Data from several groups have demonstrated that BMT combined with high dose chemotherapy and radiation therapy improves the long-term survival of poor risk ALL patients. However, despite pretransplant total body irradiation combined with high dose chemotherapy, recurrence of leukemia remains a major obstacle in BMT for ALL. In a more recent study at our institution, which compared autologous and allogeneic BMT for treatment of high risk refractory ALL, 91% of primary failures in the autologous group and 55% of primary failures in the allogeneic group were due to leukemic relapse. This high rate of relapse indicates that the residual leukemic cells in heavily treated ALL patients are resistant to chemoradiotherapy. Currently, the major challenge in BMT for ALL for the coming years is the development of novel and more effective pretransplant conditioning strategies (1). Similarly, the major challenge in the chemotherapy of ALL is the development of novel and more effective induction and maintanence protocols. We believe that the application of immunotoxins, i.e., monoclonal antibody toxin conjugates will provide a unique opportunity for highly efficient eradication of drug-radiation resistant leukemic blasts.

Immunotoxins (monoclonal antibody-toxin conjugates) represent sophisticated immunopharmacologic weaponry with a superb capacity to eradicate specific populations of target cells and provide a unique opportunity for highly efficient as well as innovative search and destroy tactics against leukemia cells bearing the target surface antigens (2, 3). The variety of toxins that have been employed by various investigators can be broadly categorized into two groups. The first group consists of intact toxins, such as intact ricin. Ricin consists of two 30 kDa subunits. The A chain is a potent catalytic enzyme that inhibits ribosomal protein synthesis. One ricin A chain molecule can inactivate as many as 1,500 ribosomes per minute, and a single molecule in the cytosol can kill a cell. The B chain of ricin recognizes non-reducing terminal galactose residues on cell surfaces and facilitates A chain entry. We have used intact ricin immunotoxins for 1) ex vivo elimination of alloreactive T cells from donor marrow grafts for GVHD prophylaxis in allogeneic BMT (4), and 2) ex vivo elimination of residual leukemic cells from autologous marrow grafts of ALL patients (5-8). Although intact ricin immunotoxins are highly effective destroyers for their target cells, they cannot be applied for in vivo treatment of leukemia because of the nonselectivity of their B chain moiety. The second group of toxins are referred to as hemitoxins. Hemitoxins are single-chain ribosome inactivating proteins that act catalytically on eukaryotic ribosomes and inactivate the 60-S subunit, resulting in an irreversible shut-down of cellular protein synthesis at the level of peptide elongation. Such polypeptide toxins have been isolated from pokeweed (Phytolacca americana), bitter gourd (Momordica charantia), wheat (Tritium vulgaris), soapwort (Saponaria officinalis), Gelonium multiflorum, and sevaral other plants. Since these ribosome inactivating proteins, unlike intact ricin, do not have a B chain subunit with nonselective cell binding capacity, they cannot easily cross the cellular membrane. Therefore, hemitoxins are practically devoid of toxicity to intact eukaryotic cells. Hemitoxins can acquire a potent and highly specific site-directed cytotoxic activity by linkage to monoclonal antibodies. The hemitoxin-containing immunotoxins bind target cells solely via the specific monoclonal antibody moiety of the conjugate and are therefore very attractive for in vivo use. Over the past six years, our laboratory has investigated the therapeutic potential of immunotoxins containing pokeweed antiviral protein (hemitoxin isolated from Phytolacca americana, PAP) in the treatment of lymphoid malignancies (9-13). Similar to other hemitoxins, PAP enzymatically inactivates the 60S subunit of eukaryotic ribosomes (14). At least 3 different species of PAP exist that are isolated from spring leaves (PAP), late summer leaves (PAP-II), and seeds (PAP-S) of pokeweed. These species differ in their amino acid compostions, are immunologically distinct, and do not cross-react with specific antibodies. They all have molecular weights of approximately 30 kDa and are equally potent inhibitors of protein synthesis in cell free translation assays. A potential problem in using immunotoxins in vivo is related to the presence of carbohydrate residues in the toxin moieties. Reticuloendothelial cells including Kupffer cells in the liver express receptors for carbohydrates which may result in rapid clearance and short activity of immunotoxins as well as a significant liver toxicity. In this regard PAP immunotoxins are of special interest because they lack carbohydrate residues. Another potential problem is the production of anti-toxin antibodies by the host. PAP immunotoxins are attractive since in case of an anti-toxin antibody response to PAP one could switch to one of the 2 remaining non-crossreactive alternative toxin species and retain the efficacy of the immunotoxin therapy.

The vast majority of ALLs are B-lineage ALL cases which are defined by their characteristic surface antigen profiles. Extensive immunological surface marker analyses using monoclonal antibodies have demonstrated that human B-lineage ALL is a heterogeneous group of diseases (15, 16).

For a candidate immunotoxin to be of therapeutic value in the treatment of B-lineage ALL, it must be reactive with the majority of self-renewing clonogenic blasts, referred to as leukemic progenitor cells. Currently, very little is known about the surface antigen profiles of leukemic progenitor cells in B-lineage ALL. Given the high degree of heterogeneity in B-lineage ALL, the immunopheno-type of the bulk population may not predict the immunophenotype of leukemic progenitor cells.

Our recent studies have provided the evidence that the bulk population of ALL blasts as well as B-lineage leukemic progenitor cells express CD19 and HMW-BCGF receptors. Herein, we report our findings to date on 1) the expression of functional CD19 and HMW-BCGF receptors in human B-lineage ALL and 2) the anti-leukemic efficacy of PAP immunotoxins directed against these progenitor cell associated molecules.

RESULTS AND DISCUSSION

Expression and Function of CD19 Receptor in B-lineage ALL: CD19 is a B-lineage specific surface receptor protein. Recently, we studied the expression of CD19 on leukemic blasts from 340 leukemia patients using B43 (anti-CD19, IgG1, kappa) monoclonal antibody (17). B43 reacted with 99.6% of B-lineage ALL cases but it did not react with T-lineage leukemias or acute non-lymphocytic leukemias (17). Using fluorescence activated cell sorting and colony assays, we have shown that the CD19 receptor is expressed on leukemic progenitor cells from B-lineage ALL patients as well as their early progeny in B-cell growth factor stimulated in vitro cell cultures (17, 18). CD19 antigen is a functionally important receptor which may play a key role in regulation of the proliferative activity of B-lineage leukemic progenitor cells. We have previously demonstrated that 1) quantitative CD19 antigen expression in B-lineage ALL correlates with the cloning efficiency of leukemic B-cell precursors (16), 2) a close correlation also exists between DNA synthesis activity in leukemic B-cell precursors and their level of surface CD19 expression (16), 3) crosslinking of the CD19 receptor with B43 monoclonal antibody induces increases in cytoplasmic free calcium in leukemic B-cell precursors and augments the B-cell growth factor induced $[Ca^{2+}]i$ responses, indicating that the putative natural ligand of the CD19 receptor may exert critical growth regulatory effects by inducing calcium mobilization (19), 4) ligation of the CD19 receptor on leukemic B-cell precursors mediates a positive proliferative signal (19). Our recent comparative studies on the functional properties of the CD19 receptor on leukemic versus normal B-cell precursors prompted the hypothesis that the CD19 receptor and/or CD19-linked signal transmission pathways may be altered during leukemogenesis in human B-lineage ALL. This hypothesis is based on two observations: 1) CD10$^+$CD19$^-$ normal B-lineage lymphoid progenitor cells do not have leukemic counterparts- i.e., CD19$^-$ leukemic B-cell precursors do not display progenitor cell characteristics and are not capable of self-renewal and proliferation, 2) crosslinking the CD19 receptor augments the proliferative activity of leukemic B-cell precursors but inhibits the proliferation of normal B-cell precursors and activated mature B lymphocytes (F. M. Uckun & J. A. Ledbetter, submitted for publication).

CD19 is not expressed on normal bone marrow progenitor cells CFU-GM, BFU-E, CFU-MK, or CFU-GEMM (17). Furthermore, B43 (anti-CD19) MoAb does not crossreact with T-lymphocytes, granulocytes, macrophages/monocytes, erythrocytes, platelets, or with normal non-hematopoietic tissues including the liver, intestine, stomach, kidney, prostate, lung, brain, thyroid, adrenal gland, ovary, breast, blood vessels, and muscles (17). These findings on the expression profile of the CD19 receptor indicate that anti-CD19 monoclonal antibodies such as B43 show considerable potential as cell-type specific carriers of toxins for selective destruction of leukemic B-cell precursors and most importantly their clonogenic fraction, i.e., leukemic progenitor cells.

Expression and Function of HMW-BCGF Receptors in B-lineage ALL: Several hematopoietic growth factors have been described that influence proliferation of human B-lineage cells. These include B-cell growth factors (BCGF) ranging in molecular weight from 10-60 kDa. BCGFs are produced by normal B and T lymphocytes, B-lineage and T-lineage lymphomas, T-cell hybridomas and clones, and EBV transformed B lymphocytes. In a recent study we analyzed the expression of BCGF receptors in B-lineage ALLs (18). The specific binding of ^{125}I labeled high molecular weight (HMW) and low molecular weight (LMW) BCGFs to leukemic B-cell precursors was investigated in standard ligand binding assays. The estimated median values for the cell-bound BCGF molecules were 3,500 molecules/cell for HMW-BCGF and 37,400 molecules/cell for LMW-BCGF (18). Although we were unable to determine the receptor numbers in Scatchard analyses because of the limited number of cells available, our findings provided direct evidence for constitutive expression of surface BCGF receptors on leukemic B-cell precursors. The proliferative responses of leukemic B cell precursors to BCGFs were determined in ^{3}H-TdR incorporation as well as colony assays to assess the function of the detected receptors. Both HMW-BCGF and LMW-BCGF stimulated the proliferative activity of leukemic B-cell precursors in the majority of B-cell precursor ALLs (18). This stimulation was mediated directly by BCGFs and not by other growth factors released from accessory cells, since the response patterns of virtually pure populations of FACS sorted leukemic B-cell precursors were essentially identical to the proliferative responses of unsorted leukemic B-cell precursors (18). Synergistic effects were observed in 80% of the cases that responded to both HMW-BCGF and LMW-BCGF contending that HMW-BCGF and

LMW-BCGF 1) most likely bind to different surface receptors on leukemic B-cell precursors, and 2) can lower the threshold for mitogenicity of each other. The ability of BCGFs to stimulate blast colony formation provided unique evidence that leukemic progenitor cells in B-lineage ALL express functional BCGF receptors. Since BCGF receptors are expressed on the bulk population as well as the clonogenic fraction of leukemic B-cell precursors, immunotoxins directed against BCGF receptors might provide an effective means of specific tumor therapy for B-lineage ALL.

Recently, Ambrus et al. described a monoclonal antibody (BA-5) which recognizes a B-lineage specific surface molecule intimately associated with the HMW-BCGF receptor (20). This antibody was produced by immunizing mice with a HMW-BCGF responsive B-cell line and initially identified by its ability to specifically block the HMW-BCGF induced proliferation of normal activated B-cells. Binding of radioiodinated HMW-BCGF to activated B cells indicated a 90 kDa receptor protein and Western blot analysis with BA-5 and an anti-HMW-BCGF monoclonal antibody provided the evidence that BA-5 recognizes this receptor protein for HMW-BCGF. Furthermore, BA-5 inhibited binding of HMW-BCGF to its receptor in both functional assays as well as ligand binding assays. Hence, BA-5-reactive epitope of the HMW-BCGF receptor is probably very close to the ligand binding site. We are currently investigating the immunoreactivity profile of BA-5 monoclonal antibody with malignant as well as normal human tissues as well as its relationship to other B-cell directed monoclonal antibodies. The availability of this novel monoclonal antibody reactive with a functional growth factor receptor on leukemic progenitor cells prompted us to prepare an anti-HMW-BCGF receptor immunotoxin containing PAP.

Immunotoxins against CD19 and HMW-BCGF Receptors: Immunotoxins against CD19 and HMW-BCGF receptors were produced by conjugation of B43 and BA-5 monoclonal antibodies to PAP. Specifically, we used the crosslinking agent SPDP to introduce a disulfide bond into the monoclonal antibodies via the primary amino groups. 2-iminothiolane was used to introduce reactive sulfhydryl groups into the toxin moieties following reaction with primary amino groups. A thiol disulfide exchange reaction between the 2-pyridyl disulfide protected groups introduced into the monoclonal antibody and free thiol groups on the modified toxin form the basis for the applied immunotoxin conjugation procedure. The composition of B43-PAP and BA-5-PAP were assessed by SDS-PAGE. As shown in Figure 1, immunotoxins contained one molecule of IgG and 1-2 molecules of PAP. No free toxin was detected and free antibody contamination was estimated to be <10% for B43-PAP and approximately 20% for BA-5-PAP (Figure 1). The ribosome inhibitory activities of B43-PAP and BA-5-PAP were analyzed in a cell-free translation system obtained from Promega Biotec. This system consists of a nuclease-treated rabbit reticulocyte lysate with the ability to translate messenger RNA into protein. Both immunotoxins were highly

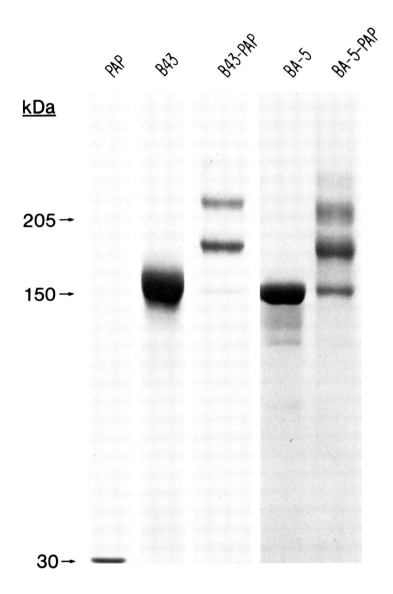

Figure 1. SDS-PAGE of B43-PAP and BA-5-PAP. Immunotoxins were electrophoresed on a 5% running gel
according to Laemmli. The gel was stained with Coomassie Blue and the positions of the molecular weight
markers are indicated on the left.

TABLE 1

BA-5-PAP AND B43-PAP EFFECTIVELY KILL BCGF-RECEPTOR POSITIVE LEUKEMIC B-LINEAGE ALL PROGENITOR CELLS

Treatment Conditions		Mean No. Blast Colonies/ 10^5 Cells Plated	
		LMW–BCGF	HMW–BCGF
No Treatment		1254	633
BA-5	5.0 μg/ml	1283	658
	10.0 μg/ml	1233	513
	25.0 μg/ml	1375	116
BA-5-PAP	0.1 μg/ml	1205	595
	0.5 μg/ml	1005	15
	1.0 μg/ml	545	3
	5.0 μg/ml	218	0
	10.0 μg/ml	214	0
B43	1.0 μg/ml	ND	ND
	5.0 μg/ml	ND	ND
	10.0 μg/ml	1351	687
B43-PAP	0.1 μg/ml	1200	575
	0.5 μg/ml	55	13
	1.0 μg/ml	0	5
	10.0 μg/ml	0	0

toxic and yielded IC$_{50}$ values of <20 pM. The immunoreactivity of B43-PAP and BA-5-PAP was evaluated by indirect immunofluorescence and flow cytometry using anti-PAP antibodies as probes for cell-bound PAP immunotoxin molecules. Both immunotoxins were highly selective in their reactivity pattern with target cells. The binding of B43-PAP to target cells was specifically blocked by excess unconjugated free B43 monoclonal antibody and similarly the binding of BA-5-PAP was blocked by excess free BA-5 monoclonal antibody (data not shown). Hence, both B43-PAP and BA-5-PAP bind their target cells via the specific monoclonal antibody moieties. The cell type specific cytotoxicity of B43-PAP and BA-5-PAP immunotoxins were first evaluated in protein synthesis inhibition assays using a CD19$^+$ HMW-BCGF-Receptor$^+$ EBV transformed B-cell line (Marbrook). Both B43-PAP and BA-5-PAP elicited >95% inhibition of the Marbrook cells (data not shown). Table 1 illustrates the effects of B43 and BA-5 monoclonal antibodies as well as their PAP toxin conjugates on the LMW-BCGF and HMW-BCGF induced proliferation of leukemic progenitor cells from one representative B-lineage ALL case. Similar findings were observed in a series of 15 B-lineage ALL patients (F. M. Uckun, unpublished data). BA-5 monoclonal antibody inhibited the HMW-BCGF induced proliferation without affecting the LMW-BCGF response of leukemic progenitor cells (Table 1). By comparison, B43 monoclonal antibody augmented the BCGF responses of leukemic progenitor cells. Both B43-PAP and BA-5-PAP were inhibitory to leukemic progenitor cell proliferation in LMW-BCGF stimulated cultures as well as in HMW-BCGF stimulated cultures, providing corroborative evidence that leukemic progenitor cells in B-lineage ALL are CD19$^+$HMW-BCGF-Receptor/BA-5$^+$LMW-BCGF-Receptor$^+$. Notably, BA-5-PAP was >50-fold more inhibitory on HMW-BCGF induced proliferation of leukemic progenitor cells than unconjugated BA-5 monoclonal antibody (Table 1). This demonstrates that the anti-leukemic efficacy of functionally inhibitory anti-HMW-BCGF-Receptor antibody BA-5 was markedly enhanced after coupling to PAP toxin. We believe that B43-PAP (anti-CD19) and BA-5-PAP (anti-HMW-BCGF-Receptor) show considerable potential for systemic treatment in B-lineage ALL. Novel immunochemotherapy / immunoradiotherapy protocols employing these B-cell specific immunotoxins may improve the poor outcome in high risk B-lineage ALL.

ACKNOWLEDGEMENTS

We thank M. Irvin for isolating and purifying PAP; K. Waddick, M. Chandan, T. Dickson, S. Swaim, V. Kuebelbeck, and K. Panger for technical assistance.

REFERENCES

1. Kersey JH, Weisdorf D, Nesbit ME, LeBien TW, Woods WG, McGlave PB, Kim T, Vallera DA, Goldman AI, Bostrom B, Hurd D, Ramsay NKC (1987) Comparison of autologous and allogeneic bone marrow transplantation for treatment of high risk refractory acute lymphoblastic leukemia. New Eng. J. Med. 317: (8): 461
2. Vitetta ES, Fulton RJ, May RD, Till M, Uhr JW (1988) Redesigning Nature's Poisons to Create Anti-Tumor Reagents. Science 238: 1098
3. Vallera DA and Uckun FM (1988). Immunoconjugates [In] Biological Response Modifiers and Cancer Research. JW Chaio, ed., Marcel Dekker, Inc. in press
4. Uckun FM, Myers DE, Kersey JH, Filipovich AH, Ramsay NC, McGlave P, Dickson TB, Vallera DA (1987) Immunotoxins in bone marrow transplantation: An updated review of the Minnesota Experience. (In) Membrane-Mediated Cytotoxicity, UCLA Symposium on Molecular and Cellular Biology, New Series, Vol. 45, pp. 231-242, B. Bonavida and R.J. Collier (eds.); Alan R. Liss, Inc., NY
5. Uckun FM, LeBien TW, Gajl-Peczalska KJ, Kersey JH, Myers DE, Anderson JM, Dickson TB, Vallera DA (1987) Ex vivo marrow purging in autologous bone marrow transplantation for acute lymphoblastic leukemia: Use of novel colony assays to test the anti-leukemic efficacy of various strategies. (In) Progress in Bone Marrow Transplantation, UCLA Symposium on Molecular and Cellular Biology, New Series, Vol. 53, pp. 759-771, R.P. Gale and R. Champlin (eds.), A.R. Liss, Inc., NY
6. Uckun FM, Stong R, Youle RJ, Vallera DA (1985) Combined ex vivo treatment with immunotoxins and mafosfamid: A novel immunochemotherapeutic approach for elimination of neoplastic T-cells from autologous marrow grafts. J. Immunol. 134:3504.
7. Uckun FM, Gajl-Peczalska K, Myers DE, Ramsay NC, Kersey JH, Colvin M, Vallera DA (1987). Marrow purging in autologous bone marrow transplantation for T-lineage acute lymphoblastic leukemia: Efficacy of ex vivo treatment with immunotoxins and 4-HC against fresh leukemic marrow progenitor cells. Blood 69:361.
8. Uckun FM, Myers DE, Ledbetter JA, Swaim SE, Gajl-Peczalska K, Vallera DA (1988) Use of colony assays and anti-T cell immunotoxins to elucidate the immunobiologic features of leukemic progenitor cells in T-lineage acute lymphoblastic leukemia. J. Immunol. 140:2103
9. Uckun FM, Ramakrishnan S, Houston LL (1985) Immunotoxin-mediated elimination of clonogenic tumor cells in the presence of human bone marrow. J. Immunol. 134:2010.
10. Uckun FM, Ramakrishnan S, Houston LL (1985) Increased efficiency of selective elimination of leukemic cells by combination of a stable derivative of cyclophosphamide and a human B cell specific

immunotoxin containing pokeweed antiviral protein. Cancer Res. 45:69.

11. Uckun FM, Gajl-Peczalska KJ, Kersey JH, Houston LL, Vallera DA (1986). Use of a novel colony assay to evaluate the cytotoxicity of an immunotoxin containing pokeweed antiviral protein against blast progenitor cells freshly obtained from patients with common B-lineage acute lymphoblastic leukemia. J. Exp. Med. 163:347.

12. Uckun FM, Ramakrishnan S, Houston LL (1985) Ex vivo elimination of neoplastic T-cells from human marrow using an anti-Mr 41,000 protein immunotoxin: Potentiation by ASTA Z 7557. Blut 50:19 (1985).

13. Uckun FM, Houston LL,Vallera DA (1987) Pokeweed antiviral protein immunotoxins and their clinical potential for systemic prophylaxis/ treatment of major complications of bone marrow transplantation in ALL. (In) Membrane-Mediated Cytotoxicity, UCLA Symposium on Molecular and Cellular Biology, New Series, Vol. 45, pp. 243-256, B. Bonavida and R.J. Collier (eds.); Alan R. Liss, Inc., NY

14. Irvin JD (1975). Purification and partial characterization of the anti-viral protein from Phytolacca americana L (pokeweed). Arch. Biochem. Biophys. 169:522

15. Greaves MF (1986). Differentiation-linked leukemogenesis in lymphocytes. Science 234:697.

16. Uckun FM, Kersey JH, Gajl-Peczalska KJ, Heerema NA, Provisor AJ, Haag D, Gilchrist G, Song CW, Arthur DC, Roloff J, Lampkin B, Greenwood M, Dewald G, Vallera DA (1987) Heterogeneity of cultured leukemic lymphoid progenitor cells from B-cell precursor ALL patients. J. Clin Invest. 80:639.

17. Uckun FM, Jaszcz W, Ambrus JL, Fauci AS, Gajl-Peczalska K, Song CW, Wick MR, Myers DE, Waddick K, Ledbetter JA (1988) Detailed studies on expression and function of CD19 surface determinant by using B43 monoclonal antibody and the clinical potential of anti-CD19 immunotoxins. Blood 71:13.

18. Uckun FM, Fauci AS, Song CW, Mehta SR, Heerema NA, Gajl-Peczalska KJ, Ambrus JL (1987) B-cell growth factor receptor expression and B-cell growth factor response of leukemic B-cell precursors and B-lineage lymphoid progenitor cells. Blood 70:1020

19. Ledbetter JA, Rabinovitch PS, June CH, Song CW, Clark EA, Uckun FM (1988) Antigen-independent regulation of cytoplasmic calcium in B-cells with 12 kilodalton B-cell growth factor and anti-CD19. Proc. Natl. Acad. Sci.85:1897

20. Ambrus JL, Jurgensen CH, Brown EJ, McFarland P, Fauci AS (1988) Identification of a receptor for high molecular weight human B-cell growth factor. J. Immunol. in press.

Human Tumor Antigens and Specific Tumor Therapy, pages 243-254
© 1989 Alan R. Liss, Inc.

IMMUNE RESPONSES TO MELANOMA ANTIGEN-POSITIVE
MOUSE FIBROBLASTS[1]

Young S. Kim, Ryszard Slomski[2], and Edward P. Cohen[3]

Department of Microbiology and Immunology
University of Illinois College of Medicine
Box 6998, Chicago, IL 60680

ABSTRACT Most spontaneously-arising tumors that form
surface antigens that might be "targets" of immune-
mediated attack do not provoke anti-tumor immune
responses even if the tumor-bearing host is fully immuno-
competent. In an attempt to augment the immunogenic
properties of B16 F1 melanoma cells ($H-2^b$) in syngeneic
C57BL/6 mice, thymidine kinase-deficient LM mouse fibroblasts ($H-2^k$) were co-transfected with genomic DNA
from B16 F1 cells, and from pTK, a plasmid carrying
the mouse thymidine-kinase gene. After selection in
HAT-medium, viable colonies of transfected cells expressing melanoma-associated antigens were identified by
erythrocyte-rosetting in situ with polyclonal anti B16
F1 antiserum followed by RBCs coupled with goat anti-
mouse $F(ab)_2$ serum. Sixteen colonies with adherent
RBCs among approximately 6000 colonies of HAT-resistant
LM cells were selectively removed. Melanoma-antigen-
expression was confirmed by flow cytometry and the
cells were used to immunize C57BL/6 mice. Reactivity
toward the melanoma was evaluated by delayed-type hypersensitivity in vivo and by cell-mediated lympholysis
in vitro. Certain melanoma-antigen-positive colonies
of transfected cells provoked anti B16 F1 immune
responses that exceeded those of (X-irradiated) B16 F1
cells. Others, although antigen-positive, were
nonstimulatory.

[1] Supported by the E.M. Bane Trust.
[2] Present address: Institute of Human Genetics, Poznan,
Poland.
[3] To whom correspondence should be addressed.

INTRODUCTION

Most spontaneously-arising tumors do not stimulate anti tumor immune responses even if tumor-associated antigens (TAA) are present. One possible explanation is the absence of a second class of determinants required for immune recognition ("associative recognition") (1). The heightened immunogenic properties of hybrids of tumor cells formed by fusion with allogeneic and xenogeneic cell-types (2-5), of tumor cells treated with enzymes such as neuraminidase (6) or with nonpathogenic viruses (7,8), is consistent with this hypothesis.

In an attempt to form tumor immunogens of augmented immunogenicity, and with defined antigenic properties, we co-transfected thymidine kinase-deficient LM mouse fibroblasts (H-2^k) with genomic DNA form B16 F1 melanoma cells (H-2^b) and the plasmid pTK, carrying the gene for thymidine kinase. After initial selection in HAT medium, we used erythrocyte-rosetting in situ to identify the small proportion of transfected fibroblasts forming melanoma-associated antigens. In C57BL/6 mice, syngeneic with the melanoma, certain clones of tumor-antigen-positive transfected cells stimulated anti melanoma immune responses that exceeded those of the (X-irradiated) tumor itself; others, although melanoma antigen-positive, were nonstimulatory.

METHODS

Cells.

B16 F1 cells, obtained originally from I. Fidler (M.D. Anderson, Houston, TX), were maintained by serial transfer in C57BL/6 mice (National Institutes of Health, Frederick, MD), histocompatible with the melanoma.

LM(TK-) cells, a thymidine kinase-deficient established mouse fibroblast cell line, were obtained originally from the American Type Culture Collection (Rockville, MD). They were maintained at 37°C in a humidified 7% CO_2/air mixture in Dulbecco's modified Eagle's medium (DMEM) (Gibco, Grand Island, NY) supplemented with 10% fetal calf serum (FCS) and antibiotics (growth medium). The cells died within seven to ten days in growth medium containing hypoxanthine, aminopterin and thymidine (HAT). Tests to determine if they were contaminated with Mycoplasma were negative. EL-4 cells, syngeneic with C57BL/6 mice, were obtained originally from the American Type Culture Collection (Rockville, MD).

Antisera.

Antiserum reactive with B16 F1 melanoma cells was raised in C57BL/6 mice injected intraperitoneally (i.p.) at weekly intervals for at least six weeks with approximately 10^7 killed (freeze-thaw) B16 F1 cells from the progressively-growing tumors of C57BL/6 mice. The antiserum (B16 F1-anti-serum) reacted in immunofluorescence tests with B16 F1 cells, but not with a variety of nonneoplastic cells from C57BL/6 mice. Normal mouse serum (NMS) was obtained from uninjected C57BL/6 mice.

Coupling of Antibodies to Human Red Blood Cells.

Chromic chloride was used to couple mouse B16 F1 anti-bodies to human red blood cells (HuRBC), according to the method described (9).

Transfection of LM(TK-) Cells with Genomic DNA from B16 F1 Melanoma.

High molecular weight DNA was isolated from B16 F1 cells as described in (10) as modified (11). The molecular weight exceeded 1.5×10^7 daltons (23,000 kbp), as determined by its rate of migration in 0.75% agarose gels using Hind III digested lambda DNA as a size marker. The calcium phos-phate coprecipitation method (12) was used to transfect LM(TK-) cells. In a representative experiment, 440 μg of DNA in TE buffer and 1 μg of plasmid DNA in 440 ml of TE buffer were added to 0.5 ml of twice concentrated HBS buffer followed by the addition of 60 μl of 2 M $CaCl_2$. The DNAs were added simultaneously to each of five 100 mm tissue culture dishes (Corning, Corning, NY) containing approximately 5×10^6 LM(TK-) cells per dish. After 4 hours incubation at 37°C, DMSO in HBS (10%, final concentration) was added for 2 minutes as a "shock", and the cells were washed once more with fresh medium and then incubated for 24 hours at 37°C after which growth medium containing HAT was added. From 30 to 40 colonies of HAT-resistant cells were obtained per μg plasmid DNA.

The Identification in situ of Transfected LM(TK-) Cells Forming B16 F1-Associated Antigens.

Viable colonies of transfected LM(TK-) cells forming antigens associated with B16 F1 cells were identified in situ by erythrocyte-rosetting.   The method described by Albino et al. (13) was adopted for this purpose.

A small glass cylinder (2 mm diameter) was carefully placed over clearly-delineated colonies of cells with adherent RBCs.   Sixteen colonies were identified from approximately 6000 colonies of cells proliferating in selective medium. They were recovered and maintained in selective medium for later analysis.

Cell Analysis by Flow Cytometry.

The flow cytofluorograph (Coulter Epics V, Coulter Electronics, Hialeah, FL) was used as further confirmation of the expression of melanoma antigens by the transfected cells.   As controls, the cells were treated in the same way and were analyzed without staining or were stained with rabbit antimouse $F(ab)_2$ serum conjugated with fluorochrome alone.

Specific Delayed Type Hypersensitivity.

Specific delayed type hypersensitivity (DTH) reactions against B16 F1 melanoma cells were evaluated in C57BL/6 female mice immunized with antigen-positive transfected cells, according to techniques described in (9). The animals were injected with 1×10^7 viable cells from various colonies of transfected cells expressing B16 F1-associated antigens or with an equivalent number of (X-irradiated, 2500 rads, ^{60}Co) B16 F1 cells.   For challenge, the mice were injected in one hind foot-pad with 1×10^5 (X-irradiated, 2500 rads, ^{60}Co) B16 F1 cells in 0.1 ml RPMI-1640 medium or with an equivalent number of (X-irradiated, 2500 rads, ^{60}Co) EL-4 cells in the other foot-pad, used as a specificity control. After 24 hours, the mean increase in foot-pad thickness was determined with a dial micrometer.

Cell-Mediated Lympholysis.

Cell-mediated lympholysis was determined according to methods described in (9). In brief, C57BL/6 female mice were injected with 5×10^6 transfected cells expressing B16

Fl-associated antigens 14 and 7 days before they were killed. Spleen cells from four mice from each group were pooled and incubated in growth medium with varying numbers of X-irradiated (2500 rads from a ^{60}Co source) transfected cells from the same colonies used for immunization. After five days, varying numbers of ^{51}Cr-labeled B16 Fl cells were added and after 4 hours the quantity of radioactivity released into the supernatant was determined.

RESULTS

The Expression of B16 Fl-Associated Antigens by Colonies of Transfected LM(TK-) Cells Selected for Melanoma Antigen Expression by Erythrocyte-Rosetting in situ.

Cells from colonies of transfected cells selected by erythrocyte-rosetting for the expression of melanoma associated antigens were analyzed by flow cytometry. The analysis of two such clones is presented (Fig. 1). To determine if the presence of bright and dull staining cells indicated a contamination of the cell population with B16 Fl-antigen-negative cells, brightly fluorescent cells (recording in channels 100 or above) were sorted directly into cell culture plates, allowed to proliferate in vitro and then analyzed again. The results were similar to those obtained at first analysis, indicating that the variation was an intrinsic property of the cells. The expression of melanoma associated antigens by the transfected cells was stable for periods in excess of eight weeks.

The staining intensity of two clones, relative to that of B16 Fl cells, is shown in Figure 2.

Delayed Type Hypersensitivity (DTH) Responses Toward B16 Fl Melanoma Cells in C57BL/6 Mice Immunized with Various Clonal Derivatives of Transfected Cells.

The immunogenic properties of the transfected cells toward B16 Fl melanoma was determined in C57BL/6 mice. Two immunizing injections were given fourteen and seven days before tumor challenge, using cells from each of six clonal derivatives of melanoma-antigen-positive transfected cells. One week later, the mice received X-irradiated (2500 rads from a ^{60}Co source) B16 Fl cells in one hind footpad and, as a specificity control, an equivalent number of X-irradiated EL-4 cells in the other hind footpad.

Mice receiving injections with cells from colony RLB-A

Figure 1 (Legend on Page 250)

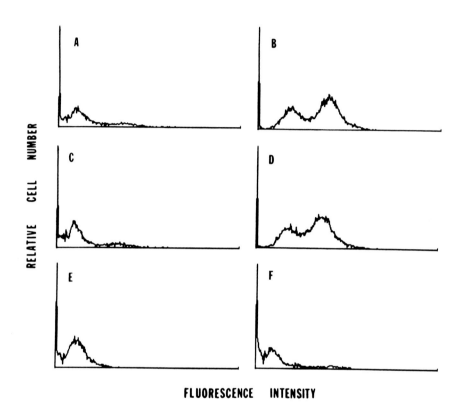

RELATIVE CELL NUMBER

FLUORESCENCE INTENSITY

Figure 2 (Legend on following page)

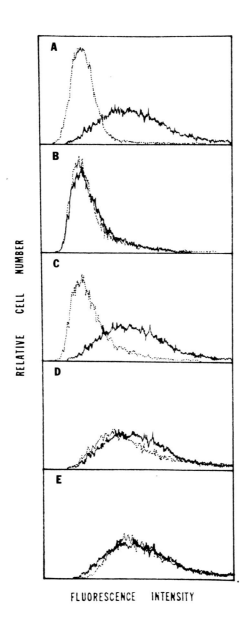

Legend to Figure 1: Flow Cytometric Analysis of Surface Antigens of Transfected LM Mouse Fibroblasts Selected for the
Expression of B16 F1- Associated Antigens.

Approximately 5 x 10^5 transfected cells, selected by erythrocyte-rosetting in situ for the expression of B16 F1-associated
antigens, were incubated for 45 min. at 4 C with 20ul of a
1:10 dilution of B16 F1 antiserum, followed by the addition
of 20ul of a 1:20 dilution of phycoerythrin-conjugated goat
anti mouse IgG (Southern Biotechnology Associates, Inc.,
Pittsburgh, PA). The incubation was continued for an additional
45 min. after which the cells were washed and analyzed in the
flow cytometer. The results of an analysis of 10,000 cells
from each group are presented.

Panel A: B16 F1 cells incubated with NMS.
Panel D: B16 F1 cells incubated with B16 F1 antiserum.
Panel B: LM cells transfected with plasmid only, incubated
         with NMS.
Panel C: LM cells transfected with plasmid only, incubated
         with B16 F1 antiserum.
Panel E: Transfected cell clone RLBA incubated with
         B16 F1 antiserum.
Panel F: Transfected cell clone TLM-6 incubated with
         B16 F1 antiserum.
All followed with phycoerythrin-conjugated goat anti mouse IgG.

Legend to Figure 2: Relative Staining Intensity of LM Mouse
Fibroblasts Selected for Melanoma Antigen-Expression after
Transfection with Genomic DNA from B16 F1 Melanoma Cells.

The analysis was performed in the flow cytometer using methods
described in the legend to Figure 1.

Panel A: B16 F1 cells stained with normal mouse serum (dotted
         line) or B16 F1 antiserum (solid line).
Panel B: Nontransfected LM cells stained with normal mouse
         serum (dotted line) or B16 F1 antiserum (solid line).
Panel C: LM cells (dotted line) or B16 F1 cells (solid line)
         stained with B16 F1 antiserum.
Panel D: Transfected clone RLBA (dotted line) or B16 F1 cells
         (solid line) stained with B16 F1 antiserum.
Panel E: Transfected clone TLM-6 (dotted line) or B16 F1
         cells (solid line) stained with B16 F1 antiserum.
All followed with phycoerythrin-conjugated goat anti mouse IgG.

stimulated tumor specific DTH reactions that exceeded ($p<.01$) those resulting from injections with an equivalent number of (X-irradiated) B16 F1 cells, (16 mil ± 4 versus 9 mil ± 2). The specific DTH reactions following injections with cells from three of the colonies, TLM-6, TLM-7 and RL-B, were approximately the same as resulted from immunizations with X-irradiated B16 F1 cells ($p > .05$). Immunizations with cells from two of the colonies, TLM-4 and TLM-1 led to DTH reactions (3 ± 3 mil; 4 ± 3 mil), ($p <.01$; $p <.05$, respectively) less than that of B16 F1 cells.

CML Responses to B16 F1 Melanoma in C57BL/6 Mice Immunized with Various Clonal Derivatives of Transfected Cells.

The capacity of various clones of transfected cells to induce antimelanoma immune responses in C57BL/6 mice was evaluated by CML. The mice received two immunizing injections; two weeks after the last injection, spleen cells from the injected animals were stimulated in vitro with cells from the same clones used for the primary immunizations, followed by ^{51}Cr-labeled B16 F1 cells.

The results (Table 1) indicate that the specific isotope release stimulated by clone RLB-A was significantly ($p <.01$) higher than that of B16 F1 cells. Cells from clone TLM-4, although positive for the expression of melanoma-associated antigens, were not immunogenic.

TABLE 1

Relative specific lysis. Cell-mediated lympholysis stimulated by spleen cells from mice immunized with B16 F1-antigen-positive transfected cells.

Clone	Relative specific lysis
TLM-1	-1.08
TLM-4	0.13
TLM-6	0.05
TLM-7	1.34
R-LB	3.79
R-LB-A	5.45
R-LB-A1	1.13
B16 F1	1.0

The data are expressed as the percent specific lysis obtained following immunizations with each colony of B16 F1-antigen-positive transfected cells relative to the specific lysis

obtained following immunizations with an equivalent number
of (X-irradiated) B16 F1 cells. (The ratio of spleen cells
to ^{51}Cr-labeled B16 F1 cells = 100.)

DISCUSSION

A small proportion of LM(TK-) mouse fibroblasts transfected with genomic DNA from B16 F1 melanoma cells stably
expressed melanoma associated antigens. Since the frequency
of transfer of single copy genes to individual recipient
cells following transfection with total cellular DNA was
expected to be low, the order of 1-10 X 10^{-7} (14), co-trans-
fection of thymidine kinase-deficient cells with the plasmid
pTK followed by preliminary selection in HAT medium was
employed. Erythrocyte rosetting in situ was used as the
second step to identify melanoma-antigen-positive colonies.
Colonies with large numbers of adherent red cells were selectively recovered for further expansion and later analysis.
Following initial selection in HAT medium, approximately
16 of 6000 colonies (frequency = 4 X 10^{-3}) were considered
positive for melanoma antigens similar to published reports
(15) in analogous systems.
Polyclonal antiserum was used to identify melanoma
antigen-positive transfected cells since more than one molecular species of TAA may be present on the melanoma cells
(16). We identified five distinguishable bands corresponding
to 118 kd, 116 kd, 85 kd, 34 kd, and 28 kd in immunoprecipitates of ^{125}I-labeled B16 F1 cells separated in SDS-PAGE
using the polyclonal antiserum (unpublished data).
Conceivably, the proportion of transfected cells expressing melanoma-associated antigens was greater than detected,
because: 1) the cells may have formed products of transfected
genes that were inaccessible to the antiserum used; 2) the
products of transfected genes may have been formed and expressed in the cell membrane, but in quantities too low to
lead to erythrocyte rosettes; and 3) the expression of genes
specifying melanoma-associated antigens might be altered by
contributions of the host cells, viz. a viz. their analogous
expression in B16 F1 cells.
The erythrocyte-rosetting method had two important
advantages. First, the viability of cells in the identified
colonies was preserved. Secondly, the resolution of the
method conveniently allowed detection of antigen-positive
transfectants at very low frequency. It is likely that the
individual colonies of transfected cells expressed each of

several melanoma-associated antigens since transfection to individual cells of unlinked genes rarely occurs (17). Final proof of this point will be dependent upon the results of more precise molecular analysis.

The varying immunogenicity of different clones of transfected cells toward the melanoma was not explained. Conceivably, each of the several melanoma-associated antigens present varied in its immunogenic properties. Others have reported (18-21) the presence of tumor-derived macromolecules that interfered with the generation of anti tumor immune responses on otherwise antigenic neoplasms, inhibiting the overall response.

REFERENCES

1. Lake P, Mitchison NA (1976). Associated control of the immune response to cell surface antigens. Immunol Commun 5:795.
2. Wang DR, Slomski R, Cohen EP (1985). Leukemia X fibroblast hybrid cells prolong the lives of leukemic mice. Eur J Can Clin Oncol 21:637.
3. Taffaletti DL, Darrow TL, Scott DW (1983). Augmentation of syngeneic tumor-specific immunity by semiallogeneic cell hybrids. J Immunol 130:2982.
4. Kim BS, Liang W, Cohen EP (1979). Tumor specific immunity induced by somatic hybrids. I. Lack of relationship between immunogenicity and tumorgenicity of selected hybrids. J Immunol 123:733.
5. Colnaghi MI (1975). Histocompatibility antigens acting as helper determinants for tumor-associated antigens of murine lymphosarcoma. Eur J Immunol 5:241.
6. Stockingen H, Majdic O, Liska K, et al. (1984). Exposure by disialylation of myeloid antigens on acute lymphoblastic leukemia cells. JNCI 73:7.
7. Cassel WA, Murray DR, Phillips HS (1983). A phase II study on the postsurgical management of Stage II malignant melanoma with a Newcastle Disease Virus oncolysate. Cancer 52:856.
8. Livingston PO, Albino AP, Chung TJC, Real FX et al. (1985). Serological response of melanoma patients to vaccines prepared by VSV lysates of autologous and allogeneic melanoma cells. Cancer 55:713.
9. Freeman WH (1980). In Mischell BB, Shigi SM (eds): "Selected Methods in Cellular Immunology.
10. Maitland N, McDougall JK (1977). Biochemical transfor-

mation of mouse cells by fragments of HSV DNA. Cell 11:323.

11. Slomski R, Hagen K, Kim YS, Cohen EP (1987). Immunity to murine leukemia induced in susceptible mice by transfected mouse fibroblasts. Leukemia 1:213.

12. Graham EL, van der Erb AJ (1973). A new technique for the assay of infectivity of human adenovirus DNA. Virology 52:456.

13. Albino AP, Graf Jr. LH, Kantor RRS, McLean W, Silazxi S, Old LJ (1985). DNA-mediated transfer of human melanoma cell-surface glycoprotein gp130: Identification of transfectants by erythrocyte rosetting. Mol Cell Biol 5:692.

14. Hsiung N, Roginski RS, Henthorn P, Smithies O, Kucherlapati R, Skoulchi AI (1982). Introduction and expression of fetal hemoglobin gene in mouse fibroblasts. Mol Cell Biol 2:401.

15. Kavathas P, Herzenberg LA (1983). Stable transformation of mouse L cells for human membrane T-cell differentiation antigens, HLA and β_2-microglobulin: Selection by fluorescence-activated cell sorting. Proc Natl Acad Sci USA 80:524-528.

16. Gersten DM, Hearing JJ, Marchalonis JJ (1983). Surface antigens of murine melanoma cells. In Cheng T (ed): "Structure of Membranes and Receptors," New York: Plenum Press, p 51.

17. Warrick H, Hsing N, Shows TB, Kucherlapati R (1980). DNA-mediated co-transfer of unlinked mammalian cell markers into mouse L cells. J Cell Biol 86:341.

18. Pellis NR, Yamagishi H, Shulan DJ, Kahan BD (1981). Use of preparative isoelectric focusing in a sepadex gel slab to separate immunizing and growth facilitating moieties in crude 3M KCl extracts of a murine fibrosarcoma. Can Immunol Immunother 11:53.

19. Sharon R, Naor D (1984). Isolation of immunogenic molecular entities from immunogenic and nonimmunogenic tumor homogenates separated by SDS-PAGE. Cancer Immunol Immunother 18:203.

20. Tom BH, Macek CM, Subramanian C et al. (1983). In vitro expression of suppressogenic and enhancing activities of human colon cancer. J Biol Respon Modifiers 2:185.

21. LaGrue SJ, Hearn DR (1983). Extraction of immunogenic and suppressogenic antigens from variants of B16 F1 melanoma exhibiting high or low metastatic potentials. Cancer Res 43:5106.

Human Tumor Antigens and Specific Tumor Therapy, pages 255–264
© **1989 Alan R. Liss, Inc.**

EXPERIMENTAL IMMUNOTHERAPY WITH A LIVING
REGRESSOR TUMOR CELL VACCINE

Hiroshi Kobayashi

Laboratory of Pathology, Cancer Institute,
Hokkaido University School of Medicine,
Sapporo, Hokkaido 060, Japan

Gene transfection experiments are now becoming common
as a method for the biological analysis of cancer. I have
been trying to transfect a xenogeneic gene to
transplantable tumor cells since 1969; but as, at that
time, no techniques for this had been reported, I used
xenogeneic antigenic viruses containing such xenogeneic
genes with which to transfect tumor cells.

As everybody knows, most viruses are cytolytic and
destroy tumor cells directly. However, the viruses used in
my experiments were nonlytic types, as well as being
xenogeneic to tumor cells.

Tumor cells infected with such xenogeneic and nonlytic
virus are capable of surviving for a long time in an
immune suppressed host but are not capable of surviving in
a normal host, since such virus-infected intact tumor cells
are antigenically xenogeneic in the normal host and will be
rejected immunologically. After the rejection of the
tumor, of course, a strong anti-tumor immunity will have
been produced to fight against the recurrence or metastasis
of the same type of tumor.

A. Living regressor tumor cell "vaccine"

In our experiments, we have used a number of different
types of tumor and virus to prepare a living tumor cell
"vaccine". We have mainly used KMT-17 fibrosarcoma cells
obtained from rats and the Friend virus derived from mouse
serum and spleen. When KMT-17 rat tumors are infected with
Friend virus, such virus-infected tumor cells can grow
initially in the local area but will eventually regress in

all cases. Such regressor tumor cells may be used as a "vaccine" for inhibiting the growth of any challenge by the same type of parental noninfected tumor cells. Such regressor tumor cell"vaccine" can sometimes grow in the area of inoculation, depending on the number of tumor cells inoculated and the tumor lines used.

From now on, whenever I use the term "the vaccine," I am always referring to the "virus-infected living regressor tumor cell vaccine."

The "vaccine" sometimes metastasizes into the local lymphnodes and the lungs. Even if it does metastasize, however, it will eventually regress (test-figure 1).

The main cause of the regression of the vaccine may be explained as a consequence of the new antigen (virus associated antigen: VAA) produced on the tumor cell surface which will be recognized as foreign and will therefore be rejected by the host.

B. Anti-tumor immunity of a living regressor tumor cell "vaccine"

Two antigens may exist on a tumor cell surface after the infection of tumor cells with a virus: that is, the pre-existing tumor-associated antigen (TAA) and a newly produced virus-associated antigen (VAA). VAA may be necessary for rejecting tumors, and TAA may play an important role in producing anti-tumor transplantation immunity against non-infected tumor cells of the same type after the regression of the "vaccine" (test-figure 2).

LTD-50 represents the number of tumor cells required to kill 50% of the animals when challenged 1-2 weeks thereafter with tumor cells, and an increase in LTD-50 may be a rather objective indication for measuring the strength of the anti-tumor immunity in the host immunized with the vaccine when it is compared to that in the non-immune control host.

The LTD-50 is approximately 2,000 times greater (sc) and more than 10,000 times greater (id) in hosts immunized with the vaccine. Such a high increase in LTD-50 is not observed in those groups immunized with formalin- or mytomycin C- treated tumor cell-vaccine, crude membrane, and irradiated tumor cell vaccine. At the same time, virus-infected destroyed tumor cells (oncolysate) which have been totally destroyed may sometimes induce a rather lower LTD-50 (table 1).

Test figure 1

Regression of Metastasis

Lymphnode metastasis

Pulmonary metastasis

* TNTC; Too numerous to count.

Test figure 2

Viral Xenogenization of Tumor Cells

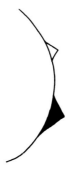

Attempts to increase antigenicity
of pre-existing tumor-associated
antigen (TAA)

Attempts to produce new
foreign virus-associated
antigen (VAA)

Table 1
TAA-immunogenicity of high immunogenic KMT-17
tumor cell achieved by various types of vaccine

Treatment of tumor cells	LTD 50 of sc tumor
Living regressor tumor cell "vaccine" (1 x)	2,000 x (sc) 10,000 x (id)
Formalin, Mitomycin C (0.2 %, 3 x)	5-10 x
Curde membrande	1- 5 x
Oncolysate	0.3-10 x
Irradiation (6,000 rad, 3 x)	200 x
None	1 x

Such strengths of LTD-50 also depend on the immunizing route and the challenging route. Intradermal immunization and intraperitoneal challenge may enable the "vaccine" to achieve its best results (table 2).

C. Mechanism of the strong anti-tumor immunity achieved by the "vaccine"

A number of explanations are available. One is the occurrence of the helper activity of newly developed VAA against pre-existing TAA. Strong anti-tumor immunity after use of the vaccine has never been observed in a VAA-tolerant rat. Both VAA and TAA must coexist on the tumor cell surface before strong immunity can be obtained. A simple mixture of living (nonirradiated) tumor cells with BCG cannot always induce the highly increased LTD-50 that is achieved by the virus-infected tumor cell vaccine.

To produce higher anti-tumor immunity, an appropriate dose of VAA and virus may be required.

The clustering of TAA on the tumor cell surface shown by immuno-ferritin conjugated anti TAA antibodies may be one of the reasons why there is a high level of anti-tumor activity.

Microvilli also disappear from the tumor cell surface, and the rather flat surface produced by the virus infection may thus be another reason for the high anti-tumor immunity.

Con-A agglutinability of the virus-infected tumor cells is high, while cytoxic sensitivity of the virus-infected cells to anti-TAA antibody is also high. All of these findings seem to indicate the strong anti-tumor immune potential of this vaccine (test-figure 3).

D. Preclinical application of the "vaccine"

Strong anti-tumor immunity is obtained after the previously described immunization with the vaccine. It is necessary, however, to begin the immunization with the vaccine after tumor development, or after tumor surgery. Since tumors needed in the experiments grow rapidly and kill the host early, we have to recognize the limitation of the vaccine effect if the vaccine is used after tumor development. The main tumor has, therefore, to be removed from the body and immunization with the vaccine has then to

Table 2
Average increase in LTD 50 of
challenged tumor after previous immunization
with living tumor cell-"vaccine" by
immunizing and challenging route

Route of Immunization	Challenge	LTD 50
–	sc	1 x
sc	sc	2,000 x
iv	sc	300 x
id	sc	> 10,000 x
–	ip	1 x
id	ip	530,000 x

Test figure 3

Cell surfaces of non-lytic virus
infected tumor cell vaccine

	TAA distribution on the cell surface (immunoferritin)	Con A agglutin-ability	Cytotoxic sensitivity
non infected tumor cell		+	+
virus-infected tumor cell (vaccine)		+++	+++

be performed. The immunization effect may result in inhibiting the growth of a metastasizing tumor, and also result in a decrease in the number of deaths and a prolonging of the number of survival days (table 3).

The therapeutic effect due to repeated immunization with the vaccine was not higher than we had expected. However, a rather better effect was observed by an initial immunization with the vaccine followed by a second immunization with the irradiated noninfected tumor cell vaccine. Repeated immunization with the irradiated tumor cell vaccine does not produce good results (table 4).

A much better therapeutic effect is obtained by immunization with the "vaccine", followed by low doses of Cyclophosphamide and Bleomycin (table 5).

For clinical approaches, tumors with low or very low immunogenic property, as is the case with most human tumors, have to be used for the vaccination. Although it is true that a vaccine from tumors with low or no immunogenic property can assist tumors to regress by themselves without recurrence, it is at present too difficult to produce such strong anti-tumor immunity as the one obtained by highly immunogenic tumors with KMT-17.

However, our living cell-vaccine can induce comparatively high immunogenicity at the rate of 1,000 x increased LTD-50, when an env gene-transfected tumor cell vaccine is used.

Summary

The living regressor tumor cell "vaccine" may be useful for clinical trials, and its application in clinical trials may be theoretically possible; but, practically, it is still difficult to achieve.

Nevertheless, such a living regressor tumor cell "vaccine" can induce the strongest anti-tumor immunity of any we have tested so far.

Table 3
Immunotherapy with living tumor cell vaccine
to lymphnode metastasis from primary tumor

Immunized* with	Metastasis*	
"vaccine" alone	20/20 (100%)	
"vaccine" after surgery	28/65 (43%)	⎤ P<0.01
Surgery alone	35/56 (68%)	⎦

* Immunized 4 hours after surgery.

Table 4
Therapeutic effects of living tumor
cell-vaccine by repeated immunization

Immunization on Day 3	Day 6	Cured/Treated (%)	p value
A	-	0/14 (0)	
A	A	2/35 (6)	
A	B	0/15 (0)	
A	C	12/39 (31) ⎤	
C	C	0/15 (0) ⎟ <0.05	
-	-	0/28 (0) ⎦	

Tumor cells (5×10^4) were sc challenged
on Day 0.
A. Living tumor cell "vaccine".
B. Irradiated tumor cell vaccine.
C. Irradiated noninfected tumor cell vaccine.

Table 5
Therapeutic effects of living
tumor cell-vaccine in combination
with bleomycin or cyclophosphamide

Living tumor cell-vaccine on Day 0	Chemotherapy on Day 3	$\dfrac{\text{Cured}}{\text{Treated}}$ (%)	p value
−	−	0/10 (0)	
+	−	0/ 9 (0)	
−	CY	3/10 (30)	⎤ <0.01
+	CY	9/ 9 (100)	⎦
−	BLM	4/10 (40)	⎤ <0.02
+	BLM	10/10 (100)	⎦

* Tumor cells (10^2) were implanted ip on Day 0.
BLM: Bleomycin (5mg/kg) ip.
CY: Cyclophosphamide (30mg/kg) iv.

REFERENCES

1. Hiroshi Kobayashi (1979). Viral Xenogenization of
    Intact Tumor Cells. In "Advances in Cancer Research,"
    Vol.30 Orland: Academic Press Inc., p.279.
2. Hiroshi Kobayashi (1982). Modification of Tumor
    Antigenicity in Therapeutics: Increase in Immunologic
    Foreignness of Tumor Cells in Experimental Model
    Systems. In Mihich E. (ed): "Immunological Approaches
    to Cancer Therapeutics" New York: John Wiley & Sons,
    Inc., p.405.
3. Hiroshi Kobayashi (1986). The Biological Modification
    of Tumor Cells as a Means of Inducing Their Regression:
    An Overview. J. of Biolog. Res. Modifiers 5:1-11.
4. Hiroshi Kobayashi, Fujiro Sendo, Toshikazu Shirai,
    Hiroshi Kaji, Takao Kodama and Hiroshi Saito (1969).
    Modification in Growth of Transplantable Rat Tumors
    Exposed to Friend Virus. J. of National Cancer Inst.
    42: 3.
5. Hiroshi Kobayashi, Eiki Gotohda, Masuo Hosokawa and
    Takao Kodama (1975). Inhibition of Metastasis in Rats
    Immunized with Xenogenized Autologous Tumor Cells after
    Excision of the Primary Tumor. J. of Nation Cancer
    Inst. 54:4.
6. Hiroshi Kobayashi, Takao Kodama and Eiki Gotohda
    (1977). Xenogenization of Tumor Cells. Hokkaido Univ.
    School of Med. Press.
7. Hiroshi Kobayashi, Noritoshi Takeichi and Noboru
    Kuzumaki: Xenogenization of Lymphocytes Erythroblasts
    and Tumor Cells. Hokkaido Univ. School of Med. Press.

Human Tumor Antigens and Specific Tumor Therapy, pages 265–275
© 1989 Alan R. Liss, Inc.

IDIOTYPIC TUMOR NETWORKS[1]

Heinz Kohler, Syamal Raychaudhuri,
Jian-Jun Chen, and Yukihiko Saeki

IDEC Pharmaceuticals Corporation
11099 N. Torrey Pines Road, Suite 160
La Jolla, California 92037

ABSTRACT   The idiotype network controlling the
response to a tumor-associated antigen (TAA) was
investigated. Evidence is presented that regulatory
idiotypes and anti-idiotypes determine the growth of
an experimental tumor in DBA/2 mice. Idiotypic
regulation was analyzed at the T helper cell level
recognizing anti-TAA idiotypes and at the serum
idiotype level. The results from this analysis
indicated different frequen-cies of idiotype (Ab1)
recognizing T helper cells at early and late stages
of tumor growth and different patterns of serum
idiotypes in anti-TAA immune and non-immune mice.
Collectively, these findings suggest that the
growing tumor induces changes in the idiotype
regulatory network which suppress anti-tumor
immunity and thus allow the tumor to grow. This
concept is supported by experimental evidence using
anti-idiotype therapy in combination with
chemotherapy.

INTRODUCTION

Anti-idiotype tumor immunotherapy is thought to work
by two conceptually different mechanisms; in one approach
anti-idiotypic antibodies are used in active immunization
protocols believed to mimic tumor-associated antigens

[1]Supported by American Cancer Society Grant IM405
and The Council for Tobacco Research Grant CTR1565R2.

(so-called internal image idiotopes) (1), the other
mechanism depends on the stimulation or suppression of
regulatory network reactions controlling the anti-tumor
host response. The latter one has been referred to as
"regulatory idiotypes" (2,3), which are part of the tumor-
associated idiotypic network (4).

Active immunotherapy can be subdivided into those
approaches which depend on tumor derived materials, such
as tumor antigens or tumor-derived materials, and into
methods which do not depend on materials derived or
extracted from tumors. The anti-idiotype manipulation is
the major tumor-specific active approach which does not
use tumor material for inducing anti-tumor immunities.

In this contribution, we will describe the idiotypic
network response induced by tumor growth and/or by
therapeutic anti-idiotypic manipulation using monoclonal
anti-idiotypic antibodies. We will discuss how tumor
progression is associated with the expression of certain
idiotopes in serum and with changes in the idiotypic T
helper repertoire. These observations lead to the
hypothesis that the tumor induces specific changes in T
and B cell idiotypic network which facilitates tumor
growth by suppressing the host anti-tumor response. In
this sense the growing tumor induces in the host an
"autocrine" idiotypic network which is conditional for its
successful establishment and continued growth.

The L1210/GZL Tumor Model.

The tumor used in these experiments, designated
L1210/GZL, is derived from DBA/2 mice and was selected as
a drug-resistant mutant (5). L1210/GZL expresses on its
surface a protein that cross-reacts with the gp52 envelope
of MMTV. This gp52 protein serves in our model as tumor-
associated antigen (TAA). Among a number of monoclonal
antibodies reacting with this gp52 protein, 11C1 has the
highest affinity. 11C1 was used as Ab1 to generate
monoclonal anti-idiotypic antibodies in non-syngeneic and
syngeneic hosts (6). Interestingly, all of these
monoclonal anti-idiotypes could inhibit binding of the
11C1 (Ab1) to the antigen tumor gp52.

Immunizing DBA/2 mice with monoclonal anti-idiotypes
induces immune responses related to the TAA on the
L1210/GZL tumor. Immunization was done after coupling to
KLH and in complete Freunds' adjuvant. The responses
induced by immunization with 2F10 or 3A4, two antigen

site-specific anti-Ids, produce anti-TAA titers and
increase the 11C1 idiotype (Ab1) expression (6). In
addition to humoral responses, the two anti-idiotypes
stimulate DTH which is specific for the L1210/GZL tumor
and cytotoxic T cells also specific for the tumor (7).
Finally, we could demonstrate the induction of T helper
cells which recognize the 2F10 and 3A4 idiotypes (8).
Collectively, these results with active anti-idiotype
immunization indicate that a TAA-like idiotope is
recognized by the tumor host on 2F10 and 3A4. However,
only immunization with 2F10 provided protection against
tumor growth (6,7). This led us to a series of experiments
designed to dissect the regulatory network which appears
to controls anti-Id-induced tumor immunity.

Serum Idiotypes in Tumor Mice

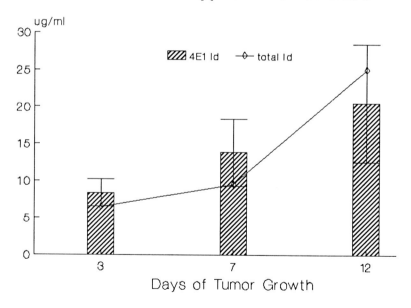

FIGURE 1.   DBA/2 mice received 10^4 live L1210/GZL
tumor cells and were bled on days 3, 7 and 12. The total
anti-11C1 anti-Id titer was measured using a polyclonal
rabbit anti-Id antibody; 4E1 idiotope was determined with
monoclonal anti-Id antibodies.

RESULTS

Regulation of the Anti-Tumor Response.

The effects of regulatory idiotypic reactions on anti-tumor immunity has been recently discussed by Kennedy and Bona (9). The first place to search for regulatory idiotypic reactions is in serum. Regulatory idiotopes are thought to be part of the idiotypic network which is involved in the regulation of immune responses. It encompasses serum idiotypes and T cell-recognizing idiotypes. By definition, regulatory idiotypes are crossreactive and not expressed by antibodies or T cells that recognize tumor targets.

We used a panel of monoclonal anti-Ids raised against 11C1 (Ab1) in Balb/c mice consisting of the antibodies 3A4, D11 and 4E1 to analyze sera from tumor-bearing mice at different times after tumor transfer. The results from 4E1 and a polyclonal rabbit anti-11C1 are shown in Figure 1. The 4E1 idiotope increases with tumor growth and represents a major portion of the total anti-11C1 anti-idiotypic response. Since the 4E1 idiotope is not expressed on anti-TAA antibodies in the tumor host strain (DBA/2) and the total anti-idiotype amount is much greater than the anti-TAA titer (7), these idiotopes which appear with the growing tumor are good candidates for being involved in regulation.

Idiotype-Specific T Help Induced by Tumor Growth.

Next, we searched in tumor bearing mice for increases of T helper cells that recognize anti-TAA idiotypes, such as 11C1 or 2B2 (Ab1s). This was done under limiting dilution and in bulk T cell cultures obtained from lymph node cells. As seen in Figure 2, the frequency of T cells recognizing 11C1 or 2B2 Ab1 taken from animals bearing growing tumors changes over time. A similarly changing pattern is seen when these T helper cells are assayed for helping TNP-specific B cells in a T-B coculture.

Collectively, these data on anti-TAA idiotypes demonstrate two points: a) the tumor induces idiotype-specific T cells that may have a regulatory role in the tumor host, and b) the specificity of these idiotype-specific T cells changes as the tumor continues to grow and to eventually kill the tumor host. A conclusion from

these data would be that idiotypic intervention in the
tumor-induced expression of regulatory T helper cells
could be beneficial for the tumor host.

The next step was to analyze the T help for anti-TAA
idiotypes (Ab1) in mice immunized with 2F10 or 3A4 anti-
idiotype. When lymph node Th cells from 2F10-immunized
mice, which resist tumor growth, are assayed for response
to anti-TAA idiotypes 11C1 and 2B2 under limiting dilution
the frequency of 11C1- responding T cells is significantly
higher than of 2B2 responding T cells, while the reverse
is seen in nonprotected 3A4 immunized mice. These
differences in 11C1- and 2B2- specific T helpers are also
seen in the T-B collaboration assay (see Figure 3). The
dominance of 11C1-recognizing helper cells

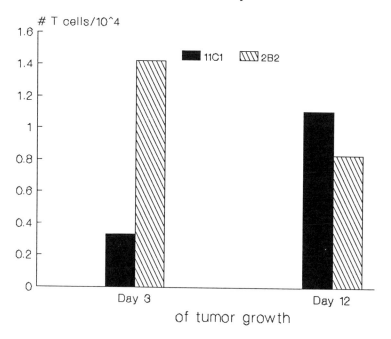

FIGURE 2. Idiotype-specific T helper cells for 11C1 and
2B2 were measured in tumor-bearing mice 3 and 12 days
after tumor transfer. On the y axis, the frequency of T
helper cells responding to 11C1 or 2B2 are shown.

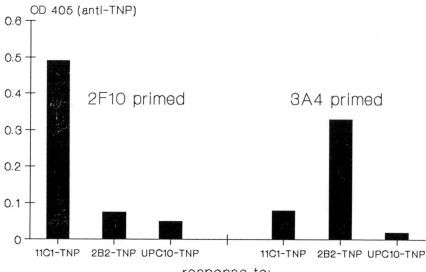

FIGURE 3. Idiotype-specific T helper cells from DBA/2 mice primed with 2F10-KLH and 3A4-KLH. The anti-TNP response from cocultures of T helper cells and TNP-primed B cells responding to TNP-11C1, TNP-2B2 and TNP-UPC10 are shown.

resembles the pattern seen in the late stage of tumor growth where 11C1 specific helpers are more frequent then 2B2 helpers (see Figure 2). The failure to establish a strong 11C1 titer by day three of tumor growth may allow the tumor to establish since this idiotype is associated with a high affinity anti-TAA antibody.

Chemo-Idiotype Therapy.

From the forgoing discussion of the idiotype network response induced by the growing tumor, it becomes evident that the tumor induces an array of different immune reactions. These can be divided into two categories: one part of the induced response is clearly directed against TAA of L1210/GZL comprising anti-TAA antibodies, TAA-specific DTH and CTLs; the other component in the response

is not directed against the tumor, but involves humoral
and cellular reactions which are part of a regulatory
network. As the tumor establishes itself, some idiotopes
increase while others decrease, and T helper cells are
stimulated which recognize idiotopes associated with anti-
TAA antibodies (Ab1s) and anti-anti-TAA antibodies (Ab2s).
A comparison of the regulatory humoral and cellular
network in anti-idiotype protected and non-protected mice
(8,10 and unpublished data) also shows significant
differences and identifies idiotopes that are present in
non-protected mice. This correlation of idiotype
expression and host anti-tumor resistance leads to the
concept of a tumor-induced autocrine idiotypic network
which then enables the tumor to overcome the host anti-
tumor response. Therefore, a rational approach for
immunotherapy of tumors would be to suppress this
autocrine idiotypic network response. While this can be
achieved by specific idiotypic manipulation, we have
approached this concept first with a general suppressive
regimen.

To test the idea that tumor induces an autocrine
network to promote growth, we developed the following
protocol: mice were given a suboptimal dose of
cyclophosphamide three days after they had received live
tumor cells. At day 7 after tumor transfer, mice were
given different amounts of 2F10 anti-Id. All groups of
mice were monitored for palpable tumor.

As can be seen in Figure 4, in mice who received 10
μg of 2F10 the tumor disappeared and the animals survived.
Mice given less than 10 μg 2F10 had a high incidence of
death. These results show that non-specific immunosuppressive treatment allows anti-idiotype manipulation to
become highly effective.

DISCUSSION

The utilization of the idiotype network in tumor
immunotherapy opens new perspectives and may enrich the
therapeutic armentarium. Basically two approaches are
feasible. The first takes advantage of the existence of
internal antigen images in the idiotype repertoire. This
approach has already been used successfully by several
investigators (11,12), and has the advantage of not being
genetically restricted (13). So-called internal image
idiotypes mimic the three-dimensional contacts between
antigen and antibody. Thus they are effective across the

Chemo-idiotype Therapy

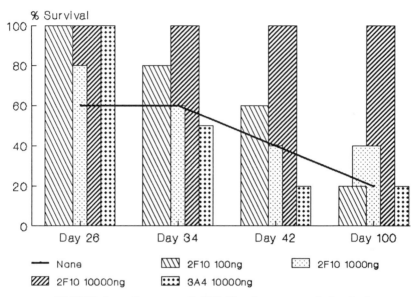

FIGURE 4. Groups of PBA/2 mice were injected intradermally with 10^4 live L1210/CZL tumor cells; on day 3 they received cyclophosphamide (80 mg/kg); on day 7 they were injected iv with different doses of 2F10, 3A4 or saline. Survival was scored.

species barrier. Because antigen is presented in a different molecular environment by anti-idiotype, the network antigens may be more effective than nominal antigens. The other method of using the idiotype network rests on the existence of so-called regulatory idiotypes (2,3,14), which are part of the regulatory network in anti-cancer responses (10). Discovering these linkages in anti-tumor responses would be important and could be the first step in using these regulatory idiotypes to control tumor growth by immunologic means.

What is intriguing in our tumor model is that, although 2F10 and 3A4 both induced CTL production substantially, only 2F10 could offer protection against tumor growth. Therefore, out of two anti-Id antibodies against an anti-TAA antibody, one is effective in controlling tumor progression, whereas the other has no

effect. The different roles of anti-Id antibodies may in
part be due to the topography of the idiotype to which
they interact and differences in affinities between anti-
Id and idiotype (17). In a separate study, we have shown
that 3A4 induces a population of regulatory T cells that
interfere with the anti-tumor effector mechanism induced
by 3A4 (data not shown). The demonstration of the
presence of both regulatory and effector T cells in anti-
Id-immunized mice is consistent with the concept that
effector and regulatory lymphocytes recognize different or
overlapping determinants on antigen. In response to a
given antigen, one cell type should be preferentially
triggered over others to govern dominance or suppression
(18).
        The experiments in the L1210/GZl tumor system
provide the first insight into a complex cascade of immune
responses, which to a large extent involve regulatory
interactions not directed against tumor-associated
antigens. These interactions can be dissected using
idiotypic and anti-idiotypic tools. The purpose of these
regulatory, tumor-induced reactions appears to be the
promotion of tumor growth. By analogy to tumor-promoting
factors released by the tumor, we introduce the term
"autocrine idiotypic network." We also show that
manipulation of this autocrine network can induce
regression of an established tumor using a combination of
idiotype-specific and non-specific intervention. These
results will be of interest in the design of idiotypic
therapies of cancer in humans (9,19).
        For the purpose of developing an anti-tumor idiotype
vaccine, our data indicate that the regulatory component
in the immune response to internal antigens plays a
critical role in determining the *in vivo* effectiveness of
such a vaccine.

REFERENCES

1.   Jerne NK (1974). Towards a network theory of the
      immune system. Ann Immunol (Inst Pasteur) 15C, 373.
2.   Bona C, Paul WE (1979). Cellular basis of regulation
      of expression of idiotype. I. T suppressor cells
      specific for MOPC 460 Id regulate the expression of
      cells secreting anti-TNP antibodies bearing 460 Id.
      J Exp Med 149:592.
3.   McNamara M, Kohler H. (1984). Regulatory idiotopes.
      Induction of idiotype-recognizing helper T cells by
      free light and heavy chains. J Exp Med 159:623.

4.   Raychaudhuri S, Saeki Y, Chen J, Kohler H. (1987). Tumor-specific idiotype vaccines: IV. Analysis of the idiotypic network in tumor immunity. J Immunol 139:3902.

5.   Rapp L, Fuji H. (1983). Differential anti-genic expression of the DBA/2 lymphoma L1210 and its sublines: Crossreactivity with C3H mammary tumors as defined by syngeneic monoclonal antibodies. Cancer Res 43:1392.

6.   Raychaudhuri S, Saeki Y, Fuji H, Kohler   H (1986). Tumor-specific idiotype vaccines I. Generation and characterization of internal image tumor antigens. J Immunol 137:1743.

7.   Raychaudhuri S, Saeki Y, Chen J-J, Iribe H, Fuji H, Kohler H (1987). Tumor-specific idiotype vaccines. II. Analysis of the tumor-related network response induced by the tumor and by internal image antigens (Ab2B). J Immunol 139:271.

8.   Raychaudhuri S, Saeki Y, Chen J, Kohler H (1987). Tumor-specific idiotype vaccines: III. Induction of T helper cells by anti-idiotype and tumor cells. J Immunol 139:2096.

9.   Kennedy R, Zhou E, Lanford R, Chanh T, Bona C (1987). Possible role of anti-idiotypic antibodies in the induction of tumor immunity. J Clin Invest 80:1217.

10.   Raychaudhuri S, Saeki Y, Chen J-J, Kohler, H (1987) Analysis of the idiotypic network in tumor immunity. J Immunol 139:3902.

11.   Koprowski H, Herlyn D, Lubeck M, DeFreitas E, Sears HF (1984). Human anti-idiotype antibodies in cancer patients: is the modulation of the immune response beneficial for the patient? Proc Natl Acad Sci USA 81:216.

12.   McNamara MK, Ward RE, Kohler H (1984). Monoclonal idiotope vaccine against Streptococcus pneumoniae infection. Science 226:1325.

13.   Auchincloss H, Bluestone JA, Sachs DH (1983). Anti-idiotypes against anti-H-2 monoclonal antibodies. V. In vivo anti-idiotype treatment induces idiotype-specific helper T cells. J Exp Med 157:1273.

14.   Gleason K, Kohler H (1982). T helper cells recognize a shared Vh idiotope on phosphorylcholine-specific antibodies. J Exp Med 156:539.

15. Frelinger J, Sign A, Infante A, Fathman CG (1984). Clonotypic antibodies which stimulate T cell clone proliferation. Immunol Rev 81:22.

16. Kaye JS, Procelli J, Tite J, Jones B, Janeway CA (1983) Both a monoclonal antibody and antisera specific for determinants unique to individual cloned helper T cell lines can substitute for antigen and antigen presenting cells in the activation of T cells. J Exp Med 158:836.

17. Stevens FJ, Jwo J, Carperos W, Kohler H, Schiffer M (1986). Relationships between liquid- and solid-phase antibody associa-tion characteristics: Implications for the use of competitive ELISA techniques to map the spacial location of idiotopes. J Immunol 137:1937.

18. Kloke O, Haubeck H-D, Kolsch E (1986) Evidence for a T suppressor cell-inducing antigenic determinant shared by ADJ PC-5 plasmacytoma and syngeneic BALB/c spleen cells. Eur J Immunol 16:659.

19. Kieber-Emmons T, Ward R, Raychaudhuri S, Rein R, Kohler H (1985). Rational design and application of idiotope vaccines. Intern Rev Immun 1:1.

Human Tumor Antigens and Specific Tumor Therapy, pages 277–286
© 1989 Alan R. Liss, Inc.

TUMOR-UNIQUE ANTIGENS ON T CELL CHRONIC LYMPHATIC[1]
LEUKEMIA (T CLL) RECOGNIZED BY MONOCLONAL ANTIBODIES.
TREATMENT OF T CLL WITH
ANTI-IDIOTYPIC MONOCLONAL ANTIBODY

Carl Harald Janson, Mahmood J. Tehrani,
Håkan Mellstedt and Hans Wigzell

Department of Immunology, Karolinska Institute,
and Departments of Oncology and
Immunology Research Laboratory,
Karolinska Hospital, Stockholm, Sweden

ABSTRACT   One approach to immunotherapy of
tumor diseases in humans is the passive transfer
of specific immunity. We have analysed the possibilities of this therapeutic modality in T cell
chronic lymphatic leukemia (T CLL).
We have produced five murine monoclonal antibodies (Mab) against the variable part (idiotypic)
of the T cell receptor for antigen TCR on the
tumor cells of two patients with T CLL (E.L.
CD3,4; I.U. CD3,8). The anti-idiotypic nature of
the Mabs was concluded from specificity, molecular
weight of antigen and CD3 comodulation and
coprecipitation. The initial Mabs were of IgG1 and
IgG2a subclasses. IgG2a spontaneous switch
variants have been selected. The Mabs mediated no
significant complement cytotoxicity and ADCC.
Patient I.U. was treated intravenously with
1+1+10 mg of Mab (IgG2a) over a period of four
weeks. An 80% reduction of total circulating tumor
cells was reached using 2 x 1 mg of Mab. 10 mg but
not 1 mg induced detectable complement activation.
Furthermore, in the process of selecting for
anti-idiotypic Mabs we have found two Mabs
reacting with tumor-unique antigens, not being the

[1]This work was supported by the Swedish
Cancer Society and the Cancer Society, Stockholm.

TCR molecule, on the membrane of a T CLL tumor
cell. One antigen has the relative molecular
weight of 74-80kD under nonreducing and 80kD under
reducing condition. The other antigen is a dimer
with a molecular weight of 74-80kD nonreduced and
38kD reduced.

INTRODUCTION

     When tumor therapy is approached with a Mab
concept, a tumor-unique, stabile and nonsecreted
tumor antigen is called for.
     Monoclonal antibodies (Mabs) have been used
therapeutically in a variety of hematological
malignancies (1,2,3,4) as well as in solid tumors
(5,6). In most cases the Mabs have been directed
against various types of antigens also expressed
on the normal counterparts of the tumor cells.
Differences in amounts expressed or expression
only in fetal cells have made them suitable for
therapy.
     The idiotypic molecules on B lymphocytes,
cell membrane bound immunoglobulin (mIg), and on T
lymphocytes, T cell receptor for antigen (TCR),
are clonaly distributed and have a variable part
(idiotypic) unique for each clone. The rearranged
idiotypic TCR seems to offer some advantages, as a
target for Mab therapy, compared to the idiotypic
B cell structure. B cells normally use somatic
hypermutation as one way of increasing diversity
of the Ig molecule. Malignant B cells retain this
mechanisms, and the tumor can become multiclonal
leading to tumor escape when treated with anti-
idiotypic Mab (7). The secretion of Ig by the
malignant B cells (blocking factor) is undesired.
Furthermore, in most B cell malignancies, the
clonal origin can be traced back to a pre-B cell
stage, not expressing membrane Ig thereby offering
another means of escape.
     T cells do not seem to use somatic
hypermutation during maturation, nor is the TCR
molecule secreted to a significant degree. Anti-
idiotypic Mabs have a direct inhibitory effect on
the growth of T cell neoplasms. These assumptions
and the close physical relation between the

malignant cells and effector systems in these
malignancies, make this, in our view, an optimal
tumor for a therapeutic trial with the monoclonal
antibody concept.
    The aim of the study was to produce and
characterize monoclonal antibodies that could be
used for specific therapy of T cell lymphoma /
leukemia.

METHODS

See schematic overview, figure 1, and reference 8.

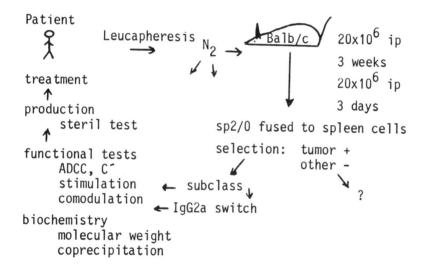

FIGURE 1. Schematic overview of procedures.

RESULTS

In vitro results:

<u>Selection and characterization of the Mabs.</u>
In order to produce monoclonal antibodies with a
restricted and maybe unique specificity for a
human T-cell leukemia, all hybridomas were
selected for binding to the relevant tumor cells

and not to any other types of cells tested.
Selection was done using micropanning or immunofluoresence assays. We have obtained a total of
seven monoclonals (D1, B8, IVH8, VD7, H2, IVF7
specific for patient E.L., and F1 for patient I.U.
tumor cells) out of more than 5000 potential
hybridomas screened.

Biochemistry: To characterize the unique
structure on the tumor cells reactive with the
Mabs, immunoprecipitation was performed using
different tumor cell lysates. Various detergents,
differing in their capacity to hold together
complexes of non-covalently associated proteins,
supported a close relationship between the D1, B8,
IVH8, VD7 and F1 antigens and CD3. The detergent
NP-40 tends to dissociate non-covalently associated proteins while chaps and digitonin keep these
complexes together.

Using NP-40, the antibodies D1, B8, IVH8, VD7
and F1 reacted with proteins with a relative
molecular weight (Mr) around 90kD under non-
reducing conditions and 40-50kD under reducing
conditions, well corresponding to the known Mr of
the TCR. OKT3 precipitated proteins with Mr of
22kD and 28kD. Using chaps or digitonin D1, B8,
IVH8, VD7 and F1 precipitated not only the
proteins detected using NP-40, but also molecules
with Mr of 22kD and 28kD. OKT3 precipitated
proteins with a similar Mr as the anti-idiotypic
Mabs using chaps or digitonin.

Two other Mabs, H2 and IVF7, with tumor-
unique reactivity did not immunoprecipitate TCR
molecular complex nor did they show any
coprecipitation tendency to CD3. The H2 reactive
antigen had the relative molecular weight of 74-
80kD under nonreducing and 80kD under reducing
condition. The IVF7 reactive antigen was a dimer
with a molecular weight of 74-80kD nonreduced and
38kD reduced.

Comodulation experiments also showed a close
relation of CD3 to D1, B8, VD7, IVH8, and F1 but
not to H2 and IVF7 Mabs.

Subclass of Mabs. D1, B8, IVH8, VD7, H2, IVF7
were all of IgG1 subclass while F1 was IgG2a.
IgG2a variants have been selected of D1, IVH8,
VD7, H2 and IVF7 by a spontaneous switch elisa.

Proliferative capacity of the Mabs. The Mabs
IVH8, VD7 and IVF7 induced a selective
proliferation in E.L. tumor cells, but not in PBL
from normal healthy donors or other T cell
leukemia cells. F1, on the other hand, stimulated
a fraction of PBL from normal donors, but not the
I.U. tumor cells.
Cytotoxic capacity in vitro. The Mabs
mediated no significant complement cytotoxicity
and ADCC.

In vivo therapy with Mab:

E.L. patient died before treatment could be
given.
I.U. patient: The tumor cells were CD3 $^+$; CD4$^-$;
CD8$^+$. Almost four years after diagnosis the
patient showed indications for therapy with
weight-loss and night-sweats, a decrease in
hemoglobin concentration, platelet count and an
increase in leukemic blood cell count. She
objected cytostatic therapy.
The treatments were given as intravenous
infusions. Before each infusion an intracutaneous
testing with Mab was done. The immediate
reactions, 30 min and 4 h, were on all occasions
negative.
The half life of F1 in plasma ($t^1/_2$) was
44 hours.
Anti-mouse antibodies were not detected prior
to the first and second infusions. At the time of
the third treatment anti-mouse IgM and IgG
antibodies were found at titers comparable to
colon tumor patients receiving 17-1A mab without
significant side effects.
I.U. was given three infusions of F1 Mab, see
figure 2. In the first two she received 1 mg and
in the third 10 mg. A rapid reduction of the
circulating leukemic cells following the
administrations was seen. 24-48 hours after
infusion there was an increase in leukemic blood
cell count to a higher level than the corresponding pre-treatment one. The numbers of
circulating leukemic lymphocytes decreased by

time. During the first four weeks a total of
two mg of anti-idiotypic Mab was administered.
This amount induced an 80% reduction in circulating leukemic cells. During the treatment period
there was an increase in neutrophil counts from
$0.6 \times 10^9/L$ to $1.7 \times 10^9/L$.

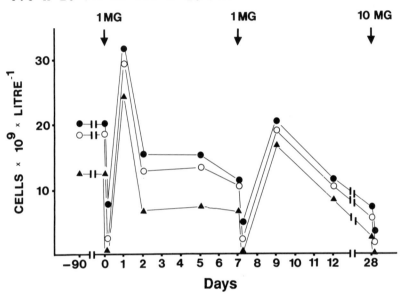

FIGURE 2. White blood cell (●), total
lymphocyte (   ) and total F1 [+] lymphocyte counts
(▲) in peripheral blood during therapy with F1
Mab in I.U. patient.

Serum complement activation was not seen
after the two first infusions. However, 2 hours
after the third infusion activation of complement
was noted, as shown by an increase of C2a and C3d,
indicating that activation occurred through the
classical pathway.

Side effects from the therapy were, chills,
fever (<38.5 °C), nausea, vomiting, diarrhea,
tachycardia (increase in heart rate with <60 beats
per minute), increase in systolic blood pressure
(<40 mm Hg), dyspnoea (increase of <12 breaths
per minute) and pain in the lumbar region. The

adverse reactions started 30-60 mins. after the
infusion and lasted for aproximately 2 hours. No
side effects on liver and kidney functions were
seen.

The therapy could not be continued as the
patient died mors subita with a clinic of cardiac
dysfunction 6 hours after the third infusion.
Autopsy showed a 3-7 days old myocardial
infarction. No other damages were seen in the
lungs, liver or kidneys. Our conclusion is that
the patient died of a myocardial infarction.
However, the third treatment with Mab may have
contributed to the fatal outcome of the myocardial
infarction.

DISCUSSION

We have shown that it is possible to produce
murine monoclonal antibodies recognizing idiotypic
determinants as well as other tumor-unique
antigens on T-cells, on a regular basis within
6-12 months. The majority of hybridomas produced
Mabs reacting with structures other than the TCR
molecule. On an average 0.1% of the clones
produced a Mab with a restricted idiotypic
reactivity.

The Mab stained the majority of PBL from the
respective leukemic patients. The Mabs also
reacted with 0-4% of PBL from non-related donors.
This reactivity could, for the anti-idiotypic
Mabs, be due to shared variable domain genes of
the TCR complex. These epitopes, if representing a
specific V, J or D gene segment, should then be
shared between different individuals, and cross-
reactivity at the T cell level would be expected
at a low frequency. A set of Mabs each of which
recognized one V gene segment or a family of gene
segments would then allow us to, at the time of
diagnosis, find an antibody suitable and
immediately available for therapy. This panel of
Mabs could also be used to study the clonal
involvement of T-cells in other diseases of
different kinds.

The Mabs H2 and IVF7 reacted with structures
not related to the TCR-T3 complex. H2 seems to

recognize a monomer of Mr 74-80kD and IVF7 a dimer
of Mr 74-80kD nonreduced and 38 kD reduced. These
have to our knowledge not previously been
described. The fact that the Mabs H2 and IVF7 also
reacted with a small percentage of PBL indicates a
normal, non neoplastic, function for these
molecules.

The results from coprecipitation and
comodulation with CD3 together with the
specificity data convince us that five of our Mabs
react with the variable part of the TCR.

When using Mab for therapy it is important to
confirm that the Mab does not induce proliferation
which may promote tumor cell growth. I.U. tumor
cells did not proliferate after in vitro
stimulation with F1 Mab.

Small amounts of F1 Mab caused a marked
immediate decrease in the number of circulating
leukemic cells. The greatest reduction was
observed after the first infusion, when the number
of tumor cells was high. The acute, temporary
increase in leukemic lymphocytes probably
represents a redistribution of cells to the
circulation from various tissue compartments. The
clear difference in tumor cell counts before the
first and third treatments indicates that a true
reduction and not only a redistribution of tumor
cells have taken place.

It has not been possible to analyze the
mechanisms of tumor reduction in I.U. patient.
Direct and rapid mechanisms for tumor cell
destruction mediated by Mab seem to be ADCC and
complement fixation. Compared to other subclasses,
IgG2a, has in vitro mediated the best ADCC
activity using human effector cells (9), binds
human complement relatively well and has in animal
systems attained a longer survival time. We have
not however seen any significant ADCC or
complement lytic capacity with neither IgG1 nor
IgG2a anti-idiotypic Mabs.

Over a longer period of time it is possible
that the administration of murine Mab (foreign
protein), that regularly gives rise to a humoral
anti mouse Ig response, would lead to a host
immunity against the tumor. This could be achieved
in different ways. Through the anti-idiotypic
network the administered Mab (ab1) could lead to

ab2 that leads to ab3 mediating a humoral anti-
tumor response. A MHC restricted "tumor specific"
immunity could conceivingly as well be achieved by
the presentation of the tumor antigen together
with the foreign murine Mab.

The cardiopulmonary side effects noted in the
patient were similar to those reported by others
using T cell reactive Mabs, indicating something
uniquely linked to T cell damage. However, such
side effects were not usually observed at the low
dosages used in this study. Patients having a
history of cardiac disease should be excluded from
this kind of therapy.

The present study shows that individual
specific (anti-idiotypic) Mab against T cell
malignancies can be produced for therapy. Such
antibodies are effective in vivo in eliminating
circulating tumor cells.

ACKNOWLEDGMENTS

This study was approved by the Ethical
Committee of the Karolinska Institute.

REFERENCES

1. Meeker TC, Lowder JN, Maloney DG, Miller RA,
   Thielemans K, Warnke R, Levy R (1985). A
   clinical trial of antiidiotype therapy for B
   cell malignancy. Blood 65:1349.
2. Dillman RO, Beauregard J, Shawler DL, Halpern
   SE, Markman M, Ryan KP, Baird SM, Clutter M
   (1986). Continous infusion of T101 monoclonal
   antibody in chronic lymphocytic leukemia and
   cutaneous T-cell lymphoma. J Biol Resp Modif
   5:394.

3. Foon KA, Schroff RW, Bunn PA, Mayer D, Abrams PG, Fer M, Ochs J, Bottino GC, Sherwin SA, Carlo DJ, Heberman RB, Oldham RK (1984). Effects of monoclonal antibody therapy in patients with chronic lymphocytic leukemia. Blood 64:1085.
4. Press OW, Appelbaum F, Ledbetter JA, Martin PJ, Zarling J, Kidd P, Thomas ED (1987). Monoclonal antibody 1F5 (anti-CD20) serotherapy of human B CLL lymphomas. Blood 69:584.
5. Frödin J-E, Biberfeld P, Christenssen B, Philstedt P, Semdelius S, Sylvén M, Wahren B, Koprowski H, Mellstedt H (1986). Treatment of patients with metastasizing colorectal carcinoma with mouse monoclonal antibodies (Moab 17-1A): a progress report. Hybridoma 5:151.
6. Oldham RK, Foon KA, Morgan AC, Woodhouse CS, Schroff RW, Abrams PG, Fer M, Schoenbergen CS, Farrel M, Kimball E, Sheriv SA (1984). Monoclonal antibody therapy of malignant melanomas: In vitro localization in cutaneous metastasis after intravenous administration. J Clin Oncol 2:1235.
7. Levy R, Levy S, Cleary ML, Carroll W, Kon S, Bird J, Sklar J (1987). Somatic mutation in human B-cell tumors. Immunological Reviews 96:43.
8. Janson CH, Tehrani M, Mellstedt H, Wigzell H (1987). Three kinds of tumor-unique surface molecules on a human T-cell chronic lymphocytic leukaemia (T-CLL) detected by monoclonal antibodies. Scand J Immunol 26:237.
9. Kipps TJ, Parham P, Punt J, Herzenberg LA (1985). Importance of immunoglobulin isotype in human antiboby-dependent, cell-mediated cytotoxicity directed by murine monoclonal antibodies. J Exp Med 161:1.

Human Tumor Antigens and Specific Tumor Therapy, pages 287–296
© 1989 Alan R. Liss, Inc.

THE BASIS FOR GANGLIOSIDE VACCINES IN MELANOMA

Philip O. Livingston
Memorial Sloan-Kettering Cancer Center
New York, N.Y. 10021

ABSTRACT   The gangliosides GM2, GD2, and GD3 are differentiation antigens largely restricted to cells of
neuroectodermal origen. They are expressed on most
melanomas, astrocytomas, and neuroblastomas and have
been shown to function as effective targets for monoclonal antibody therapy. The immunogenicity of these
gangliosides has been explored in the mouse and in man
by analyzing the humoral immune response after
vaccination. In the mouse, vaccination with GM2
combined with Salmonella minnesota mutant R595 or BCG,
but not with GM2 alone or whole cells expressing GM2,
results in frequent production of anti-GM2 IgM, and
similar vaccines containing GD3 (in place of GM2)
result in higher antibody titers than seen with GM2.
Pretreatment of the mice with low dose cyclophosphamide (to decrease suppressor cell activity)
significantly increases the frequency and titers of
anti-ganglioside antibodies. Based on these findings,
my collaborators Drs. L.J. Old and H.F. Oettgen, and
I have treated disease-free patients with metastatic
melanoma with a series of vaccines and used ELISAs on
purified gangliosides to detect the serologic
response. The specificity of observed reactions was
further defined by immune staining of thin layer
chromatography plates. Vaccines containing GM2 alone
resulted in no antibody responses, vaccines containing
R595/GM2 resulted in occasional antibody responses and
those containing BCG/GM2 resulted in high titer antibodies in most patients. Pretreatment with low dose
cyclophosphamide (200 mg/M^2) significantly increased
the immunogenicity of R595 and BCG/GM2 vaccines.
Cimetidine (1 gram/day PO) did not further augment the
immunogenicity of GM2 vaccines in Cy pretreated
patients. Nineteen of 24 patients immunized with Cy-

BCG/GM2 produced high titer IgM antibodies (>1/80) and 8 produced high titer IgG antibodies. Disease progression was found to be significantly delayed in patients with high titer anti-GM2 antibody response after vaccination. Cy-BCG/GD2 or GD3 vaccines, however, resulted in no high titer antibody responses in the 12 patients immunized with each ganglioside. While GM2 is significantly more immunogenic than GD3 in man, the reverse is true in the mouse. This reflects the expression of these gangliosides on normal tissues, i.e. GD3>GM2 in man GM2>GD3 in the mouse.

INTRODUCTION

Although several thousand patients have been injected with tumor cell preparations in this country and elsewhere over the past 25 years (1), the complexity of the studies has made an assessment of the value of this approach to cancer therapy impossible. Even under the most favorable clinical circumstances, and with a most carefully designed trial, the testing of human cancer cell vaccines is fraught with difficulties arising from the uncertainty of whether the vaccines contained in fact tumor-specific antigens, and whether the patients responded immunologically to these antigens. What is required for the development of an immunogenic cancer vaccine are methods to assess effectiveness that are both rapid and objective and that can be used to guide the process of vaccine construction and testing step by step. With regard to vaccines against infectious diseases, serological responses to bacterial or viral antigens have served this purpose. With the development of serological typing systems for defining cell surface antigens of melanoma and other cancers, we now have serological tests of requisite sensitivity and specificity that are comparable to those used for monitoring vaccines against infectious diseases. This is not to say that we think cell-mediated immunity is less important in the host's defense against cancer, on the contrary, just that at present serological techniques are more precise and better suited to screening approaches to vaccine construction.

The basis for clinical trials with vaccines designed to augment the antibody response against poorly immunogenic antigens is a considerable body of experimental evidence supporting the approach. These studies have identified several important aspects of vaccine construction and administration. In this regard, prior to conducting clinical trials with tumor vaccines, three components must be selected: the antigen(s), the adjuvant and the method for decreasing suppressor cell activity.

CHOICE OF ANTIGEN

The most important single decision in planning a clinical trial with active specific immunotherapy is the choice of antigen. My collaborators, Drs. L.J. Old, H.F. Oettgen, and I have emphasized gangliosides and in particular GM2, in our recent studies for the following 4 reasons. 1) The importance of cell surface gangliosides as targets for cancer therapy has been suggested by regression of melanoma and neuroblastoma metastases in patients treated with monoclonal antibodies against GD3 (2), GD2 (3) and GM2 (4), and by our recent findings (described below) that melanoma patients with high titer anti GM2 antibodies appear to have an improved prognosis (5). 2) We have tested the reactivity of sera from 75 melanoma patients on autologous melanoma cells and identified 5 sera with reactivity largely restricted to autologous and allogenic melanoma cells (6). Four of the five shared melanoma antigens identified by these sera are gangliosides related to GM2 and GD2. 3) We have previously described a series of clinical trials with nine different tumor cell vaccines consisting of various autologous or allogeneic melanoma cell lines mixed with BCG or C parvum, or "xenogenized" in various ways, and injected intradermally to patients with early stage metastatic melanoma (7-10). While consistent high titer antibody responses against HLA, fetal calf serum or viral antigens on the immunizing melanoma cells were detected, only occasional serologic reactions against melanoma antigens were seen, and most of these were against gangliosides related to GM2 and GD2. Similar findings have been reported by Tai et al. (11). 4) We have used an anti GM2 mouse monoclonal antibody to identify GM2 as a cell surface antigen largely restricted to cells of neuroectodermal origin, including tumors such as melanoma (12).

CHOICE OF ADJUVANT AND ANTI SUPPRESSOR CELL REAGENT

There was little information available on the relative potency of different approaches to augmenting the immunogenicity of tumor antigens (i.e. adjuvants/cell surface modification/suppressor cell inhibition). Consequently, we studied the effect of immunization with a variety of vaccination approaches on the serological response to the unique cell surface antigen of Meth A sarcoma in the mouse (13,14). Some of these results are shown in Table 1. Endotoxin and monophosphoryl lipid A (Ribi Immunochem) were the most successful adjuvants tested, and the immunogenicity of all vaccines were further increased by pretreatment of the mice with low (anti suppressor cell) dose cyclophosphamide (Cy).

Table 1

THE SEROLOGICAL RESPONSE TO IMMUNIZATION WITH IRRADIATED METH A CELLS:
EFFECT OF ADJUVANTS AND PRETREATMENT WITH CYCLOPHOSPHAMIDE-(CY)

ADJUVANT	NO. METH A CELLS	CY (25 mg/kg)	NO. MICE VACCINATED	NO. MICE MAKING ANTIBODY	MEDIAN ANTI METH A TITER BY CDCX
NONE	5×10^6	-	15	0	
NONE	5×10^6	+	9	9	160
NONE	10^5	-	15	0	
NONE	10^5	+	40	8	80
BCG	10^5	-	8	0	
BCG	10^5	+	14	6	120
*CFA	10^5	-	4	0	
CFA	10^5	+	5	2	240
ENDOTOXIN	10^5	-	8	4	160
ENDOTOXIN	10^5	+	18	15	160
MPLA	10^5	+	28	21	320
MPLA + CWS	10^5	+	20	12	160

* CFA = Complete Freund's Adjuvant: MPLA = Monophosphoryl Lipid A (Ribi Immunochem)
  CWS = Cell Wall Skeletons (Ribi Immunochem)

We have also studied approaches to augmenting the antibody response against the ganglioside GM2 in C57BL/6 x BALB/c F1 mice. We found that vaccines containing GM2 alone were poorly immunogenic, resulting in only occasional low titer antibody responses. A variety of approaches for increasing the immunogenicity of GM2 were identified (15). Salmonella minnesota mutant R595 was the most effective adjuvant, but BCG and liposomes also significantly increased the antibody response and Cy further increased the immunogenicity of these vaccines (15). We have also used Cy plus R595/ganglioside to compare the relative immunogenicity of the gangliosides GM1, GM2, GM3, GD2 and GD3 in these mice (17). Antibody titers were significantly higher against GM1 and GD3 then against GM2, GM3 or GD2, confirming the applicability of this approach to a variety of different antigens. Based on this experience in experimental models we selected R595 and BCG as the adjuvants and Cy as the antisuppressor cell reagent to be tested in clinical trials.

Prior to initiating these trials, however, it was necessary to determine the optimal Cy dose and Cy-vaccine interval. For this purpose we conducted a Phase I trial with three low doses of Cy (100, 300 or 500 mg/M2 IV) to determine the effect on suppressor cell activity in melanoma patients (16). Delayed hypersensitivity to dinitrochlorobenzene and other recall antigens, and the serologic response to primary immunization with pneumococcal or influenza virus antigens were found to be normal and were not changed by Cy treatment. In contrast, in vitro assays for production of antibodies against sheep red blood cell (SRBC) antigens, reactivity in the mixed lymphocyte culture reaction, and induction of suppressor cells by conconavalin A were shown to be abnormal as a consequence of increased suppressor cell activity in many patients and these abnormalities were found to respond to low dose Cy. No difference could be detected between the three doses of Cy, but examining all patients as a group, a statistically significant effect was seen with peak effect on day 21 but clear effects persisting between days 7 and 35. The results obtained in a single patient with the plaque forming cell assay are charted in Figure 1. Figure 1 shows the number of anti SRBC plaque forming cells induced by a one week culture in the presence of SRBC of a melanoma patient's peripheral lymphocytes cultured unseparated or after separation over a sephadex G-10 column to remove suppressor cells. Decreases in suppressor cell activity such as that shown here was largely restricted to patients with increased suppressor cell activity prior to treatment with Cy (16). Our results suggest that increased

suppressor cell activity in patients with malignant
melanoma does not effect immune reactions generally but is
selective, and that the anti suppressor cell effect of Cy
is restricted to reactions with increased suppressor cell
activity prior to treatment. It is not yet possible to
determine which patients have, or would have after
vaccination, high suppressor cell activity against
GM2.Therefore, based on these results, we selected a Cy
dose of 200 mg/M^2 to be administered to all patients, and
days 5-35 after Cy treatment as the optimal interval for
vaccine administration.

FIGURE 1
ANTIGEN SPECIFIC PLAQUE FORMING CELLS IN PERIPHERAL BLOOD OF PATIENT 15 BEFORE AND AFTER TREATMENT WITH CYCLOPHOSPHAMIDE

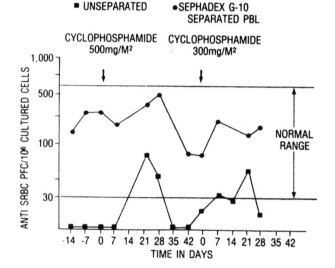

RESULTS OF CLINICAL TRIALS WITH GM2 IN AJCC STAGE III
MELANOMA PATIENTS

The results of 12 trials with 8 different vaccines are
presented in Table 2. GM2 or GM2 attached to R595 in the
absence of Cy was not immunogenic. Pretreatment with Cy
resulted in occasional high titer serologic responses in
R595/GM2 treated patients. N-glycolyl GM2 was not more
immunogenic than standard GM2 (N-acetyl GM2). BCG was a

significantly more immunogenic carrier-adjuvant than R595
and the immunogenicity was further increased by Cy. The
combination of Cy + BCG/GM2 resulted in high titer

Table 2

ANTI GM2 TITERS (ELISA) OF NORMAL INDIVIDUALS, UNTREATED MELANOMA

PATIENTS, AND MELANOMA PATIENTS AFTER IMMUNIZATION WITH PURIFIED GM2 VACCINES

	GM2 DOSE (mcg)	TOTAL NO. PATIENTS	NO. PATIENTS WITH A GIVEN TITER (Reciprocal)					
			0	20	40	80	160	320
NO TREATMENT								
Normal Individuals		44	37	4	2	1	0	0
Stage III Melanoma Patients		50	37	8	3	0	0	0
TREATMENT *								
GM2 Alone	100	5	4	1	0	0	0	0
GM2/R595	100	5	3	2	0	0	0	0
Cy + GM2/R595	100	6	0	1	3	0	2	0
Cy + GM2/R595	300	6	1	1	2	2	0	0
Cy + NG GM2/R595	100	6	1	2	2	1	0	0
GM2/BCG	100	5	0	1	1	1	1	1
Cy + GM2/BCG	100-300	28	2	3	1	7	11	4
Cy + Ci + GM2/BCG	200	12	3	0	0	3	6	0

* NG, N-glycolyl; Cy, cyclophosphamide; Ci, cimetidine.

serologic reactivity (>1/40) in 22 of 28 patients. Addition
of another anti suppressor T cell reagent, Cimetidine (1
gram/day beginning 3 days before the initial immunization
and extending until 2 weeks after the initial series of
immunizations was completed), had no demonstrable effect on
serological titer or duration of titer. The specificity of
all reactions for GM2 was confirmed by immune staining of
thin layer chromatography plates as previously described
(5).

We have previously reported that evaluation of 31
vaccinated patients with resected locally metastatic
melanoma observed for 15 months showed a significantly
improved disease free interval in patients with serologic
titers of 40 or greater (5). We have now followed these and
33 additional patients for at least 2 years after

immunization. Figure 2 shows a comparison of the time to melanoma progression in patients with titers of 40 or greater and those with titers of 20 or less. The significantly improved prognosis in patients with anti GM2 antibody may reflect improved prognosis as a consequence of vaccination, or antibody production may identify patients destined to do well irrespective of vaccination. We have recently initiated a randomized immunization trial comparing non-specific immunotherapy (low dose Cy and BCG applied intradermally) with specific immunotherapy (Cy and BCG/GM2) to address this question.

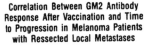

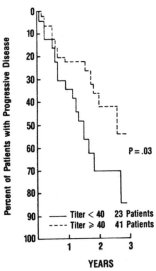

Correlation Between GM2 Antibody Response After Vaccination and Time to Progression in Melanoma Patients with Ressected Local Metastases

P = .03

Titer < 40   23 Patients
Titer ≥ 40   41 Patients

Tumor heterogeneity, antibody synergism and the possibility that immune responses against other melanoma antigens may have greater protective value, provide strong motivation for the development of a multivalent tumor vaccine. Consequently, 12 patients have been immunized with Cy plus BCG/GD2 and 12 patients with Cy plus BCG/GD3, resulting in 3 antibody titers of 40 against GD2 and none over 20

against GD3. We continue to search for new immunogenic
melanoma antigens and improved approaches for augmenting
the immunogenicity of GD2 and GD3.

HORROR AUTOTOXICUS

The greater immunogenicity of GM2 than GD3 in man
contrasts sharply with the ease of inducing a serologic
response against GD3 in the mouse and the difficulty of
inducing anti GM2 antibodies. When ganglioside expression
on normal (non-brain) tissues in man and mouse are compared
however (17), antibody titers vary inversely with
ganglioside expression. GM2 expression in human kidney,
liver and spleen is less than 3% of total gangliosides in
each case as compared with greater than 50% of total
ganglioside in murine liver and greater than 10% in murine
spleen and erythrocytes. In contrast, GD3 expression is
19% on human kidney and there is significant expression of
GD3 on human T cells, while GD3 is not expressed more than
3% on any murine tissues. This emphasizes the importance of
selecting tumor antigens for vaccine construction and
clinical testing based on previously detected antibody
production in patients or detailed immunohistologic or
extraction data showing low expression of the antigen on
normal tissues.   This is consistent with the concept of
"horror autotoxicus" which dates back to 1900 when it was
first expressed by Ehrlich (18).

Our studies suggest that there is a window between the
level of antigen expression on normal tissues permitting
antibody induction after appropriate vaccination and the
level resulting in immune rejection in the presence of
these antibodies. The level of GM2, GD2 and GD3 expressed
in human melanoma cells is at least 10-fold higher than in
the major organ systems (excluding brain) that we reviewed
(17,19). The basis for our continuing studies with GM2,
GD2 and GD3 ganglioside vaccines in melanoma patients,
then, rests on these three findings: 1) this apparent
window of opportunity between the quantity of GM2, GD2 and
GD3 ganglioside in normal (nonbrain) tissues and the
greater amount in melanomas, 2) the proven value of GM2,
GD2 and GD3 as targets for immune therapy in melanoma
patients, and 3) our ability in these initial trials to
induce a consistent antibody response against GM2, with no
detectable toxicity.

BIBLIOGRAPHY

1. Livingston PO et al (1982). In Immunologic
   Approaches to Cancer Therapeutics, E Mihich, Ed.,
   John Wiley & Sons, Inc., New York, 364.
2. Houghton AN, et al (1985). PNAS 82: 1242.
3. Cheung N-K V, et al (1987). J Clin Oncol 5: 1430.
4. Irie RF & Morton DL (1986). PNAS 83: 8694.
5. Livingston PO, et al (1987). PNAS 84: 2911.
6. Old LJ (1981). Cancer Res 41: 361.
7. Livingston PO, et al (1982). Int J Cancer 30: 413.
8. Livingston PO, et al (1983). Int J Cancer 31: 567.
9. Livingston PO, et al (1985). Cancer 55: 713.
10. Livingston PO, et al (1985). In Monoclonal
    Antibodies and Cancer Therapy, UCLA Symposia
    on Molecular and Cellular Biology, New Series,
    Vol. 27, eds. R.A. Reisfeld and S. Sell, Alan
    R. Liss, Inc., New York, N.Y.
11. Tai T, et al (1985). Int J Cancer 35: 607-612.
12. Natoli Jr EJ, et al (1986). Cancer Res 46: 4116.
13. Livingston PO, et al (1983). J. Imm 131: 2601.
14. Livingston PO, et al (1985). J. Imm 135: 1505.
15. Livingston PO, et al (1987). J. Imm 138: 1524.
16. Livingston PO, et al (1987). J. Biol Resp Mod 6:
    392.
17. Livingston PO, et al (1988). J. Imm (in press).
18. Ehrlich, P (1900). Proc. R. Soc. Lond. (Biol.) 66B:
    424.
19. Tsuchida T, et al (1987). J Natl Cancer Inst 78:
    55.

Human Tumor Antigens and Specific Tumor Therapy, pages 297–306
© 1989 Alan R. Liss, Inc.

IMMUNOTHERAPY OF MELANOMA WITH AUTOLOGOUS TUMOR VACCINE PRECEDED BY LOW DOSE CYCLOPHOSPHAMIDE

David Berd[1]

Division of Medical Oncology, Thomas Jefferson University, Philadelphia, Pa. 19107

ABSTRACT   Cyclophosphamide (CY), can augment immune responses in experimental animals and humans. We have shown that administration of CY to patients with metastatic melanoma is followed by a reduction in the number of circulating CD4+ T cells expressing the antigen, 2H4, a marker for inducers of T suppressor function. Treatment of these patients with CY + autologous melanoma vaccine can induced delayed-type hypersensitivity to autologous tumor cells, which is sometimes associated with clinically-important regression of metastases. Finally, these experiments have provided evidence that antigenic heterogeneity of melanoma cells is an important limitation of this therapeutic approach.

INTRODUCTION

It is now generally recognized that the cytotoxic drug, cyclophosphamide (CY), can augment immune responses in both experimental animals and humans.

[1]This work was supported by Grant CA39248 from the National Cancer Institute

The initial animal experiments were reported by Maguire and Ettore (1). In the course of their studies of the modulation by CY of the induction and expression of allergic dermatitis, these investigators made an unexpected observation: Guinea pigs treated with CY and then contact-sensitized developed much more intense and prolonged allergic contact dermatitis reactions than did control guinea pigs that had received sensitizer alone. This finding was soon confirmed: CY was observed to immunopotentiate the acquisition of delayed-type hypersensitivity (DTH) to a variety of conventional antigens (2) and even to syngeneic testicular tissue (3). The critical factor determining whether CY depressed or potentiated an immune response in experimental animals was the timing of administration of CY and antigen. Thus, the administration of CY to guinea pigs 2 days before sensitization to an antigen increases the DTH response three- to fourfold, whereas administration of CY after sensitization completely suppresses it (2).

Our laboratory first demonstrated this phenomenon in humans. In two studies, we sensitized advanced cancer patients with the primary antigen, keyhole limpet hemocyanin (KLH), either alone or 3 days after administration of CY, 1000 mg/M^2 or 300 mg/M^2 (4,5). DTH was tested by injecting 0.1 mg KLH intradermally and measuring the mean diameter of induration at 48 hours. Pretreatment of patients with CY, at either "high" or "low" dose, significantly augmented the development of DTH to KLH; the median DTH responses were as follows: KLH alone = 0 mm, KLH + CY 1000 mg/M^2 = 18 mm, KLH + CY 300 mg/M^2 = 27 mm. DTH responses to microbial recall antigens (trichophyton, mumps, candida) were not augmented by CY administration, indicating that immunopotentiation was not due to CY alone but to CY administered at the proper interval before cutaneous injection of antigen.

It has become apparent that CY immunopotentiation in rodents is due to selective inhibition of T suppressor function.

This has been demonstrated directly in the
studies of Kaufmann et al (6), who showed that T
cells capable of transferring antigen-specific
suppression were much more sensitive to CY than
T cells capable of transferring DTH. This
principle was subsequently extended to
experimental tumor systems. For example,
North (7) showed that established tumors could
be cured by adoptive transfer of immune
lymphocytes if, and only if, mice were depleted
of suppressor T cells by administration of CY.

RESULTS

Reduction in Suppressor T Cell Function After CY

Work from our laboratory indicates that
administration of CY causes reduction of T cell-
mediated suppressor function, possibly by
selective toxicity for a subset of T lymphocytes
that is necessary for the induction of
suppressor activity. Thus in two studies (8,9)
we demonstrated that the generation of
concanavalin A-inducible T suppressor cells was
significantly impaired in PBL from tumor-bearing
patients treated with CY - either 1000 mg/M^2 or
300 mg/M^2. Suppressor function was
significantly reduced by day 3, and declined
progressively through day 21. In parallel, PBL
were tested for their proliferative response to
phytohemagglutinin (PHA). In contrast to its
effect on Con A suppressors, CY caused no
significant changes in PHA reactivity.
Initially, we hypothesized that the
reduction in suppressor function would be
paralleled by a selective loss of the CD8+
subset of T cells, with relative sparing of CD4+
(helper-inducer) T cells, but that model proved
to be incorrect: Neither high dose nor low dose
CY caused any significant changes in the
relative proportions of these two subsets
(8,9,10).
However, treatment of melanoma patients
with CY + autologous melanoma vaccine (described
below) did result in a gradual fall in the

number of CD4+ T cells expressing the 2H4
antigen (10). This CD4+,2H4+ subset is required
for the induction of suppressor function in CD8+
cells (11). It is noteworthy that the reduction
of CD4+, 2H4+ T cells did not become apparent
until day 28 after the first dose of CY and
reached statistically significance only on days
49 (21 days after the second dose) and 105 (21
days after the fourth dose). In contrast, there
was no change in the number of CD4+ T cells
expressing the antigen 4B4, which are considered
to function as true helper cells (11).

We considered the possibility that these
changes could be attributed solely to
progression of metastatic disease. However, a
comparison of patients with progressive
metastases with patients who remained disease-
free showed no significant differences in the
reduction of the percentage of CD4+ T cells
expressing 2H4+. In addition, we were able to
study lymphocytes from 5 patients who had
received the vaccine on the same schedule, but
without CY pretreatment, all of whom had
progressive metastases, and found that the
percentage of CD4+ T cells expressing 2H4
actually increased.

Augmentation of DTH to Autologous Melanoma Cells

Our findings on CY potentiation of cell-
mediated to KLH suggested that a similar
approach could be used to induce a meaningful
immune response to autologous tumor cells. To
address this question, we treated 19 patients
with advanced melanoma with an autologous
melanoma vaccine, consisting of 25×10^6
irradiated tumor cells mixed with BCG, either
alone, or 3 days after administration of CY,
300 mg/M^2 (12). The DTH responses of CY-
pretreated patients were significantly greater
than those of controls (medians: vaccine alone =
4 mm, CY + vaccine = 11 mm, p<.05, 2-tailed
Mann-Whitney U test). At the completion of two
vaccine treatments, 7/8 CY patients, but only

2/7 controls had DTH reaction greater than 5 mm (p=.034, Fisher's exact test).

This initial study was performed with tumor cells that had been dissociated with enzymes (collagenase and DNAse). It soon became apparent CY-pretreated patients developed strong DTH to residual enzymes on the immunizing tumor cells. Therefore, in subsequent studies we skin-tested patients with autologous melanoma cells that had been obtained by mechanical dissociation. Prior to immunotherapy, DTH to enzyme-free tumor cells was minimal (mean = 2.7 mm). Statistically significant increases in DTH were observed after 2 course of CY + vaccine (49 days) with progressive increases measured on days 154, 210, and 266 (Figure 1).

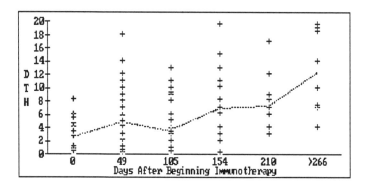

FIGURE 1. DTH to autologous melanoma cells. Each mark represents the DTH response (diameter of induration, mm) of an individual patient. The line represents the mean.

After two treatments (49 days), 44.1% of patients had "positive" DTH reactions (>5 mm induration); of patients who received at least 10 treatments, 90.0% were "positive". Thus, it appears that patients receiving CY + vaccine developed DTH to tumor-associated antigens and that the magnitude of the reaction increased with repeated immunizations.

DTH to Different Tumor Preparations from the
Same Patient

Seven patients who developed DTH to
melanoma cells in their vaccine preparation
subsequently developed new metastases from which
tumor cells were obtained and tested for ability
to elicit DTH. As shown in Figure 2, 5/7 cases,
the DTH response to the "new" tumor was
considerably less than the DTH response to the
"old" tumor. In the other 2 cases, DTH to the
two preparations was similar.

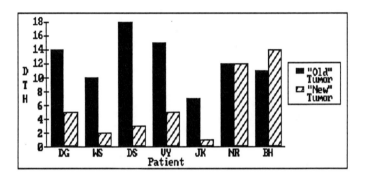

FIGURE 2. Comparison of DTH responses of
individual patients to "old" and "new" melanoma
cells.

Although the sample size is small, these
observations support the hypothesis that
metastases that developed after immunization
were antigenically different from the original
tumors used for immunization.

With two patients we were able to retest
the DTH response to a "new" tumor before and
after immunizing with that tumor. In both
cases, immunization with the "old" tumor
resulted in the development of DTH to those
cells but not to cells from the "new" tumor.
Subsequent immunization with the "new" tumor was

followed by the development of DTH to those
cells as well.

Anti-Tumor Responses

   In some patients, the development of DTH to
melanoma cells following treatment with CY +
vaccine was associated with regression of
metastatic disease. Thus, of 35 evaluable
patients, 3 had complete remissions (CR) and 2
had partial remissions (PR). The metastatic
sites and remission durations were as follows:
1)CR - multiple cutaneous and a single pulmonary
metastases, 65+ months; 2)CR - cutaneous and
liver metastases, 39 months; 3)CR - single
nodal metastasis, 15 months; 4)PR - lung
metastasis, 10 months; 5)PR - complete
regression of skin metastases with concomitant
radiation therapy of a solitary bone metastasis,
8 months. In addition, 3 patients exhibited
minor degrees of tumor regression with complete
regression of some lesions followed by the
development of new metastatic sites.

DISCUSSION

   In a series of experiments performed over
the past 6 years, we have demonstrated that CY
can augment human immune responses, thus
corroborating the results reported previously
reported with experimental animals.
Pretreatment of advanced cancer patients with CY
3 days before injection of antigen resulted in
significant augmentation of the development of
DTH to both KLH and to autologous melanoma
cells. As predicted by the animal data, CY
caused potentiation of DTH at both "high"
(1000 mg/M^2) and "low" (300 mg/M^2) doses.
   Although we have not yet determined the
specificity of the immune response elicited by
melanoma cells, it seems likely that the
response was directed against melanoma-
associated antigens, because: 1)Clinically
significant regression of metastases occurred in

5 patients following CY + vaccine;
2)Immunotherapy was often followed by the
development of DTH to autologous melanoma cells
that were not contaminated with enzymes,
antibiotics, or other artifacts; 3)Patients who
developed "new" metastases while receiving
immunotherapy exhibited less DTH to the "new"
tumor cells that to the "old" tumor cells to
which they had been putatively immunized; 4)In
three cases, we have demonstrated lymphocytic
infiltration of metastatic masses following
immunotherapy (13).

The mechanism of CY immunopotentiation in
humans has not been clearly defined, but our
data suggest that it is due to reduction of T
suppressor function and, possibly, to depletion
of the 2H4+ subset of CD4+ T cells that is
required for induction of suppression. A
tentative model suggested by these findings is
that CY's selective toxicity for inducer T cells
results in impaired generation of antigen-
specific suppression, and thus more efficient
production of T cells that mediate DTH and
provide help for antibody production. This
model is also supported by in vitro experiments
previously reported by Ozer et al (14).

It seems likely that more effective
immunization of tumor-bearing patients against
tumor-associated antigens could be accomplished
by intelligent manipulation of the immune
system. If so, there is reason to be optimistic
that such approaches will eventually lead to
immunologically-mediated cures of human cancer.

ACKNOWLEDGMENTS

The author wishes to acknowledge the
assistance of Carmella Clark and Ellen Hart, RN,
whose skills and dedication were essential to
the completion of this work.

REFERENCES

1. Maguire, HC Jr, Ettore VL (1967).
    Enhancement of dinitrochlorobenzene (DNCB)
    contact sensitization by cyclophosphamide
    in the guinea pig. J Invest Dermatol,
    48:39-42.
2. Turk JL, Parker D (1982). Effect of
    cyclophosphamide on immunological control
    mechanisms. Immunol Rev 65:99-113.
3. Yoshida S, Nomoto K, Himeno K, Takeya K
    (1979). Immune response to syngeneic or
    autologous testicular cells in mice.
    I.Augmented delayed footpad reaction in
    cyclophosphamide-treated mice. Clin Exper
    Immunol 38: 211-217.
4. Berd D, Mastrangelo MJ, Engstrom PF, Paul
    A, Maguire H (1982). Augmentation of the
    human immune response by cyclophosphamide.
    Cancer Res 42:4862-4866.
5. Berd D, Maguire HC Jr, Mastrangelo MJ
    (1984). Potentiation of human cell-mediated
    and humoral immunity by low-dose
    cyclophosphamide. Cancer Res 44: 5439-5443.
6. Kaufmann SHE, Hahn H, Diamantstein T
    (1980). Relative susceptibilities of T cell
    subsets involved in delayed-type
    hypersensitivity to sheep red blood cells
    to the in vitro action of
    4-hydroperoxycyclophosphamide. J Immunol,
    125:1104-1108.
7. North RJ (1982). Cyclophosphamide-
    facilitated adoptive immunotherapy of an
    established tumor depends on elimination of
    tumor-induced suppressor T cells. J Exp
    Med, 55:1063-1074.
8. Berd D, Maguire HC Jr, Mastrangelo MJ
    (1984). Impairment of concanavalin A-
    inducible suppressor activity following
    administration of cyclophosphamide to
    patients with advanced cancer. Cancer Res
    44:1275-1280.

9.   Berd D, Mastrangelo MJ (1987). Effect of low dose cyclophosphamide on the immune system of cancer patients. Reduction of T suppressor function without depletion of the CD8+ subset. Cancer Res, 47:3317-3321.

10.   Berd D, Mastrangelo MJ (1988). Effect of low dose cyclophosphamide on the immune system of cancer patients: Depletion of CD4+, 2H4+ suppressor-inducer T cells. Cancer Res, 48:1671-1675.

11.   Morimoto C, Letvin NL, Distaso JA, Aldrich WR, Schlossman SF (1985). The isolation and characterization of the human suppressor inducer T cell subset. J Immunol 134:1508-1515.

12.   Berd D, Maguire HC Jr, Mastrangelo MJ (1986). Induction of cell-mediated immunity to autologous melanoma cells and regression of metastases after treatment with a melanoma cell vaccine preceded by cyclophosphamide. Cancer Res 46:2572-2577.

13.   Berd D, Mastrangelo MJ (1988). Active immunotherapy of human melanoma exploiting the immunopotentiating effects of cyclophosphamide. Cancer Invest, in press.

14.   Ozer H, Cowens JW, Colvin M, Nussbaum-Blumenson A, Sheedy D (1982). In vitro effects of 4-hydroperoxycyclophosphamide on human immunoregulatory T subset function. I. Selective effects on lymphocyte function in T-B collaboration. J Exp Med 155:276-290.

Human Tumor Antigens and Specific Tumor Therapy, pages 307–315
© 1989 Alan R. Liss, Inc.

VACCINE IMMUNOTHERAPY OF HUMAN MALIGNANT MELANOMA:
RELATIONSHIP BETWEEN METHOD OF IMMUNIZATION,
IMMUNOGENICITY,
AND TUMOR PROGRESSION (1)

J-C. BYSTRYN, M. DUGAN, R. ORATZ, J. SPEYER,
M.N. HARRIS, AND D.F. ROSES.

Kaplan Cancer Center
New York University School of Medicine
560 First Avenue
New York, New York 10016

ABSTRACT   63 patients with surgically resected Stage
II malignant melanoma were immunized to a polyvalent melanoma antigen vaccine using one of 4 immunization procedures.   There was a relationship between the ability of
the procedure to augment delayed type hypersensitivity
(DTH) responses to the vaccine and delay in tumor progression.   Overall, DTH responses to the vaccine were augmented in 25 (40%) of the patients.   The median disease-free
interval was 2 years longer in responding than in non-
responding patients.   Though this represents a 3 fold pro-
longation in disease-free interval, it is not yet statistically significant by log rank analysis.   The median disease-free interval has not been reached for responding patients, so that these numbers are subject to change.
These results suggest that the progression of melanoma in
man may be delayed in patients who develop a DTH response
to vaccine immunization.   Measuring the DTH response to
tumor vaccines may also provide an early indication of
their clinical effectiveness.

(1)This work was supported by a USPHS Research Grant
CA34358, and by grants from the Fred P. Goldhirsh Foundation, the Skin Cancer Foundation, Pardee Foundation and
the Culpepper Foundation.

INTRODUCTION

Tumor vaccines are conceptually attractive as immunotherapy for cancer. They have the potential to be very
specific in their effect, of stimulating both humoral and
cellular immune responses to tumors, and of inducing long
lasting immunity. A unique feature of vaccines is their
potential application to prevent cancer in persons without
the disease.The rational and results of vaccine immunotherapy of melanoma have recently been reviewed (1,2). The
most convincing evidence vaccines can be effective is that
they can prevent melanoma in animals (3-5). In man, they
appear to be safe to use and immunologically active (6-
11), but their immunogenicity is generally poor. There is
an intense interest in measures that can potentiate vaccine immunogenicity and in identifying immune parameters
of vaccine activity that relate to clinical effectiveness.
The aim of this study was to examine the relationship
between methods of immunization, vaccine immunogenicity,
and tumor progression. The study was conducted in patients with minimal tumor burden but poor prognosis using
a partially purified, polyvalent, melanoma antigen vaccine
which in prior studies has been shown to be safe to use
and able to augment humoral and/or cellular immune responses to melanoma in some patients (10).

METHODS

Melanoma Vaccine:

Vaccine was prepared from material shed into serum-
free   culture medium by 4 lines of melanoma cells, as
previously described (7).   Three of the cell lines were
human and one was of hamster origin. The cells were selected because they expressed different patterns of cell-
surface melanoma associated antigens (MAA's). The   cells
were adapted to grow, and were maintained, in serum-free
medium to prevent contamination of the vaccine with fetal
calf serum proteins.

For vaccine production, shed material was collected,
concentrated by vacuum dialysis, pooled, treated with 0.5%
NP-40 to break up aggregates, and ultracentrifuged at
100,000 x g for 90 minutes to remove transplantation alloantigens. The supernatant was filter sterilized, adjusted

to a protein concentration of 200 ug/ml, dispensed into sterile glass vials, and frozen at -70C until used. Some lots of vaccine were bound to alum. Aggregated vaccine was prepared as above but omitting the NP-40, ultracentrifugation, and filtration steps.

All lots of vaccine were tested for aerobic and anaerobic bacteria, fungi, and pyrogens and injected into mice and guinea pigs for general safety tests. The melanoma cells used for vaccine production were tested and found free of HIV and hepatitis virus, and were negative for other virus infections by culture on human embryo cells.

Patients and Immunization Procedures:

The vaccine was used to treat 63 patients with surgically resected stage II melanoma. All had intact cellular immunity as evidenced by skin test reactivity to recall antigens or ability to be sensitized to DNCB. Patients were entered sequentially into one of 4 immunization protocols (Table 1).

TABLE 1

IMMUNIZATION PROTOCOL	VACCINE	DOSE ug (a)	ADJUVANT	SCHEDULE (b)	NO PTS TREATED
A	soluble	1-160(c)	none	I	11
B	soluble	40	none	II	12
C	soluble	40	alum	II	24
D	aggregated	40	none	II	16
TOTAL					63

a) indicated dose split into 4 aliquots and administered in 0.05 ml of saline into each extremity.
b) I= immunization weekly x 8 with escalating dose vaccine
   II=   "   q 2wks x 4   "   fixed   "
   subsequently, all pts immunized monthly x 3, q3 months x 2, and q6 months to disease recurrence.
c) 1 ug/wk x 2; 10 ug/wk x 2; 40 ug/wk x 2; 160 ug/wk x 2.

Immune Studies:

Cellular immune response to the vaccine was evaluated by delayed type hypersensitivity (DTH) reactions to intra-dermal skin tests to 10ug of vaccine. This was measured before and 6-10 weeks after initiation of treatment. DTH was considered to have been augmented by immunization if the average diameter of induration post-immunization was at least 10 mm greater than the pre-immune measurement in the same patient.

Evaluation of Tumor Progression and Statistical Analysis:

All patients were followed at regular intervals. Disease-free interval was calculated as the number of months between initiation of vaccine therapy and first documented evidence of tumor recurrence. The median disease-free interval was calculated by Kaplan-Meier analysis and the significance of differences in these intervals calculated by the log rank test.

RESULTS

Immunogenicity Of Melanoma Vaccine:

The vaccine augmented cellular immune responses to melanoma, as measured by DTH response to the vaccine, in 25 (40%) of the 63 patients entered into the study (Table 2). Different immunization protocols differed in their effectiveness. The most effective was protocol C, i.e. immunization with a fixed dose of vaccine (40 ug) bound to alum as an adjuvant. It augmented DTH responses to mela-noma in 54% of 24 patients.

TABLE 2
IMMUNOGENICITY OF MELANOMA VACCINE

IMMUNIZATION PROTOCOL	NO PTS	CELLULAR(a) RESPONSE No (%) pts
A	11	2 (18%)
B	12	5 (42%)
C	24	13 (54%)
D	16	5 (32%)
TOTAL	63	25 (40%)

a)b)>10 mm increase in DTH response
to vaccine post-immunization.

To evaluate the antigenicity of the individual melanoma cell line used to construct the vaccine, (7) patients
with a DTH response to the vaccine were skin tested concurrently to the complete vaccine and to vaccine prepared
similarly from each individual cell line.   Various patterns of reactivity were seen.   Most patients reacted to
more than one cell line; and all reacted to at least one
of the human cell lines.   In some cases reaction to the
single cell vaccine was stronger than to the complete vaccine. We suspect this is because the concentration of the
reactive cell line in the complete vaccine was only one
quarter that in the single cell vaccine.

Tumor Progression In Immunized Patients:

The progression of melanoma seemed to be delayed in
patients in whom immunization augmented DTH response to
the vaccine in comparison to those who did not respond.
Two years post immunization there were 28% fewer recurrences in responding than in non-responding patients (recurrences in 60% of 30 non-responding patients at risk vs
in 43% of 21 responding patients at risk).   The median-
disease free interval was 2 years longer in responders

than in non-responders (>38 vs 13.5 months respectively).
Though there was a 3 fold difference in disease-free interval between responding and non-responding patients, the
difference is not statistically significant by log rank
analysis (p<0.1). The median disease-free interval for
patients with a DTH response to the vaccine has not yet
been reached, so that these numbers are subject to change.

The differences in progression of melanoma between
patients with and without DTH response to the vaccine did
not appear to result from differences in disease severity.
There was no major difference in the incidence of risk
factors which are known to influence the progression of
stage II melanoma between the two groups i.e. age greater
than 50, stage II at presentation, nodes clinically positive, 2 or more histologically positive nodes, and primary
lesions greater than 1.7 mm in size.

Relationship Between Immunization Protocol, Cellular
Immune Response To Immunization, and Tumor Progression:

There was a relationship between the ability of immunization protocols to augment cellular responses to the
vaccine and tumor progression (Table 3). Recurrences were
least frequent and the median disease-free interval longest in patients immunized to the protocol that most often
induced cellular responses (protocol C). The reverse was
true for the immunization protocol that least often augmented DTH responses to immunization (Protocol A).

TABLE 3

RELATIONSHIP BETWEEN IMMUNIZATION PROTOCOL, CELLULAR
RESPONSE TO IMMUNIZATION, AND PROGRESSION OF MELANOMA.

IMMUNIZATION PROTOCOL	NO PTS	% WITH DTH RESPONSE	DISEASE PROGRESSION disease-free interval(a)
A	11	18%	11 months
D	16	32%	12.5 "
B	12	42%	26 "
C	24	54%	34.5 "

a)by Kaplan-Meier life table analysis

DISCUSSION:

The most important result of this study is that the progression of early metastatic malignant melanoma in man seems to be delayed in patients who develop a cellular immune response to immunization to a polyvalent melanoma antigen vaccine. There was a relationship between the ability of different immunization procedures to stimulate delayed cutaneous hypersensitivity reactions to the vaccine and delay in tumor progression.

The current study was conducted with a partially purified, polyvalent, melanoma antigen vaccine which was designed to circumvent some of the problems associated with prior vaccines (7). The important features of the vaccine are that: a) it contains multiple MAA's to augment the chance of containing antigens expressed by the tumor to be treated, b) it is enriched in surface antigens which are more likely to be biologically relevant, c) it is prepared from cultured cells to ensure a continued and reproducible source of material for vaccine preparation, d) the cells have been adapted to grow in serum-free medium to minimize contamination of vaccine by these undesirable and highly immunogeneic proteins, e) the biochemical and antigenic properties of the vaccine have been partially characterized (7).

The results of this study suggest that a melanoma vaccine may be able to slow the progression of melanoma if able to augment cellular immunity to melanoma as measured by DTH response to the vaccine. The median disease-free interval in 25 pts with stage II disease who developed a DTH response to the vaccine was 2 years longer than in 38 similar patients who failed to respond. Though there is a 3 fold difference in disease-free interval between responding and non-responding patients, this difference is not yet statistically significant by log rank analysis ($p < 0.1$). The median disease-free interval for patients with a DTH response to the vaccine has not yet been reached, so that these numbers are subject to change. Our results also suggest that the method of immunization has an impact both on the immunogenicity and clinical effectiveness of vaccines. The most effective of 4 immunization protocols we examined was immunization with a constant dose of antigen bound to alum which augmented DTH responses to the vaccine in 54% of patients. There was a relationship between increasing effectiveness of an immunization protocols as estimated by ability to increase DTH responses to the vaccine and clinical effectiveness as measured by delay in tumor progression.

The differences in progression of melanoma in patients with and without cellular responses to immunization are unlikely to be due to differences in severity of disease between the two groups. There was no significant difference in the major risk factors that influence the prognosis of stage II melanoma between the two groups.

However, we have not excluded the possibility that the difference in outcome between the two groups reflects the selection of patients with a more active immune system who do well because of that and not because the vaccine has induced an antimelanoma immune response. We believe this possibility is unlikely as all patients entered into the study had intact cellular immunity as evidenced by ability to respond to recall antigens or to be sensitized to DNCB.

The nature of the antigens responsible for the induction of cellular responses to immunization is not clear. They seem to be melanoma related since none of 17 patients with a DTH reaction to the melanoma vaccine reacted to an equal amount of a control vaccine prepared from pooled allogenenic peripheral leukocytes or to human albumin (10).

Though the vaccine contains hamster melanoma products, we found by skin testing 7 patients to single cell line vaccines that the responses which were induced were all directed, at least in part, to human melanoma.

Lastly, our results must be interpreted with caution since they are derived from studies conducted in relatively small numbers of patients.

The relationship that we have observed between methods of immunization, stimulation of delayed type hypersensitive responses to vaccine, and delay in tumor progression suggest that measuring DTH response to melanoma vaccine may provide an early indication of vaccine's clinical effectiveness. The development of melanoma vaccines should be guided in part by their ability to potentiate cellular immunity to this cancer.

REFERENCES

1.   Bystryn J-C, (1988). "Vaccine immunotherapy of melanoma." Springer-Verlag: In S. Ferrone, "Human Melanoma: Immunology, Diagnostic, and Therapy", Springer-Verlag, Berlin. In Press.

2. Dugan M, Bystryn J-C, (1988). "Immunotherapy in the treatment of malignant melanoma." In Friedman R.J., Rigel D.R., Kopf A.W., Harris M.N., Baker, D.(eds): "Cancer Of The Skin", Saunders, New York. In Press.

3. Bystryn J-C (1978). Antibody response and tumor growth in syngeneic mice immunized to partially purified B16 melanoma-associated antigens.   J Immunol 120:96-101.

4. Avent J, Vervaert C, Seigler HF (1979). Non-specific and specific active immunotherapy in a B16 murine melanoma system.   J Surg Oncol 12:87-96.

5. Livingston PO, Calves MJ, Natoli EJ (1987). Approaches to augmenting the immunogenicity of the ganglioside GM2 in mice, purified GM2 is superior to whole cells.   J Immunol. 138:1524-1529.

6. Seigler HF, Cox E, Mutzner F, et al: (1979). Specific active immunotherapy for melanoma.   Ann Surg 100:366-372.

7. Bystryn J-C, Jacobsen S, Harris M et al: (1986). Preparation and characterization of a polyvalent human melanoma antigen vaccine.   J Biol Response Modifier 5:211-224.

8. Berd D, MaGuire HC Jr, Mastrangelo MJ (1986). Induction of cell-mediated immunity to autologous melanoma cells and regression of metastases after treatment with a melanoma cell vaccine preceded by cyclophosphamide.   Cancer Res. 46:2572-2577.

9. Livingston PO, Natoli EJ, Calves MJ (1987). Vaccines containing purified GM2 ganglioside elicit GM2 antibodies in melanoma patients.   Proc Natl Acad Sci (USA) 84:2911-2915.

10. Bystryn J-C, Oratz R, Harris MH et al: (1988). Immunogenicity of a polyvalent melanoma antigen vaccine in man.   Cancer 61:1065-1070.

11. Wallack MK, Bash JA, Leftheriotis E, et al: (1987). Positive relationship of clinical and serologic responses to vaccinia melanoma oncolysate.   Arch Surg. 122:1460-1463.

Human Tumor Antigens and Specific Tumor Therapy, pages 317–334

HUMAN TUMOR REGRESSION-ASSOCIATED
ANTIGENIC DETERMINANTS

George C. Fareed, Jar-How Lee,
Pradip Gosh-Dastidar and Alvin Liu

International Genetic Engineering, Inc. (INGENE)
1545 17th Street
Santa Monica, CA 90404

and

Guy J.F. Juillard, William H. McBride,
Thomas H. Weisenburger, Daniel Padua
and Danilo Canlapan

Immunotherapy Section
Department of Radiation Oncology
UCLA School of Medicine
Los Angeles, CA 90024

ABSTRACT The use of active specific
immunotherapy in cancer patients has demonstrated in a growing number of investigations the ability to elicit regressions
in solid tumors, decreased incidences of
tumor recurrences and increased survival
rates in malignancies with high recurrence
rates. We have attempted to define the
components in crude human tumor cell
vaccines which are eliciting anti-tumor
responses after intralymphatic infusion of
irradiated, whole cell preparations. Our
approach has been to examine antibody
responses in immunized patients by
immunoblot assays on human tumor cell
extracts and cellular immune responses
directed against human tumor cell targets.

These studies have revealed specific
antibody responses in different responding
patients most commonly to antigens of
approximately 22, 38, 43 and 70 kDa. These
antigenic determinants can be detected on
human tumors and are shared by different
malignancies. Preliminary findings on
cellular immune responses using both
cytostasis and cytotoxicity assays indicate
significantly enhanced cellular immunity in
responding patients.

INTRODUCTION

Various forms of active specific
immunotherapy of cancer have been used for years
(2-4,7,8,11,12,16A,19-23,27,28,32,38,42,49,53,
55). In brief, studies in animal models have
definitively demonstrated that adjuvant plus
antigen can be used to induce a immune response
effective in controlling microscopic
transplantable tumor in rodents and a variety of
other animals. While these studies have proven
reproducible in these animal tumor models, there
translation to the clinic has been difficult.
Some of the clinical studies seem to indicate
minor effects but most have proven negative.
While a variety of mechanisms have been proposed
for active specific immunotherapy including
induction of antibody, activation of
macrophages, induction of cytotoxic T-cells and
activation of NK cells, none of these mechanisms
have been demonstrated as a unifying hypothesis
for specific immunotherapy (7,16,37,40,42).
More recent studies using active specific
immunotherapy have indicated some mechanisms by
which this modality might work (4,8). The
disruption of the cellular architecture of the
tumor so that other factors (chemotherapy,
biotherapy, etc.) may become active has been
proposed (8). There is now increasing evidence
that the active specific immunotherapy of human
cancer may be of value both for its direct
effects on activating immune responses in the
patient as well as through its effects on
activating B-cells for human antibody production

in vitro (4,9). Thus, there is increasing
rationale for the use of active specific
immunotherapy in man and while it is unclear
whether this active specific immunotherapy
should be in the form of viral oncolysates, BCG
plus autologous tumor cells, purified tumor
antigen plus adjuvant or autologous and/or
allogeneic human tumor cells formulated based on
specific monoclonal antibody typing profiles
from frozen sections of each patient's tumor
(39,42,52).

One major limitation of the efforts in
active specific immunization has been the
undefined nature of the tumor cell preparations
(generally, intact autologous or allogeneic
irradiated cell suspensions or mechanically
disrupted lysates). Cells from autologous tumor
cells grown in tissue culture or continuously
passaged tumor cell lines may undergo
significant changes in their antigen expression
profiles during growth in laboratory culture
(6,17,27,29,30,39). Membrane proteins may be
lost during irradiation of cells and antigens
may be degraded by proteolytic enzymes during
the preparation of cell lysates. Different
preparations used in the previous studies may,
therefore, have had variable efficacies even
when the same investigating group used similar
processes and cell types to prepare the
immunogens. Reagents or tests to standardize
the preparations for antigen(s) presence and
potency have not been available. Furthermore,
the means of monitoring an individual patient's
immune response was not available to tailor the
immunization dose and schedule for optimal
response.

A systematic search for antibodies against
tumor cell-associated components raised in
patients undergoing tumor regression may lead to
the identification of regression-associated
antigens (RAAs), immunogens with great potential
for cancer prevention as well as active specific
immuotherapy of various cancers (35). We have
recently identified tumor cell antigens using
antibodies developed in patients immunized by
the intralymphatic route with irradiated human
tumor cell lines and characterized by

significant tumor regression (4). These human
tumor cell antigens and antibodies directed
against them offer the possibility of novel
approaches in the biotherapy of human cancers
and are also intriguing candidates for cancer
prevention. Sera from immunized patients have
been used in sensitive immunoblots to screen
extracts of normal and tumor-derived cells as
well as normal and tumor tissue extracts to
identify specific antigens in tumor cells and
tissues. These tumor-associated antigens have
been further grouped based on their sizes, their
ability to react with antibodies from patients
regressing different malignancies, and their
presence on different human cancer cell types.
The putative involvement of these immunogens in
tumor regression was based on the following
findings:

1. The majority of patients who responded
with tumor regression following intralymphatic
immunization with a mixture of intact allogeneic
tumor cell lines without any adjuvant produced
antibodies against a limited number of antigenic
molecular species referred to as RAAs. Similar
specific antibody response has also been
observed in a different group of patients
immunized with intradermal injections of
allogeneic cell lysates containing DETOX
(produced by Ribi Immunochem) as an adjuvant.

2. None of the patients who had tumor
progression in either of the above immunotherapy
programs produced strong antibody titers against
any RAA, although antibody responses against
other antigens present in the immunizing cells
were observed.

METHODS

All procedures for intralymphatic
immunotherapy using irradiated human tumor
cells, clinical response evaluations, and
analyses of patient sera by immunoblotting and
of peripheral blood lymphocytes for cytostasis
activity have been published (4,23,35A,55).

RESULTS

Serum samples obtained before, during the course of therapy, and after termination of immunotherapy in patients with a variety of advanced malignancies were analysed for their ability to detect specific antigens in various cultured human tumor cells, including those used for treatment. Immunoblots performed with postimmune sera from two patients are shown in Figure 1. Lanes 1 and 2 in each filter strip contain, respectively, fractionated proteins from A375 melanoma cells or the conditioned media from these cells. Antigens of 38, 43 and 70 kDa are readily detected in the cell extract with the 38 kDa species also detected in conditioned media. Patient 1 had been immunized with ovarian tumor cells whereas patient 2 had received subcutaneous immunizations with a lysate mixture of two melanoma cell lines in a study conducted by Dr. Malcolm Mitchell (these Proceedings).

Figure 1. Immunoblot detection of antibodies to regression-associated antigens.

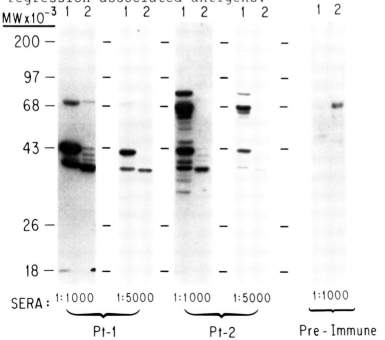

Occasionally, a responding patient's sera has also detected a 22 kDA species in this assay. These antibody responses of patient 1 are representative of many the patients in the present investigation who achieved clinical regressions or prolonged (greater than 4 months duration) tumor stabilization as summarized in Table 1. Patients with strong (greater than 1:500 titers) antibody responses experienced partial or complete regressions at a significantly greater frequency than those with negative responses (less than 1:50 titers). Clinical responses in patients with weak antibody levels (titers between 1:50 and 1:500) were increased in the regression category compared to the antibody negative group but also had a comparable percentage of tumor progressions to those in the negative titer group.

Table 1.

ANTIBODY AND CLINICAL RESPONSES FOLLOWING ACTIVE SPECIFIC INTRALYMPHATIC IMMUNOTHERAPY				
Antibody Response	Number of Patients	Clinical Response (%)		
		Regression	Stabilization	Progression
Strong	10	40	60	0
Weak	16	25	18	57
Negative	27	11	33	56

Partial purification of concentrated
conditioned medium from A375 melanoma cells
using DEAE-cellulose step NaCl elution allows
for the detection of the 22 kDa antigen in the
50 mM NaCl eluate of the column shown in Figure
2, lane 1. Post immune sera from patient 1
faintly reacts with this species in the "load"
conditioned media (lane 6).

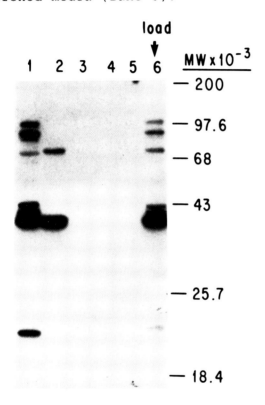

Figure 2.   Immunoblot detection of 22 kDa RAA.

We have also evaluated cellular immune
responses in immunized patients. Both
cytotoxicity and cytostasis assays on peripheral
blood lymphocytes from responding patients
indicate enhancement of specific cellular
immunity after intralymphatic immunizations. A
representative cytostasis analysis before and
after three immunizations with autologous

melanoma cells in patient T.H. is presented in
Table 2 and Figure 3.   Prior to ILI
(intralymphatic immunotherapy) this patient's
lymphocytes were inactive in suppression to [3]H-
thymidine incorporation into the patients own
tumor cells (T.H.) whereas after 3 ILIs
substantial inhibition is observed at effector
to target cell ratios of 20:1 and 40:1.
Cytostatic activity is also observed against an
allogeneic melanoma cell line, A375, but not
against two other allogeneic melanoma cell
lines, RO-E81-1 and M14.

DISCUSSION

Evaluable tumor regressions were associated
in this study with detection of antibodies
against human tumor cell antigens of 22, 38, 43
and 70 kDa. We have previously shown these
antigens to be distinguishable from HLA antigens
and fetal calf serum contaminants of cultured
human cells. The production of pure
preparations of these antigens should allow for
their definitive characterization as well as the
assessment of their immunogen potential in
cancer patients. It is reasonable and rational
to continue investigations in this area to
attempt to further define the use of active
specific immunotherapy both for the stimulation
of in vivo immune responses as well as for the
induction of immune responses which might be
augmented in vitro. Tumors are likely to be
heterogeneous for regression-associated antigens
among which may well be found antigens detected
with murine monoclonal antibodies. Tumor cell
lines generated from the patient's tumor may
have lost certain of these antigens and thereby
may not be the most effective sources of
immunogens for specific immunization.
There is a rapidly growing list of tumor
specific antigens identified using murine
monoclonal antibodies (5,15,34,43,45,46,50,51).
The basis for selection of monoclonal antibodies
against human tumor markers is not necessarily
relevant to tumor regression. In contrast, the
selection of human-human hybridomas producing

Table 2.

CYTOSTASIS ANALYSIS - T.H.				
AFTER 3 ILI 4/2/88				
Effector to target cell ratio	T.H.	A375	RO-E81-1	M14
40:1	44.20%	98.20%	5.70%	-163%
20:1	40.50%	41.10%	4.10%	-85.60%
10:1	27.90%	22.00%		-71.00%
05:1	15.80%	16.20%		
BEFORE ILI 1/29/88				
20:1	-4.90%			
10:1	-5.40%			

Figure 3.

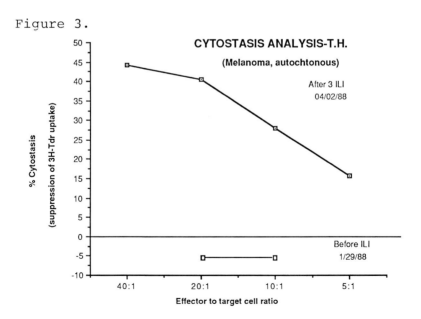

CYTOSTASIS ANALYSIS-T.H.
(Melanoma, autochtonous)
After 3 ILI
04/02/88
Before ILI
1/29/88

% Cytostasis
(suppression of 3H-Tdr uptake)

Effector to target cell ratio

tumor cell reactive monoclonal antibodies from
actively immunized cancer patients or the
production of human monoclonal antibodies from
fusions with draining lymph node cells for
particular malignancies may yield antibodies
having specificities associated with tumor
regression (1,10,18,24,25).
    Perhaps the most intriguing antigenic
candidates for cancer epitope vaccines use are
those surface antigens identified with
monoclonal antibodies on specific malignant
human cells. There are a growing number of such
antigens which have been localized in vivo using
intravenous infusion of monoclonal antibodies
(41,50). The precise molecular characterization
of these antigens such as the melanoma p97 (47)
or p250 (45) and the ability to produce pure
forms of these antigens or selected epitopes
derived from them through genetic engineering
techniques, offers extremely attractive
possibilities for highly-specific immunogens.
As a promising indication of these
possibilities, the melanoma p97 antigen has
recently been expressed in a vaccina virus
vector and both vaccinated mice and monkeys have
developed strong humoral and cellular immunity
to human melanoma cells (Brown, J.P. et al.,
these Proceedings). Specific gangliosides, GD2
and GD3, have been associated with certain human
melanomas and, despite their very limited
efficacy as active melanoma immunogens (53),
dramatic regression of cutaneous metastatic
melanoma was recently described after
intralesional injection with a human monoclonal
antibody to the ganglioside GD2 (19). More
recently, Livingston and his colleagues (33, and
these Proceedings) have demonstrated the
feasibility of generating significant cytotoxic
antibody responses in melanoma patients after
immunization with purified GM2 ganglioside
preparations.
    Several anti-tumor monoclonal antibodies
have been described with relatively broad range
of carcinoma reactivities. Two examples of
these are monoclonal antibodies to L6, a human
carcinoma-specific lipid structure (13,14), and
to a ras oncogene associated gp74 antigen (48).

These antigens or epitopes derived from them may also be meaningfully evaluated as described above for p97; however, much broader immunization potential may exist with these offering protection potentially against different human carcinomas. As a complement to immunization with the purified anti-cancer epitopes, anti-idiotypic antibodies (anti-Id Ab) mimicking the tumor antigens could be exploited for vaccine use (44). During the onset of an immune response, auto-anti-idiotypic antibody complementary to the antigen combining site of the idiotype plays a major role in determining whether a suppressive or inductive response will take place. There have been several reports of the utility of anti-idiotype antibodies (those expressing an idiotypic determinant that mimics the structure of the antigen for the original antibody) as vaccines for different pathogens. Anti-Id Ab has been applied in the treatment of B cell lymphoma, but in many cases the success may be limited due to spontaneous generation of somatic variants (36). Despite this possible outcome, anti-Id Abs have been shown to induce protective immunity in animal tumor models (26,31).

ACKNOWLEDGEMENTS

We are indebted to Karima Hambey, Tomas Totanes, John Robert, and David Ewing for their excellent assistance and to Dr. Malcolm Mitchell for sera and vaccine lysate samples from his immunotherapy study.

REFERENCES

1.   Andreasen, R.B., Olsson, L. Antibody-producing human-human hybridomas III. Derivation and characterization of two antibodies with specificity for human myeloid cells. The Journal of Immunology. 137, 1083-1090, 1986.
2.   Berd, D., Maguire, H.C., Jr., and Mastrangelo, M. J., Induction of cell-mediated immunity to autologous melanoma cells and regression of metastases after

treatment with melanoma cell vaccine preceded by cyclophosphamide. Cancer Res. 46, 2572–2577, 1986.

3. Bystryn, J.-C., Jacobsen, S., Harris, M., Roses, D., Speyer, J., and Levin, M., Preparation and characterization of a polyvalent human melanoma antigen vaccine. J. Biol. Resp. Modifiers 5, 211–224, 1986.

4. Fareed, G.C., Mendiaz, E., Sen, A., Juillard, G.J.F., Weisenburger, T.H., and Totanes, T., Novel Antigenic Markers of Human Tumor Regression. J. Biol. Resp. Modifiers 7,11–23, 1988.

5. Fradet, Y., Cordon-Cardo, C., Thomson, T., Daly, M.E. et al. Cell surface antigens of human bladder cancer defined by mouse monoclonal antibodies. Proc. Natl. Acad. Sci. USA. 81, 224–228, 1984.

6. Giacomini, P., Imberti, L., Adriano, A., Fisher, P.B., Trinchieri, G., Ferrone, S. Immunochemical analysis of the modulation of human melanoma-associated antigens by DNA recombinant immune interferon. The Journal of Immunology. 135, 2887–2894, 1985.

7. Hanna, Jr., M.G., et al., these Proceedings.

8. Hanna, Jr., M.G., Key, M.E., Oldham, R.K., Biology of cancer therapy: some new insights into adjuvant treatment of metastatic solid tumors. J. Biol. Resp. Modif. 4: 295–309, 1983.

9. Hanna, Jr., M.G., McCabe, R.P. and Oldham, R.K., Immunotherapy of Cancer. Clin. Immunol. Newsletter, 1985.

10. Haspel, M.V., McCabe, R.P., Pomato, N., Janesch, N.J., Knowlton, J.V., Peters, L.C., Hoover, H.C., Jr., and Hanna, M.G., Jr. Generation of tumor cell reactive human monoclonal antibodies using peripheral blood lymphocytes from actively immunized colorectal carcinoma patients. Cancer Research 45, 3951–3961, 1985.

11. Hearing, V.J., Gersten, D.M., Montague, P.M., Viera, W.D., Galetto, G., and Law, L.W., Murine melanoma-specific tumor rejection activity elicited by a purified,

melanoma-associated antigen. J. Immunol. 137, 379-384, 1986.

12. Heicappell, R., Shirrmacher, V., von Hoegen, P., Ahlert, T., et al. Prevention of metastatic spread by postoperative immunotherapy with virally modified autologous tumor cells. I. Parameters for optimal therapeutic effect. Int. J. Cancer. 37, 569-577, 1986.

13. Hellstrom, I., Horn, D., Linsley, P. et al. Monoclonal mouse antibodies raised against human lung carcinoma. Cancer Research 46, 3917-3923, 1986.

14. Hellstrom, I., Beaumier, P.L., and Hellstrom, K.E. Antitumor effects of L6, an IgG2a antibody that reacts with most human carcinomas. Proc. Nat. Acad. Sci. USA 83, 7059-7063, 1986.

15. Heyderman, E., Chapman, D.V, Richardson, T.C. Rosen, S.W. Human chorionic gonadotropin and human placental lactogen in extragonadal tumors. Cancer 56, 2674-2682, 1985.

16. Herberman, R.B., and Oldham,R.K., Cell-mediated cytotoxicity against human tumors: lessons learned and future prospects. J. Biol. Resp. Modif. 1:217-231, 1983.

16A. Hollinshead, A., Elias, E.G., Arlen, M., Buda, B., Mosley, M., and Scherrer, J. Specific active immunotherapy in patients with adenocarcinoma of the colon utilizing tumor-associated antigens (TAA). Cancer 56, 480-490, 1985.

17. Hostetler, L.W., Ananthaswamy, H.N., Kripke, M.L. Generation of tumor-specific transplantation antigens by UV radiation can occur independently of neoplastic transformation. The Journal of Immunology. 137, 2721-2725, 1986.

18. Imam, A., Mitchell, M.S., Modlin, R.L., Taylor, C.R. et al. Human monoclonal antibodies that distinguish cutaneous malignant melanomas from benign nevi in fixed tissue sections. The Journal of Investigative Dermatology. 86,145-148, 1986.

19. Irie, R.F., Morton, D.L. Regression of
     cutaneous metastatic melanoma by
     intralesional injection with human
     monoclonal antibody to ganglioside GD2.
     Proc. Natl. Acad. Sci. USA. 83, 8694-8698,
     1986.
20. Jarrett, W., Jarrett, O., Mackey, L.,
     Laird, H., Hood, C., and Hay, D.
     Vaccination against felie leukemia virus
     using a cell membrane antigen system.
     Int. J. Cancer 16, 134-141, 1975.
21. Jeglum, K.A., Mangan, C., Wheeler, J.E.
     Enhanced antitumor effects with
     intralymphatic delivery using bacillus
     calmette-guerin in animal models. Cancer
     Drug Deliv. 2, 127-132, 1985.
22. Jessup, J.M., McBride, C.M., Ames, F.C.,
     Guarda, L., Ota, D.M., et al. Active
     specific immunotherapy of Dukes B2 and C
     colorectal carcinoma: Comparison of two
     doses of the vaccine. Cancer Immunol
     Immunother. 21, 233-239, 1986.
23. Juillard, G.J.F., Boyer, P.J.J., and
     Yamashiro, C.H., A phase I study of
     active specific intralymphatic
     immunotherapy (ASILI). Cancer 41,
     2215-2225, 1978.
24. Kan-Mitchell, J., Imam, S., Kempf, R.A.,
     Taylor, C.R., and Mitchell, M.S. Human
     monoclonal antibodies directed against
     melanoma tumor-associated antigens.
     Cancer Res 46, 2490-2496, 1986.
25. Kan-Mitchell, J., Kempf, R.A., Imam, A.,
     Reisfeld, R.A., and Mitchell, M.S.,
     Monoclonal antibodies in the development
     of active specific immunotherapy for
     melanoma in Monoclonal Antibodies and
     Cancer Therapy, Reisfeld and Sell, Eds.,
     523-536, 1985 Alan Liss, Inc., pub.
26. Kennedy, R.C., Dreesman, G.R., Butel, J.
     S., and Lanford, R.E., Suppression of in
     vivo tumor formation induced by simian
     virus 40-transformed cells in mice
     receiving antiidiotypic antibodies. J.
     Exp. Med. 161, 1432-1441, 1985.
27. Key, M. D., Brandhorst, J. S. and Hanna,
     M. G., More of the relevance of animal

tumor models: immunogenicity of
transplantable leukemias of recent origin
in syngeneic strain 2 guinea pigs. J.
Biol. Resp. Modifiers 3, 359-365, 1984.

28. Key, M. E., Hoover, H. C. and Hanna, M.
G., Active specific immunotherapy as an
adjunct to the treatment of metastatic
solid tumors: present and future
prospects. Adv. Immun. Cancer Ther.,
1:195-219, 1985.

29. Holden, H. T., Oldham, R.K., Ortaldo,
J.R., Herberman, R.B. Cryopreservation of
the functional reactivity of normal and
immune leukocytes and of tumor cells.
Bloom, B.R., and David, J.R. (eds.): in:
In Vitro Methods in Cell Mediated and
Tumor Immunity. Academic Press, New York,
pp. 723-729, 1976.

30. Oldham, R.K., Dean, J., Cannon, G.B.,
Graw, R., Dunston, G., Applebaum, r.,
McCoy, J, Djeu, J., and Herberman, r.B.
Cryopreservation of human lymphocyte
function as measured by in vitro assays.
Int. J. Cancer. 18, 145-155, 1976.

31. Lee, V.K., Harriott, T.G., Kuchroo, V.J.,
Halliday, W.J., Helstrom, I., and
Hellstrom, K.E. Monoclonal antiidiotypic
antibodies related to a murine oncofetal
bladder tumor antigen induce specific
cell-mediated tumor immunity. Proc. Nat.
Acad. Sci. USA 82, 6286-6290, 1985.

32. Livingston, P.O., Takeyama, H., Pollack,
M.S., Houghton, A.N. et al. Serological
responses of melanoma patients to vaccines
derived from allogeneic cultured melanoma
cells. Int. J. Cancer 31, 567-5752, 1983.

33. Livingston, P.O., Natoli, E.J., Calves,
M.J., Stockert, E., Oettgen, H.F., and
Old, L.J., Vaccines containing purified
GM2 ganglioside elicit GM2 antibodies in
melanoma patients. Proc. Natl. Acad. Sci.
USA 84, 2911-2915, 1987.

34. Luner, S.J., de Vellis, J.
Immunoprecipitation of a MR 64,000 GLIAL
tumor-associated antigen by monoclonal
antibody 217C. Cancer Res. 46, 863-865,
1986.

35. Mattes, M.J., Real, F.X., Furukawa, K.,
     Old, L.J., and Lloyd, K.O. Class I
     (unique) tumor antigens of human melanoma:
     partial purification and characterization
     of the FD antigen and analysis of a mouse
     polyclonal antiserum. Cancer Res. 47,
     6614-6619, 1987.
35A. McBride, W.H., Notes on the use of in
     vitro techniques for the assessment of
     cellular reactivity against tumours. In
     Handbook of Experimental Immunology. D.M.
     Weir, ed.. Blackwell Scientific Pub.,
     Oxford. 3rd edition, chapter 36.
36. Miller, R.A., Maloney, D.G., Warnke, R.,
     and Levy, R. Treatment of B-cell lymphoma
     with monoclonal anti-idiotype antibody. N.
     Engl. J. Med. 306, 517-522, 1982.
37. Milstein, C. From the structure of
     antibodies to the diversification of the
     immune response. The EMBO Journal 4,
     1083-1092, 1985.
38. Moy, P.M., Golub, S.H., Calkins, E., and
     Morton, D.L., Effects of intralymphatic
     immunotherapy on natural killer activity
     in malignant melanoma patients. J. Surg.
     Oncol. 29, 112-117, 1985.
39. Natali, P.G., Giacomini, P., Bigotti, A.,
     Imai, K. et al. Heterogeneity in the
     expression of HLA and tumor-associated
     antigens by surgically removed and
     cultured breast carcinoma cells. Cancer
     Research. 43, 660-668, 1983.
40. Oldham, R.K., Natural killer cells:
     history and significance. J. Biol. Resp.
     Modif. 1, 217-231, 1982.
41. Oldham, R.K., Foon, K.A., Morgan, A.C. et
     al. Monoclonal antibody therapy of
     malignant melanoma: in vivo localization
     in cutaneous metastasis after intravenous
     administration. J. Clin. Oncol. 2,
     1235-1243, 1984.
42. Oldham, R.K., and Smalley, R.V.,
     Immunotherapy: the old and the new. J.
     Biol. Resp. Modif. 2, 1-37, 1983.
43. Philben, V.J., Jakowatz, J.G., Beatty,
     B.G., Vlahos, W.G. et al. The effect of
     tumor CEA content and tumor size on tissue

uptake of indium 111-labeled anti-CEA
monoclonal antibody. Cancer 57, 571-576,
1986.

44. Raychaudhuri, S., Saeki, Y., Fuji, H.,
Kohler, H. Tumor-specific idiotype
vaccines I. Generation and
characterization of internal image tumor
antigen. The Journal of Immunology. 137,
1743-1749, 1986.
45. Reisfeld, R.A., Schulz, G., and Cheresh,
D.A. Approaches for immunotherapy of
malignant melanoma with monoclonal
antibodies. in Monoclonal Antibodies and
Cancer Therapy, pages 173-191. Reisfeld
and Sell, editors, 1985 Alan R. Liss, Inc.
46. Rettig, W.J., Cordon-Cardo, C., Koulos,
J.P., Lewis, J.L. Jr., et al. Cell surface
antigens of human trophoblast and
choriocarcinoma defined by monoclonal
antibodies. Int. J. Cancer. 54, 469-475,
1985.
47. Rose, T.M., Plowman, G.D., Teplow, D.B.,
Dreyer, W.J. et al.Primary structure of
the human melanoma-associated antigen p97
(melanotransferrin) deduced from the mRNA
sequence. Proc. Natl. Acad. Sci. USA. 83,
1261-1265, 1986.
48. Roth, J.A., Ames, R.S., Restrepo, C.,
Scuderi, P. Monoclonal antibody 45-2D9
recognizes a cell surface glycoprotein on
a human c-Ha-ras transformed cell line
(45-342) and a shared epitope on human
tumors. The Journal of Immunology. 137,
2385.
49. Savage, H.E., Rossen, R.D., Hersh E.M.,
Freedman, R.S. et al. Antibody development
to viral and allogeneic tumor cell-
associated antigens in patients with
malignant melanoma and ovarian carcinoma
treated with lysates of virus-infected
tumor cells. Cancer Res. 46, 2127-2133,
1986.
50. Schlom, J. Basic principles and
applications of monoclonal antibodies in
the management of carcinomas: The Richard
and Hinda Rosenthal foundation award

lecture., Cancer Research. 46, 3225-3238, 1986.

51. Sell, S., Cancer markers: past, present and future. in Monoclonal Antibodies and Cancer Therapy, pages 3-21, Eds. Reisfeld, R.A., and Sell, S., A.R. Liss, Inc., N.Y. 1985.

52. Stewart-Tull, D.E.S. Immunopotentiating conjugates. Vaccine 3, 40-44, 1985.

53. Tai, T., Cahan, L.D., Tsuchida, T., Saxton, R.E., Irie, R.F. et al. Immunogenicity of melanoma-associated gangliosides in cancer patients. Int. J. Cancer. 35, 607-612, 1985.

54. Watt, K.W.K., Lee, P-J., Timkulu, T.M., Whan, W-P. et al. Human prostate-specific antigen: Structural and functional similarity with serine proteases. Proc. Natl. Acad. Sci. USA. 83, 3166-3170, 1986.

55. Weisenburger, T. H., Jones, P.C., Ahn, S.S., Irie, R.F., and Juillard, G.J.F., Active specific intralymphatic immunotherapy in metastatic malignant melanoma: evidence of clinical response. J. Biol. Resp. Modifiers 1,57-66, 1982.

Human Tumor Antigens and Specific Tumor Therapy, pages 335–344
© 1989 Alan R. Liss, Inc.

Coming Full Circle in the Immunotherapy
of Colorectal Cancer: Vaccination with
Autologous Tumor Cells - to Human Monoclonal
Antibodies - to Development and Application
of a Generic Tumor Vaccine

Martin V. Haspel, Richard P. McCabe,
Nicholas Pomato, Herbert C. Hoover[1],
and Michael G. Hanna, Jr.

Organon Teknika/Bionetics Research Institute,
1330-A Piccard Drive, Rockville, Maryland 20850.
and [1]Massachusetts General Hospital,
Boston, Massachusetts 02114.

ABSTRACT Treatment of postsurgical colorectal
patients with an autologous vaccine consisting
of viable nontumorigenic cells admixed with
BCG resulted in significant increases in
disease-free status and survival. Peripheral
blood lymphocytes obtained from these patients
were used to develop human monoclonal
antibodies (MCA) reactive with colon tumor
associated antigens (TAA). The MCA have been
successfully used for the radioimaging of
disseminated colon cancer. The MCA are
nontoxic, nonimmunogenic, and able to
effectively localize metastases. The
antibodies have also been used as probes to
isolate the cognate antigens. These TAA are
currently being evaluated for relevance as
cell-mediated immunogens for possible
inclusion in a generic vaccine to supplement
or ultimately replace the autologous tumor
cell vaccine.

INTRODUCTION

Specific immunotherapy, because of the
exquisite sensitivity of the immune system, is a
desirable alternative to the generalized toxicity

of chemotherapy or radiation therapy. A number
of theoretical arguments have been presented
which question the rationale behind specific
immunotherapy. Do TAA exist and are they
immunogenic? Does putative antigenic
heterogeneity result in antigen-negative tumor
cells escaping immune-mediated destruction?
Finally, would active specific immunotherapy
(ASI) evoke suppression rather than a protective
immune response resulting in enhanced growth of
the tumor? The gratifying successes of ASI in
the treatment of colorectal carcinoma and the
development of human MCA to TAA of colon cancer
have virtually rendered these theoretical
objections to immunotherapy moot.

ASI IN A GUINEA PIG TUMOR MODEL

The rationale, methods of vaccine
preparation and the regimen for ASI of colorectal
CA are based upon our previous studies with the
transplantable syngeneic L-10 heptocarcinoma of
inbred strain 2 guinea pigs. The L-10 tumor is
weakly antigenic, and hence represents a
realistic model for the immunotherapy of human
cancer. Although effective, intratumoral
administration of BCG would not have broad
applications to the majority of human tumors,
because they are not easily accessible to direct
injection. Consequently, a tumor cell vaccine
consisting of dissociated tumor cells admixed
with BCG was developed and shown to be successful
in stimulating systemic tumor immunity (1,2).
However, to be effcctive, careful control of such
variables as the number of viable but nontumorigenic cells (10^7 optimal), the ratio of
viable BCG organisms to tumor cells (1:1), and
the vaccination regimen (3 weekly vaccinations)
was required. The efficacy of the vaccine was
strongly correlated with the percentage of viable
cells. Vaccines with requisite cell viability
are obtained when the optimal procedures for
enzymatic dissociation and cryopreservation are
rigorously adhered to.
The anatomical characteristics of tumor foci
may restrict interactions of the host with the
tumor, thus protecting tumors not only from some
forms of immunotherapy, but also from other forms

of treatment. Studies with an MCA directed
against L-10 tumor cells revealed that
intravascular-administered antibodies did not
penetrate uniformly into all areas of the solid
tumor but were restricted to those areas that
were highly vascularized or hemorrhagic (3).
Chemotherapeutic drugs may encounter similar
barriers, thus limiting their access to all
portions of the tumor. During the course of ASI,
the tumor is infiltrated by mononuclear cells
resulting in significant disruption of the
otherwise highly compact micrometastatic nodules.
Penetration of the MCA was significantly
increased in tumors disrupted by ASI.

These results prompted investigation of
possible synergism between immunotherapy and
chemotherapy (4). Tumor-bearing animals were
treated with cyclophosphamide, ASI, or a
combination of immunotherapy and chemotherapy.
The immunotherapy was delayed until 10 days after
inoculation; at this point the metastases are 0.1
to 0.2 mm in diameter, and the ASI cure rate is
substantially reduced. Chemotherapy alone had no
protective effects, while guinea pigs treated
with immunotherapy alone had a 33% survival rate.
In contrast, the survival rate increased to 74%
when a single injection of cyclophosphamide was
administered after completion of ASI. These
findings suggest that a successful therapeutic
approach for metastatic solid tumors might be a
process that would disrupt anatomic barriers and
deliver cytotoxic agents to the tumor. Thus, a
multimodal approach to the treatment of cancer
would be most successful. One can envision ASI
followed by treatment with MCA conjugated with
toxins, chemotherapeutic drugs, or radioisotopes
as a means of increasing the specificity and
efficacy of these treatments, while minimizing or
eliminating problems of generalized toxicity.

CLINICAL STUDIES OF ASI

Our favorable experiences with the guinea
pig model motivated us to translate the
methodology to a prospectively randomized,
controlled clinical trial of ASI for colorectal
carcinoma (5,6). Surgical specimens were
expeditiously dissociated and cryopreserved using

precisely the same techniques developed for the
animal model. Patients received two weekly
intradermal injections of 10^7 viable irradiated
tumor cells admixed with 10^7 BCG and a third
immunization of 10^7 tumor cells alone (the same
dose and regimen used in the guinea pig model!).
One question that could be addressed relatively
early was whether or not autologous immunization
resulted in an enhanced cellular immune response
to tumor cells. Immunized patients developed
significant ($p < 0.01$) delayed cutaneous
hypersensitivity to autologous tumor cells
compared to autologous normal colonic mucosal
cells that persisted for at least 6 months. By
contrast, the nonimmunized control patients
failed to develop measurable responses to their
tumor cells. This latter finding demonstrates
that nonimmunized cancer patients are tolerant,
as measured by delayed cutaneous
hypersensitivity, to their tumor cells. The
patients were, however, responsive to a series of
recall antigens.

As of December 1987, 74 patients (44 with
colon cancer and 30 with rectal cancer) had a
minimum of three years follow-up study (median
follow-up time of 56 months). Using the Cox
model and actuarial estimates, there was a
significant benefit in disease-free status
($p < .037$) and survival ($p < .031$) for colon and
rectal carcinoma patients combined. Patients
with rectal carcinoma were treated with radiation
therapy 1 week after completion of ASI.
Interestingly, the actuarial estimate for 6-year
survival for colon cancer patients is
substantially higher (approximately 75%) than
rectal carcinoma patients (approximately 20%).
Thus, the figures given above for both colon and
rectal patients have higher statistical
significance when only patients with colon
carcinoma are analyzed.

Another interesting outcome was an analysis
of the qualitative aspects of the recurrence in
the control and immunized patients. When
analyzed with respect to focal resectable
metastases as compared with diffuse surgically
nontreatable metastases, the majority of the
recurrences among immunized patients (60%) were
focal whereas most of the recurrences in the

control group (80%) were diffuse. Thus, most of
the recurrences in the immunized patient group
could be treated by repeat surgery and the
patients are now again considered to be free of
tumor.

It is clear that ASI has a significantly
beneficial impact in delaying both death and
recurrence. The toxicity from the immunization
is minimal. Although the techniques for the
preparation of vaccines are demanding, they can
be readily translated to appropriately equipped
and trained personnel. Thus, ASI should be able
to serve as a cornerstone of a rational
multimodal therapy for cancer.

STUDIES OF HUMAN MONOCLONAL ANTIBODIES REACTIVE WITH TUMOR ASSOCIATED ANTIGENS

The use of murine MCA for immunotherapy is
greatly limited by the widely documented HAMA
(human anti-mouse antibody) response. The
development and application of human MCA to the
therapy of cancer have been previously limited by
the general unavailability of suitably sensitized
lymphocytes, instability of antibody production,
and major technical problems associated with
large-scale production and purification. We
formulated a different strategy for the
production of human MCA to TAA: lymphocytes were
obtained from actively immunized patients (7).
No suitable MCA were obtained prior to
immunization. Optimal results were with
lymphocytes obtained 1 week after the first and
second immunizations, with a marked decrease in
frequency after the third immunization.

The antibodies were characterized by
immunohistochemistry using both indirect and
direct techniques. In general, the patchy
labeling reported frequently with the mouse MCA
was not observed, but rather a more homogenous
type of labeling was seen. In addition, no
single antibody reacted with all of the
colorectal tumors tested. The matrix of
reactivity of the antibodies tested indicated
that individual antibodies reacted with between
40 to 80% of the tumor specimens tested. Thus, a
cocktail of several carefully chosen MCA could
cover the spectrum of colon tumors. As

increasing numbers of antibodies have been
isolated and their reactivities determined, it is
becoming increasingly clear that there is a
relatively small number of TAA. That is, many
antibodies from different patients (either colon
or lung cancer) react, as determined by Western
blot analysis, with the same antigen(s). This
finding has major implications concerning the
logistics of formulating a generic tumor vaccine
consisting of genetically engineered peptides.

Specificity testing of the antibodies has
eliminated CEA and normal erythrocyte and
lymphocyte antigens from consideration. Through
extensive immunohistochemical study, it is clear
that the antigens recognized by the antibodies
under consideration, exhibit, at the very least,
substantial quantitative (if not qualitative)
differences when compared to normal cells.

Since our initial report was published, we
have developed human MCA using peripheral blood
lymphocytes obtained from patients who were
treated by ASI for lung cancer, pancreatic cancer
or melanoma. Thus, these techniques have broad
application. We have developed more efficient
and stable fusion partners, and have altered our
screening techniques in order to detect a wide
diversity of human MCA.

Specificity aside, the major obstacles to
application of human MCA in clinical practice are
large scale production and purification. We have
developed proprietary hollow fiber technology
which permits us, with minimal capital
expenditure and labor, to produce half a kilogram
of purified pharmaceutical-grade antibody
suitable for parenteral administration. Process
development is currently underway for routine
production of over 5 kilograms of purified
antibody.

**Preclinical Evaluation of the Radioimmuno-
detection of Colon Carcinoma by Human Monoclonal
Antibodies.**

Two first-generation IgM MCA, 16-88 and
28A32, were chosen for further study because of
their specificity, range of reactivity, and
levels of antibody production. THO, a human
colon tumor, was passaged as a xenograft in nude

mice; it reacts strongly with both antibodies.
The antibodies were radiolabeled with ^{125}I to a
specific activity of approximately 1 mCi/mg, and
50 µg were administered intravenously to the
tumor-bearing nude mice (8). The radiolabeled
MCA were cleared from circulation of both
nontumor and tumor-bearing nude mice with a 6-8
hour half-life. The half-life of the antibodies
in tumor tissues was 48-72 hours as compared to
8-12 hours for normal tissue. Maximum tumor-to-
normal-tissue ratios were achieved 4-7 days after
injection, with colon tumor to blood ratios of
10:1 to 12:1 (28A32 and 16-88, respectively) were
obtained.

Experiments were carried out with two other
xenograft colon tumors, EPP and ATK. Both
antibodies react well, as detected by indirect
immunohistochemistry, with ATK but react poorly
with EPP. Localization, comparable to THO, was
seen in the ATK tumor. By contrast, both
antibodies localized poorly in the EPP tumor.
Comparable amounts (2%) of the ^{125}I-labeled
antibody were taken up by the EPP and THO tumors.
Subsequently, the EPP tumors cleared the antibody
at the same rate as normal tissues, whereas the
THO xenografts cleared the antibody much more
slowly. Results of radioimmunoscintigraphic
studies with ^{125}I-labeled 16-88 and 28A32
antibodies of mice bearing the THO and
contralateral EPP xenografts confirm the
localization studies. At day 8, the thyroid was
the only detectable normal tissue and the THO
tumors were clearly labeled. The EPP xenograft
was poorly visible at day 8 in the animals
administered 16-88, and was not detected at all
in the animals given 28A32 antibody.

These studies clearly demonstrate that IgM
MCA, despite their large size, are able to
localize in human colon tumor xenografts. The
specificity of the antibody binding was
demonstrated by an inability to image an antigen-
poor tumor.

Clinical Studies of the Immunoscintigraphic Detection of Colon Tumors.

Phase I clinical study of the two MCA
labeled with ^{131}I was initiated to determine the

optimal dose levels, pharmacokinetics, radioimaging capabilities and possible therapeutic
benefits in patients with metastatic colon
carcinoma (9).

Patients with disseminated colon carcinoma
were prescreened for immunoreactivity on paraffin
sections of the primary tumor with the two
antibodies; only those patients whose primary
tumor reacted well with an antibody were eligible
for this study. Prior to the administration of
antibody, each patient was skin tested with 10 μg
of antibody; a patient showing any response
within 2 hours was excluded from the study.
During the first week of the five week study, 8
mg of ^{131}I-labeled (5 mCi) was administered
intravenously as a 2-hour infusion. One week
later, the patient again received the same dose
of radiolabeled antibody together with a dose of
unlabeled antibody. During weeks 3 to 5, the
patient received only unlabeled antibody. The
dose of unlabeled antibody was 10 mg for the
first group of three patients, 50 mg for the
second, 100 mg for the third, and 200 mg for the
fourth group.

Tumor images have been obtained in 9 of 11
patients treated with 16-88, and 13 of 15
patients treated with 28A32, with optimal
contrast between tumor and nontumor after 5 days.
^{99m}Tm sulfur colloid administered after the
radiolabeled antibody confirmed localization of
the antibody in liver metastases. The smallest
lesions detected thus far have been 1.5 cm
nodules with 16-88 and 2.0 cm lesions with 28A32.
Tumor was imaged in liver, lung, bone, and the
pelvic area. No clear antibody-related toxicity
was observed with any of the patients treated
with 16-88, even at the 200 mg dose level. One
patient developed a rash when receiving the first
200 mg dose of 28A32 and was removed from the
study. A second patient developed urticaria
after the second 50 mg dose, the symptoms did not
recur after subsequent injections.

No evidence of induction of immunoreactivity
to either 16-88 or 28A32 was observed in any
patient up to 1 month after completion of the
5-week study. No correlation between immune
complex levels and imaging results or other
clinical observations was made.

These studies indicate that human IgM MCA are able to detect metastasis of colon cancer as well as murine IgG MCA. More significant is the finding that these antibodies are nontoxic and nonimmunogenic and hence would lend themselves to **repeat** administrations for in vivo diagnosis and therapy of cancer.

PROSPECTIVES FOR THE DEVELOPMENT OF A GENERIC COLON TUMOR VACCINE

The rigorous methodology for the preparation of an autologous tumor vaccine can be transferred to and implemented by well-trained, dedicated personnel. However, the logistics of treating 137,000 cases of colon cancer annually in the U.S. alone make wide-scale availability of this highly successful therapeutic procedure unlikely. Thus, the development of a generic vaccine is the most probable solution. It is becoming increasingly clear that there are a finite number of tumor associated antigens. Our current approach is to use the human MCA as probes to isolate and characterize these antigens (10). The relevance of individual antibodies is being screened in an in vitro assay using T cells from tumor-immunized patients; subsequently, ASI patients will be skin tested with purified antigens. Those antigens which appear to be involved in cellular immunity can then be considered for inclusion in a generic vaccine, consisting of no more than 8 to 10 antigens presented with a carrier that elicits protective immune responses. It is likely that native antigens eventually will be replaced by genetically engineered peptides.

REFERENCES

1. Peters, LC, Brandhorst, JS, and Hanna, MG, Jr (1979). Preparation of immunotherapeutic autologous tumor cell vaccines from solid tumors. Cancer Res 39:1353.
2. Peters, LC and Hanna, MG, Jr (1980). Active specific immunotherapy of established metastasis: Effect of cryopreservation procedures on tumor cell immunogenicity in guinea pigs. J Nat Cancer Inst 64:1521.

3. Key, ME, Bernard, MI, Hoyer, LC et al (1981).
    Guinea pig line 10 hepatocarcinoma model for
    monoclonal antibody serotherapy. In vivo
    localization of a monoclonal antibody in
    normal and malignant tissues. J Immunol
    130:1451.
4. Key ME, Brandhorst, JS and Hanna, MG, Jr
    (1983). Synergistic effects of active
    specific immunotherapy and chemotherapy in
    guinea pigs with disseminated cancer. J
    Immunol 130:2987.
5. Hoover, HC, Jr, Surdyke, M, Dangel, RB, et al
    (1984). Delayed cutaneous hypersensitivity
    to autologous tumor cells in colorectal
    cancer patients immunized with autologous
    tumor cell-bacillus Calmette-Guerin vaccine.
    Can Res 44:1671.
6. Hoover, HC, Jr, Surdyke, M, Dangel, RB et al
    (1985). Prospectively randomized trial of
     adjuvant active-specific immunotherapy for
    human colorectal cancer. Cancer 55:1236.
7. Haspel, MV, McCabe, RP, Pomato, N, et al
    (1985). Generation of tumor cell-reactive
    human monoclonal antibodies using peripheral
    blood lymphocytes from actively immunized
    colorectal carcinoma patients. Cancer Res
    45:3951.
8. McCabe, RP, Peters, LC, Haspel, MV, et al,
    (1988). Preclinical studies on the
    pharmacokinetic properties of human
    monoclonal antibodies to colorectal cancer
    and their use for detection of tumors.
    Cancer Res, 48:4348.
9. Steis, R, et al (1988). Manuscript in
    preparation.
10. Pomato, N, Murray, JH, Bos, et al, (1988).
    Identification and characterization of a
    human colon tumor antigen, CTAA 16-88,
    recognized by a human monoclonal antibody.
    In Metzger, R, Mitchell, M (eds): "Human
    Tumor Antigens and Specific Tumor Therapy,"
    New York: Alan R. Liss, (in press).

Human Tumor Antigens and Specific Tumor Therapy, pages 345–358
© 1989 Alan R. Liss, Inc.

COMBINING CHEMOTHERAPY AND BIOMODULATION
IN THE TREATMENT OF CANCER[1]

Malcolm S. Mitchell, M.D.

Departments of Medicine and Microbiology, USC School of
Medicine and Comprehensive Cancer Center,
Los Angeles, California 90033

INTRODUCTION

Biological response modifiers, which we have
abbreviated as "biomodulators", have emerged as an
important new class of agents for treating cancers. While
a great deal more remains to be learned about the full
range of effects and the precise mechanisms of action of
these agents, several have already demonstrated efficacy
in Phase II trials against disseminated human tumors. The
term biomodulator should imply far more than simply
"immunotherapy", although the latter is subsumed under the
new broader term. In particular, "biomodulator" should
also connote an agent that can modify the host's ability
to tolerate cytotoxic therapy, promote increased
incorporation of or sensitivity to cytotoxic chemicals or
radiation, decrease metastasis, or by means other than
direct immunological stimulation tip the balance between
tumor and host in favor of the latter. A classification
of these new agents appeared in an article in a recent
volume (1), and so we will not repeat the categorization
here. It is important however to take the broad view of
biomodulation in order to appreciate the many ways in
which it can potentially interact with and aid
chemotherapy against cancers.
By the same token, it is important to recognize that
most, but not all, chemotherapy is immunosuppressive. If

[1]Supported by USPHS grant CA36233, the Concern Foundation
for Cancer Research, Mr. Alan Gleitsman, USC Cancer
Research Associates and Ribi ImmunoChem Research Inc.

two modalities are to be used together the schedule of administration must be carefully chosen at least to avoid one's negating the effects of the other, and preferably with the aim of obtaining additive or synergistic effects. This seems obvious, but too often "empiricism" here has meant simply giving two agents together without regard for differences in their mechanisms of action, which is a crucial consideration for agents as different as biomodulators and chemotherapeutic drugs.

Since most of the clinical trials using combinations of chemotherapeutic agents and a biomodulator have been performed with nonspecific immunotherapy, such as the immunological "adjuvants", it may be more productive to consider the principles underlying the construction of such combinations rather than dwelling on the clinical results.

DIFFERENTIAL EFFECTS ON IMMUNOGENIC AND NONIMMUNOGENIC TUMORS

With highly immunogenic tumors in animals, the most effective chemotherapeutic agents are those that are the least immunosuppressive. For example, in a comparison of DNR and ADR, closely related congeners, Spreafico and colleagues (2) found that for the immunogenic SL2 tumor ADR, a drug causing little if any immunosuppression, was far more effective than the immunosuppresive DNR. However, for other tumors that were much less immunogenic in the autologous host, both drugs were of comparable effectiveness. It is likely that for immunogenic human tumors, it would be important to choose the least immunosuppressive drug to obtain maximal effectiveness, whereas with poorly immunogenic tumors the property of immunosuppression is irrelevant. Melanoma is among the most immunogenic human tumors, as is renal cell carcinoma, judging from a variety of studies on the immune response they elicit in the autologous patient, but what percentage of human tumors will prove to be immunogenic is uncertain. The representation of HLA Class I antigens may prove to be very important in determining which human tumors are immunogenic, extrapolating from work by Jay and collaborators in mice (3), perhaps playing a major role in determining whether tumor-associated antigens are discerned as "foreign" by the host. Since interferons can induce Class I and II histocompatibility antigens, they may find increasing use as an adjunct to other forms of immunotherapy that require that the tumor be immunogenic. If all human tumors could be made more immunogenic by such a means, a knowledge of the immunosuppressive properties of each chemotherapeutic drug would become far more central in determining our choices of agent.

CATEGORIZATION OF CHEMOTHERAPEUTIC AGENTS ACCORDING TO THEIR EFFECTS ON IMMUNITY

Table 1 lists those chemotherapeutic agents that have been demonstrated to have potent immunosuppressive activity in animals and/or man. There are several reviews on this subject which can be consulted for further details about this immunosuppression and its various mechanisms (4; 5; 6). On the list in Table 1 are many of the agents commonly used in cancer chemotherapy, such as cyclophosphamide (CY), methotrexate (MTX), 5-fluorouracil (5-FU), daunorubicin (DNR), and cytosine arabinoside (cytarabine, ara-C). The doses at which these agents are immunosuppressive are generally those used therapeutically against tumors. A number of cytotoxic agents are relatively less immunosuppressive. Table 2 indicates several of those agents with little or no immunosuppressive potency except at toxic doses, such as the antibiotics bleomycin (7), mithramycin, and ADR (2; 7). Dimethylbusulfan, busulfan (myleran), and DTIC (dacarbazine) (8), all members of the usually potent immunosuppressive alkylating agent group, also appear on the list. It is noteworthy that ADR, the hydroxy- analogue of DNR, has far less immunosuppressive activity than the latter (9), which is nicely exemplified in tumor models such as the immunogenic SL2 mouse tumor (2) mentioned earlier, and the Moloney virus-induced rat osteosarcoma (10).

TABLE 1: Chemotherapy with Demonstrated
Immunosuppressive Properties

Alkylating agents: Cyclophosphamide, Nitrosoureas (e.g., BCNU)
Purine analogues: 6-Mercaptopurine, Azathioprine (imuran)
Pyrimidine analogues: 5-Fluorouracil, Cytosine Arabinoside
Folate antagonists: Methotrexate
Vinca alkaloids: Vincristine, Vinblastine
Antibiotics: Daunorubicin
Corticosteroids

348   Mitchell

TABLE 2: Chemotherapy with Relatively Little
Immunosuppressive Activity

Antibiotics: Bleomycin, Mithramycin, Doxorubicin
Alkylating agents: Busulfan, Dimethylbusulfan, Dacarbazine
(DTIC)

Table 3 shows agents that have immunoaugmentative
effects at selected schedules. These include such diverse
agents as CY, cis-platin, bleomycin, colchicine and ADR.
Note that Table 3 contains several of the same agents
listed previously, which at specific doses and schedules
act not to suppress immunity, their most usual effect, but
instead to increase it. The mechanisms by which
augmentation of immunity occurs differ with each agent,
and none may exclude others. CY has been shown in animals
and man to inhibit suppressor T cells selectively at low
doses (approximately 15 to 20 mg/kg in mice (11), and 300-
500 mg/m^2 in man (12; Hengst,J.C.D. and Mitchell, M.S.,
unpublished data). Our own work in mice (13) has
indicated that the locus of action of CY is the precursor
of the suppressor-inducer T cell, i.e., the Lyt 1+, Lyt 2-
(L3T4+) cell analogous to the human CD4+ T cell. It is
conceivable, as our preliminary data suggest, that the
inhibition of soluble suppressor substances, such as
alpha-1 acid glycoprotein, may also be an important
mechanism of action of CY in man (Oh, S.K., Harel, W. and
Mitchell, M.S., unpublished data). ADR has been shown to
increase immunity mediated by IL-2 dependent cells, which
seems to be explainable by ADR-induced IL-2 release (14).
Similarly cis-platin can increase immunity (15), but by
the more direct mechanism of increasing the potency of
nonspecifically cytotoxic macrophages(16; 17).

TABLE 3: Chemotherapy with Immunoaugmentative
Effects

Cyclophosphamide at low doses
Cis-platin
Bleomycin
Colchicine
Doxorubicin
Prostaglandin antagonists

SCHEDULING OF COMBINED MODALITY TREATMENT

Despite the range of effects of chemotherapy we have noted, it is a good general rule that chemotherapy should generally be given before the biomodulator, to permit recovery from any agent with immunosuppressive effects to occur before attempting to stimulate the immune system. Those agents that selectively eliminate suppressor influences will obviously improve the effectiveness of subsequent immunotherapy. A special property of several chemotherapeutic agents is that they affect the cell membrane of the tumor cells, making the cells more susceptible to immune lysis (18) (Table 4). Included here are the antibiotics dactinomycin, ADR and mitomycin C, the alkylating agent BCNU, and the antifolate MTX. Alterations in membrane fluidity by chemotherapy through effects on lipid metabolism, as shown by Schlager and colleagues (16;17) can consequently increase the sensitivity of the tumor cell to antibody-dependent cell-mediated cytotoxicity or complement-mediated lysis by (monoclonal) antibodies.

TABLE 4: Chemotherapy that Affects the Cell Membrane, Increasing Susceptibility to Immune Lysis

Antibiotics: Dactinomycin, Doxorubicin, Mitomycin C
Alkylating agents: BCNU, Dacarbazine (?hapten)
Folate antagonists: Methotrexate
Guanazole

Several chemotherapeutic agents can alter the immunogenicity of the tumor cells, perhaps by acting as a hapten or by selecting immunogenic drug-resistant mutants. DTIC and guanazole are typical of this group of agents, which appears to be very limited in number (19; 20; 21).

Another obvious reason for giving chemotherapy first is to reduce the number of tumor cells with which the immune system has to contend, i.e., lowering the tumor burden through cytoreductive therapy. It has been amply demonstrated, as well as being intuitively obvious, that immunotherapy is most effective against small numbers of tumor cells, in mice approximately 10^3 to 10^4, although our recent experience has shown that relatively large metastatic masses are also amenable to treatment by biomodulation (22; Mitchell, M.S., Kan-Mitchell, J.,

Kempf, R.A., et al., Active specific immunotherapy for melanoma, submitted for publication). It has been suggested that some forms of chemotherapy can arrest tumor cells in G_0 or G_1, during which phases the cells are more susceptible to immune lysis (23). Merely slowing the growth of the tumor cells without killing them can also be helpful by giving the immune response sufficient time to develop and respond to the tumor.

Virtually the only concomitant chemotherapy and immunotherapy that seems logical is with nonimmunosuppressive or weakly immunosuppressive agents, such as DTIC (8;24). DTIC in particular has been shown not to affect the immune response to melanoma tumor-associated antigens, in a trial that also showed significant immunosuppression of that response by a nitrosourea, BCNU (24). One potentially harmful effect of chemotherapy on subsequent immunotherapy is that a massive release of tumor antigens might serve as a component of the soluble immune complexes that can act as "blocking factors". The latter elicit suppressor T cells and thus inhibit cell-mediated immunity (25). This may actually be more a theoretical than a real objection, since there has been no conclusive evidence that chemotherapy has enhanced the growth of human tumors by any means, including this type of immunosuppression. Profound and prolonged diminution of lymphocytes, such as by CY, could also prevent subsequent active immunotherapy from being effective, by removing the cells that must be stimulated in the host.

There are reports in which biomodulation was used before chemotherapy to achieve a defined goal. Hanna and co-workers (26) have found that active immunotherapy with line 10 hepatoma combined with BCG in guinea pigs led to disorganization of vascular barriers in the tumor, which made subsequent chemotherapy with cyclophosphamide more effective than chemotherapy alone. However, validation of these findings in human beings has not yet been achieved. Sensitization of tumor cells by biomodulators such as IFN-alpha and tumor necrosis factor (TNF) to the cytotoxic action of subsequent chemotherapy is another reason to use a "reverse" sequence of administration. In our in vitro experiments (Shau and Mitchell, unpublished data), pretreatment with TNF caused a higher percentage of melanoma cells to be killed by chemotherapy than with chemotherapy alone.

Protection of the host's bone marrow against the

cytotoxic effects of chemotherapy or irradiation has often required pretreatment with nonspecific stimulants of macrophages, such as azimexon or BCG, which elicit macrophage-derived colony stimulating factors. Continued treatment with the biomodulators throughout the course of the cytotoxic therapy was required in this application. Genetically cloned colony stimulating factors now available can be used for the same purpose. In mice, BCG can protect against some but not all of the immunosuppressive effects of ara-C (27;28) when given before, but not after, the chemotherapy. Yet, these examples notwithstanding, one generally should not cause immunologically active lymphocytes to undergo proliferation before chemotherapy is administered, to avoid making them highly vulnerable to the cytotoxic chemicals. In fact, recent work by Stolfi and Martin (29) has shown that interferon(IFN)-alpha given during a 2-day period after 5-FU in mice protected against leukopenia and mortality. The same effect was produced by IFN inducers such as poly I:C. Inhibition of the normal cycling of the normal tissues, protecting against the antiproliferative action of 5-FU, was a likely explanation for this activity of IFN.

EXAMPLES OF SUCCESSFUL COMBINED MODALITY THERAPY WITH CHEMOTHERAPY AND A BIOMODULATOR

Cyclophosphamide or Adriamycin and Interleukin-2

We have recently described a regimen for treating melanoma that is successful in 25% of patients with advanced disease (22), in a group that now comprises 40 patients. This treatment, with low-dose CY (350 mg/m^2)and low-dose IL-2 (3.6 million units/m^2/day as a daily bolus, x 10 days), was designed to reduce or eliminate precursors of suppressor T cells before administration of the IL-2, which could stimulate that subset as well as more clinically helpful cytolytic T cells, helper T cells and lymphokine activated killer (LAK) cells. Remissions have now been noted in 9 of 35 patients, including 2 complete remissions in patients with subcutaneous and pulmonary nodules, respectively, and complete resolution of liver lesions in 2 patients whose overall response was a partial remission. Two other patients with liver disease had partial remissions, for a total of 4 responders of 8 who had involvement of that organ. The toxicity of the regimen was tolerable, with no more than twenty per cent sustaining severe (Grade III) toxicity and none with lifethreatening problems. In fact, the regimen was administered entirely in an outpatient ("day-hospital") setting.

A variation on this regimen has included DTIC 850 mg/m^2 followed in 2 weeks by IL-2, the latter given in the same dose and schedule as in our regimen, and has yielded results at least as good as those with our CY + IL-2 treatment thus far (30). In a recent update of those results, Flaherty has found that of the first 20 21 patients with melanoma one had a complete response and 7 had partial remissions, with responses in the lung, liver and bone among other sites (Flaherty, personal communication). DTIC was used for its effects on the tumor rather than for immunomodulation, but it seems likely that its relatively low degree of immunosuppression that we have already discussed made it particularly suitable for use in this combined modality setting.

Rosenberg and colleagues have used CY in higher, therapeutic doses in order to provide lebensraum for reinfused LAK cells or tumor-infiltrating lymphocytes (TIL). Their regimen involves the use of IL-2 at a higher dose, approximately 3 times that used in ours or Flaherty's studies. In animal experiments and early investigations in the clinic, Rosenberg and colleagues noted that each of their regimens that contained CY appeared to be superior to the corresponding regimen without it (31). Whether CY had any direct effect on the tumors was uncertain, nor can a potentiating effect of IL-2 on the effectiveness of the CY be ruled out.

Recent work by Wiltrout and colleagues (32) has shown that ADR can act synergistically with IL-2 and LAK cells in the adoptive chemoimmunotherapy of an advanced experimental mouse renal cell carcinoma. Sixty seven percent of the mice were cured with the combined regimen of ADR on day 7, IL-2 and LAK cells on days 8-10, whereas longterm survivors were rare with any of the agents given singly or in other combinations. Here the ADR reduced the volume of the tumor masses directly, but also improved the localization of cytolytic lymphocytes into the sites of tumor, both of which contributed to the success of the regimen. Adverse (or beneficial) effects of ADR on immunity were not apparent in this work.

Yu et al (33) reported that ADR augmented the effects

of recombinant IL-2 on survival in mice inoculated with a syngeneic (EL-4) lymphoma. In their experiments, ADR was confirmed not to be significantly immunosuppressive on the effects of IL-2 in producing cytolytic lymphocytes, extending the observations made by Spreafico et al. and by our group (2; 10).

Cyclophosphamide and Active Immunotherapy

As described by Berd et al elsewhere in this volume, low dose CY can potentiate the delayed hypersensitivity response to melanoma cells, when given before irradiated autologous melanoma cells in an active immunization regimen (see also 12). There were only 5 of 35 responses in that study, but the practical implications of a potentiation of the immunogenicity of autologous melanoma cells are extremely important. In our own study of allogeneic melanoma lysates (Mitchell, M.S., Kan-Mitchell, J., Kempf, R.A. et al., Cancer Res., In Press), we treated half of each group of 6 or more patients with 300 mg/m^2 of CY 3 days before beginning a 5-injection course of immunization. Eight of 11 patients who received CY had an increase in the frequency of cytolytic lymphocytes, while only 3 of 11 who received lysates alone showed an increase. However, skin test reactivity and antibody formation, as well as the clinical results, were unaffected by pretreatment with the drug. There were many responders in the group not receiving CY as in that receiving only the active immunotherapy, including our longest responder. Nevertheless, it will be worthwhile for us to examine this issue more carefully in subsequent studies.

Chemotherapy and Interferons

There are many examples of the potentiation of chemotherapy by interferon-alpha in clonogenic (stem cell) assays in vitro (34; 35), but very little substantiation in vivo. In fact, only an increase in toxicity (severe leukopenia) was found in one study, although the numbers were rather limited (36). This of course is directly opposite to predictions made from the Stolfi-Martin mouse model (29) cited above. Further work with such agents as ADR, CY and FU combined in various sequences with IFN-alpha are in process at several centers and should help to clarify this important issue.

OTHER BIOMODULATIONS OF POTENTIAL IMPORTANCE
IN FUTURE TRIALS

The broader category of biomodulation, as opposed to immunotherapy, contains agents that can increase the maturation of tumor cells, such as retinoids, inhibit metastasis (e.g., antibodies to glycolipid GD-3 or GD-2 (37) or promote the increased uptake into or decreased egress of chemotherapy from the tumor cell, such as amphotericin B (38) or immunoconjugates. These agents, some of which are described in other communications at this symposium, all promise to work effectively with chemotherapy in the treatment of difficult tumors. A multipronged attack on the tumor cell, acting not only against its synthesis of DNA or proliferation but also other aspects of its complex biology, will surely be more effective than the more limited approach that we have of necessity taken in the past.

In summary, an understanding of the actions and mechanisms of actions of specific chemotherapeutic agents and specific biomodulators is crucial to the rational development of combinations. Such combinations may be additive, in some cases may be synergistic, but at the very least will not cancel each other's activity.

REFERENCES

1. Mitchell MS (1985). Biomodulation: a classification and overview. In Reif AE and Mitchell MS (eds): "Immunity to Cancer," Orlando: Academic Press, pp 401-411.

2. Spreafico F (1980). Heterogeneity of the interaction of anticancer agents with the immune system and its possible relevance in chemoimmunotherapy. Oncology 37(supp.1):9-18.

3. Hayashi H, Tanaka K, Jay F, Khouri G, Jay G (1985). Modulation of the tumorigenicity of human adenovirus-12-transformed cells by interferon. Cell 43:263-267.

4. Kempf RA, Mitchell MS (1985). Effects of chemotherapeutic agents on the immune response. Cancer Invest 2: 459-466; 3:23-33.

5. Braun DP, Harris JE (1981). Modulation of immune responses by drugs. Pharmacol Therap 14:89-122.

6. Mitchell MS, Fahey JL (eds) (1984). Immune suppression and modulation. In: "Clinics in Immunology and Allergy," London: WB Saunders, 4, no. 2.

7. Dlugi AM, Robie KM, Mitchell MS (1974). Failure of bleomycin to affect humoral or cell-mediated immunity in the mouse. Cancer Res 34:2504-2507.

8. Bruckner HW, Mokyr MB, Mitchell MS (1974). Effect of imidazole-4-carboxamide, 5-(3,3-dimethyl-1-triazeno) on immunity in patients with melanoma. Cancer Res 33:181-183.

9. Cohen SA, Ehrke MJ, Mihich E (1980). Selectivity of immunomodulation by adriamycin. Adv Enzyme Regul 18:335-346.

10. Kempf RA, Cebul RA, Mitchell MS (1980). Antitumor effects of doxorubicin against a virally-induced rat osteosarcoma with minimal immunosuppression. J Immunopharmacol 2: 509-525.

11. Askenase PW, Hayden B, Gershon RK (1975). Augmentation of delayed-type hypersensitivity by doses of cyclophosphamide which do not affect antibody synthesis. J Exp Med 141: 697-702.

12. Berd D, Maguire HC, Jr, Mastrangelo MJ (1984). Potentiation of human cell-mediated and humoral immunity by low-dose cyclophosphamide. Cancer Res 44: 5439-5443.

13. Rao VS, Bennett JA, Shen FW, Gershon RK, Mitchell MS (1980). Antigen-antibody complexes generate Lyt 1 inducers of suppressor cells. J Immunol 125:63-67.

14. Ehrke MJ, Maccubbin D, Ryoyama K, Cohen SA, Mihich E (1986). Correlation between adriamycin-induced augmentation of interleukin-2 production and of cell-mediated cytotoxicity in mice. Cancer Res 46:54-60.

15. Kleinerman ES (1980). The enhancement of naturally occurring spontaneous monocyte-mediated cytotoxicity by cis-diamine-dichloroplatinum (II). Cancer Res 40: 3099-3102.

16. Schlager SI (1981). Relationship between cell mediated and humoral immune attack on tumor cells: I. Drug and hormonal effects on susceptibility to killing and macromolecular synthesis. Cell Immunol 58:398-414.

17. Schlager SI (1982). Relationship between cell mediated and humoral immune attack on tumor cells: II. The role of cellular lipid metabolism and cell surface charge in the outcome of immune attack. Cell Immunol 66:300-316.

18. Borsos T (1976). Induction of tumor immunity by intratumoral chemotherapy. Ann N Y Acad Sci 276:565-580.

19. Fuji H, Mihich E (1979). Differential tumor immunogenicity of DBA/2 mouse lymphoma L1210 and its sublines: II. Increased expression of tumor-associated antigens on subline cells recognized by serologic and transplant methods. J Natl Cancer Inst 62:1503-1510.

20. Fuji H, Mihich E (1977). Differential tumor immunogenicity of L1210 and its sublines. I. Effect of an increased antigen density on tumor cell surfaces on primary B cell responses in vitro. J Immunol 119:983-986.

21. Ciampietri A, Bonmassar A, Puccetti P, Circolo A, Goldin A, Bonmassar E (1981). Drug-mediated increase of tumor immunogenicity in vivo for a new approach to experimental cancer immunotherapy. Cancer Res 41:681-687.

22. Mitchell MS, Kempf RA, Harel W, Shau H, Boswell WD, Lind S, Bradley EC (1988). Effectiveness and tolerability of low-dose cyclophosphamide and low-dose interleukin-2 in the treatment of disseminated melanoma. J Clin Onc 6:409-424.

23. Mathé G (1977). Effectiveness of murine leukemia chemotherapy according to the immune state. Cancer Immunol Immunother 2:139-141.

24. Mitchell MS, Mokyr MB, Davis JM (1977). Effect of chemotherapy and immunotherapy on tumor-specific immunity in melanoma. J Clin Invest 59:1017-1026.

25. Mitchell MS, Rao VS (1981). Interrelationship of immune complexes and suppressor T cells in the suppression of macrophages. In Daniels JC, Serrou B, Rosenfeld C and Denney CB (eds): "Fundamental Mechanisms in Human Cancer Immunology," New York, Amsterdam, Oxford: Elsevier-North Holland, pp 243-258.

26. Hanna MG, Jr, Key ME (1982). Active specific immunotherapy of metastases enhances subsequent chemotherapy. Science 217:367-369.

27. Murahata RI, Mitchell MS (1982). Modulation of cell-mediated alloimmunity by BCG: antagonism and potentiation of immunosuppression caused by cytarabine. J Natl Cancer Inst 69:607-612.

28. Murahata RI, Mitchell MS (1982). Modulation of cell-mediated alloimmunity by BCG. II. Induction of specific, nonadherent, non-T killer cells by BCG and alloantigen. J Natl Cancer Inst 69:613-618.

29. Stolfi RL, Martin DS (1985). Modulation of chemotherapeutic drug activity with polyribonucleotides or with interferon. J Biol Resp Modif 4:634-639.

30. Flaherty L, Redman B, Chabot G, Martino S, Valdivieso M, Bradley E (1988). Combination of Dacarbazine (DTIC) and Interleukin-2 (IL-2) in Metastatic Malignant Melanoma (MMM). Proc Amer Assoc Clin Onc 7:254.

31. Papa MZ, Yang JC, Vetto JT, Shiloni E, Eisenthal A, Rosenberg SA (1988). Combined Effects of Chemotherapy and Interleukin 2 in the Therapy of Mice With Advanced Pulmonary Tumors. Cancer Res 48:122-129.

32. Wiltrout RH, Salup RR (1988). Adoptive immunotherapy in combination with chemotherapy for cancer treatment. In: "Prog Exp Tumor Res," Basel: Karger, 32, pp 128-153.

33. Yu PP, Paciucci PA, Holland JF (1986). Activity of recombinant human interleukin-2 (rIL-2) and doxorubicin in tumor bearing BL/6 mice. Proc Amer Assoc Cancer Res 27:317.

34. Aapro MS, Alberts DS, Salmon SE (1983). Interactions of human leukocyte interferon with vinca alkaloids and other chemotherapeutic agents against human tumors in clonogenic assay. Cancer Chemother Pharmacol 10:161-166.

35. Welander CE, Morgan TM, Homesley HD, Trotta PP, Spiegel RJ (1985). Combined recombinant human interferon alpha 2 and cytotoxic agents studied in a clonogenic assay. Int J Cancer 35:721-729.

36. Ashford R, Priestman T, Mott T, Bottomley JM (1986). Combining interferon with cytotoxic chemotherapy in patients with advanced breast cancer. Cancer Immunol Immunother 23:217-219.

37. Cheresh DA (1988). Human melanoma cell attachment involves an arg-gly-asp-directed adhesion receptor and the disialoganglioside GD2. In Mitchell, MS (ed): "Immunity to Cancer II." New York: Alan R. Liss, in press.

38. Medoff G. (1981). Antitumor effects of amphotericin B. In: Hersh EM, Chirigos MA, Mastrangelo MJ (eds): "Augmenting Agents in Cancer Therapy," New York: Raven Press, pp 479-496.

Index

366 **Index**